The Healing Arts

The Healing Arts

HEALTH, DISEASE AND SOCIETY IN EUROPE

1500–1800

—————— Edited by Peter Elmer ——————

 The Open University   MANCHESTER

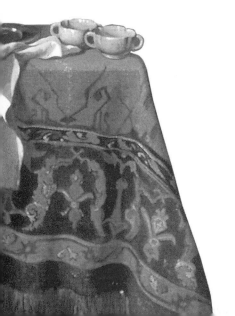

This publication forms part of an Open University course: A218 *Medicine and Society in Europe, 1500–1930*. The complete list of texts that make up this course can be found in the Preface. Details of this and other Open University courses can be obtained from the Course Information and Advice Centre, PO Box 724, The Open University, Milton Keynes MK7 6ZS, United Kingdom: tel. +44 (0)1908 653231; e-mail general-enquiries@open.ac.uk

Alternatively, you may visit the Open University website at http://www.open.ac.uk where you can learn more about the wide range of courses and packs offered at all levels by The Open University.

To purchase a selection of Open University course materials, visit the webshop at www.ouw.co.uk, or contact Open University Worldwide, Michael Young Building, Walton Hall, Milton Keynes MK7 6AA, United Kingdom for a brochure: tel. +44 (0)1908 858785; fax +44 (0)1908 858787; email ouwenq@open.ac.uk

Published by Manchester University Press; written and produced by The Open University

Manchester University Press
Oxford Road, Manchester
M13 9NR
www.manchesteruniversitypress.co.uk

The Open University
Walton Hall, Milton Keynes
MK7 6AA

Distributed exclusively in the USA by Palgrave, 175 Fifth Avenue, New York, NY 10010, USA

Distributed exclusively in Canada by UBC Press, University of British Columbia, 2029 West Mall, Vancouver, BC, Canada V6T 1Z2

First published 2004

Edited, designed and typeset by The Open University

Printed and bound in the United Kingdom by The Bath Press, Bath

Colour plates printed in the United Kingdom by Nicholson & Bass Ltd

British Library Cataloguing in Publication Data: data available

Library of Congress Cataloging in Publication Data: data available

ISBN 0 7190 6734 0 paperback

1.1

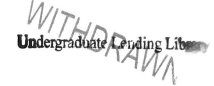

Contents

Preface ix

List of contributors x

Acknowledgements x

Introduction xi
Peter Elmer

1 Medicine in western Europe in 1500 1
Sachiko Kusukawa
1.1 Introduction 1
1.2 Rome and Europe in 1500 1
1.3 The organization of medical practice 3
1.4 The medical knowledge of the ancient Greeks 4
1.5 The making of the learned doctor in medieval Europe 12
1.6 Christianity and healing 18
1.7 The old and the new 20
1.8 Conclusion 24

2 The sick and their healers 27
Silvia De Renzi
2.1 Introduction 27
2.2 Medical care: its economy and control 28
2.3 The maintenance of health 32
2.4 Women as healers 34
2.5 Leonardo Fioravanti: a sixteenth-century itinerant healer 38
2.6 Barber-surgeons, surgeons and apothecaries 43
2.7 The skills and career of a physician: Girolamo Cardano 47
2.8 Conclusion 55

3 The medical renaissance of the sixteenth century: Vesalius, medical humanism and bloodletting 58
Sachiko Kusukawa
3.1 Introduction 58
3.2 The Renaissance and medical humanism 59
3.3 Bloodletting 61
3.4 Humanism, bloodletting and a new medical controversy 66
3.5 Andreas Vesalius 68
3.6 The *Fabrica* 74
3.7 Vesalius' legacy 79

4	**Medicine and religion in sixteenth-century Europe** *Ole Peter Grell*	**84**
4.1	Introduction	84
4.2	Medicine and religion in the later Middle Ages	85
4.3	Medicine and the Reformation	86
4.4	The Reformation, the Counter-Reformation and attitudes to popular and sacred healing	91
4.5	Paracelsus and Paracelsianism	93
4.6	Religion and epidemics	99
4.7	Health care	100
4.8	Conclusion	105

5	**Chemical medicine and the challenge to Galenism: the legacy of Paracelsus, 1560–1700** *Peter Elmer*	**108**
5.1	Introduction	108
5.2	The Paracelsian revolution, 1560–1640	109
5.3	The new challenge of Helmontianism, 1650–1700	121
5.4	Conclusion	131

6	**Policies of health: diseases, poverty and hospitals** *Silvia De Renzi*	**136**
6.1	Introduction	136
6.2	Diseases and society	137
6.3	Hospitals	150
6.4	Public health in the eighteenth century: the Habsburg territories and the German lands	160
6.5	Conclusion	162

7	**Old and new models of the body** *Silvia De Renzi*	**166**
7.1	Introduction	166
7.2	Harvey and the circulation of the blood	168
7.3	The mechanical body	173
7.4	Glands everywhere: the body according to Malpighi	176
7.5	The body expressed in numbers	181
7.6	The power of patients	184
7.7	The sensible body	187
7.8	Conclusion	192

8	**Women and medicine**	**196**
	Silvia De Renzi	
8.1	Introduction	196
8.2	A different body?	197
8.3	Questions of generation	205
8.4	Childbirth: from female ceremony to male medical practice	215
8.5	Conclusion	224

9	**The care and cure of mental illness**	**228**
	Peter Elmer	
9.1	Introduction	228
9.2	Richard Napier and his patients: a case study	230
9.3	Caring for the mad in eighteenth-century Europe: a 'psychiatric dark age'?	245
9.4	Conclusion	253

10	**War, medicine and the military revolution**	**257**
	Ole Peter Grell	
10.1	Introduction	257
10.2	Changes to warfare in the early modern period	258
10.3	New wounds and old diseases	260
10.4	Surgical treatment of gunshot wounds	263
10.5	Wounds to the head and the disappearance of the helmet	265
10.6	Treatment of burns	266
10.7	Amputations	267
10.8	Foot rot and shell shock	275
10.9	Scurvy	276
10.10	Hygiene	278
10.11	Military hospitals	280
10.12	Conclusion	282

11	**Environment, health and population**	**284**
	Mark Jenner	
11.1	Introduction	284
11.2	Airs, waters, places	285
11.3	Analysing places, analysing populations	295
11.4	Changing populations? The case of inoculation	301
11.5	Changing places? Hygiene and improvement	305
11.6	Conclusion	310

12   **Medicine and health in the age of European colonialism**   **315**
Andrew Wear

12.1   Introduction   315

12.2   The biological effects of European colonialism   316

12.3   Climate, place and health   318

12.4   Perceptions of health and new environments in the early English settlements of North America   321

12.5   Systems of medical care in the Spanish and English colonies   327

12.6   Remedies and medical contact between the old and new worlds   329

12.7   The exchange of medical knowledge   331

12.8   Medicine and slavery   334

12.9   Conclusion   341

13   **Organization, training and the medical marketplace in the eighteenth century**   **344**
Laurence William Brockliss

13.1   Introduction   344

13.2   The organization of licensed medical practice   346

13.3   The distribution of licensed medical practitioners: the case of France   352

13.4   Medical training   356

13.5   The medical marketplace   371

13.6   Conclusion   378

Glossary   **382**

Index   **395**

Preface

This is the first of two books of specially commissioned essays that form the main teaching texts of a Level 2 Open University course: A218 *Medicine and Society in Europe, 1500–1930*. The course aims to demonstrate how social, political and cultural contexts shaped medical thought and practice between 1500 and 1930. This way of approaching the history of medicine is relatively new, and differs from traditional accounts, which in the main have focused on the achievements of individuals. In both books, the contributors engage with this new approach, and guide readers through some recent debates provoked by it. The books are intended to appeal to as wide an audience as possible, including students of history or medicine and the interested general reader.

A feature of the main teaching texts is the inclusion of exercises designed to allow readers to explore a selection of primary and secondary source materials. Each teaching text has a companion volume, in which these source materials can be found. For convenience, these companion volumes are referred to as 'Source Book 1' and 'Source Book 2'. For general readers who do not have access to the companion volumes, a bibliographical list of relevant source materials is supplied at the end of each chapter.

The four books that make up the series are:

> *The Healing Arts: Health, Disease and Society in Europe, 1500–1800*, edited by Peter Elmer (Book 1)

> *Health, Disease and Society in Europe, 1500–1800: A Source Book*, edited by Peter Elmer and Ole Peter Grell (Source Book 1)

> *Medicine Transformed: Health, Disease and Society in Europe, 1800–1930*, edited by Deborah Brunton (Book 2)

> *Health, Disease and Society in Europe, 1800–1930: A Source Book*, edited by Deborah Brunton (Source Book 2)

Readers are not required to have undertaken any previous historical or medical study; all concepts are explained in the text, and, as a further aid to understanding, we have included a glossary at the end of the book. Entries in the glossary are emboldened in the text, usually on their first appearance. The convention for dating adopted is to use CE (Common Era) and BCE (Before Common Era) in preference to the more traditional AD and BC.

I would particularly like to thank all those who have been involved in the production of this volume. Special thanks are due to my colleagues at The Open University, Deborah Brunton, Silvia De Renzi and Ole Peter Grell, and to our consultant authors, Sachiko Kusukawa, Mark Jenner, Andrew Wear and Laurence William Brockliss. Behind the scenes, the contributions of Robert Doubleday and Adrian Roberts (course managers), Jane Lea and Audrey Linkman (visual resources), Liliana Torero de Clements, Janet Fennell and Kerry Lawrence (course secretaries), Ray Munns (cartographer), Pam Higgins (graphic designer) and

Charles Harris (compositor) have been indispensable. Above all, however, I would like to thank our editors, Hazel Coleman and Christine Considine, whose tireless pursuit of editorial clarity and comprehension was an object lesson for anyone wishing to edit an academic text such as this.

Peter Elmer

Contributors

Laurence William Brockliss is Professor of Early Modern French History at the University of Oxford and Fellow of Magdalen College

Silvia De Renzi is Wellcome Lecturer in the Department of the History of Science, Technology and Medicine at The Open University

Peter Elmer is Senior Lecturer in the Department of the History of Science, Technology and Medicine at The Open University

Ole Peter Grell is Reader in the Department of History at The Open University

Mark Jenner is Lecturer in the Department of History at the University of York

Sachiko Kusukawa is Fellow in History and Philosophy of Science at Trinity College, Cambridge

Andrew Wear is Reader in the History of Medicine at the Wellcome Trust Centre for the History of Medicine at University College London

Acknowledgements

Grateful acknowledgement is made to the following sources for permission to reproduce material in this book.

Tables

Table 13.1: Brockliss, L. and Jones, C. (1997) 'Table 8e: Number of physicians, surgeons, and apothecaries in selected French towns in the 1780's', *The Medical World of Early Modern France*, Clarendon Press. Reprinted by permission of Oxford University Press.

Table 13.2: Brockliss, L. and Jones, C. (1997) 'Table 8d: Number of physicians, surgeons, and apothecaries in eighteenth-century France', *The Medical World of Early Modern France*, Clarendon Press. Reprinted by permission of Oxford University Press.

Table 13.5: Brockliss, L. and Jones, C. (1997) 'Table 10b: Users of Jean Ailhaud's poudres purgatives 1724–1754', *The Medical World of Early Modern France*, Clarendon Press. Reprinted by permission of Oxford University Press.

Every effort has been made to trace all the copyright owners, but if any have been inadvertently overlooked, the publishers will be pleased to make the necessary arrangements at the first opportunity.

Introduction

Peter Elmer

In the spring of 2002, a travelling exhibition, seen by millions across Europe, opened in an East End gallery in London. Among the many exhibits were the preserved bodies of recently deceased people that were presented to the public in a number of authentic and realistic poses. All had been cut, dissected or flayed in order to show the interior workings of the body. Thus it was possible to see the exposed brain of a man engaged in a game of chess, or the skinless body of a horseman riding the skeleton of a horse. Most provocatively of all, a pregnant woman was cut to reveal an eight-month-old foetus. Not surprisingly, the exhibition, 'Body Worlds', met with a storm of popular and official disapproval, much of it orchestrated by the media. The Conservative MP, Teddy Taylor, probably summed up the general mood when he opined 'What possible benefit can any normal person gain from looking at dead bodies?' (quoted in the *Guardian*, *G2*, 19 March 2002, p.3).

The organizer of the exhibition was a German professor, Gunther von Hagens, an anatomist and the man behind the groundbreaking invention of 'plastination', which made the realistic modes of preservation possible. In response to critics like Taylor, von Hagens came up with an interesting and original rationale for his work. He claimed that his prime motive in assembling such shocking exhibits was to challenge the supremacy of the medical profession in matters relating to the human body. For too long, he argued, the medics had monopolized such issues and in the process had deprived the general public of the opportunity to know their own bodies and thus to assume greater responsibility for their health. Instead, von Hagens wished to return to the 'heady days' of the Renaissance, when, according to one commentator, 'anatomists and artists explored the workings of the human body as never before and made their workings public at anatomical theatres' (*Guardian*, *G2*, 19 March 2002, p.3). Von Hagens reaffirmed his challenge to the medical status quo when on 20 November 2002 he conducted the first public autopsy in Britain for over 170 years. The event was televised live on Channel 4 and drew an audience of some 1,800,000 – an extraordinarily large viewing figure for a late-night programme.

Von Hagens's resort to history to justify his 'art' is indicative of a growing interest, in both public and academic circles, in the early history of western medicine. In reminding his audience of the spectacle of public dissections in Renaissance Europe, for example, von Hagens was reflecting a large body of recent scholarship devoted to uncovering the exact conditions under which the early anatomists carried out their work. This work, in turn, constitutes only part of a vast field of historical research concerned with exploring the medical world of the past in all its varied forms. Indeed, so great has been the growth of academic interest in the subject since the 1970s that it has given birth to its own specialized sub-discipline – the social history of medicine. This new approach to the subject paints a fascinating picture of what it was like to experience illness, suffer pain and seek a cure in earlier times. Above all, it seeks to demonstrate how medical knowledge and practice in the past did not exist or evolve in a vacuum, but was rather the product of the wider social and cultural forces prevalent at any given moment. As such, it has benefited greatly from the insights of academic historians working in related fields, such as social and cultural history, as well as borrowing concepts and ideas derived from the social sciences and anthropology. The end result is a discipline that approaches the history of medicine from a variety of perspectives and emphasizes the importance of critical analysis, rather than mere description, in discussing the medical past.

In this volume, the various contributors – all specialists in the discipline – actively engage with this new approach, and with some of the most recent debates that it has stirred, in relation to medicine in early modern Europe (that is, broadly speaking, the period between 1500 and 1800). Before embarking on these essays, however, it might be useful to say a little more about both the origins of the new social history of medicine and the corresponding growth of public interest in the subject. The two developments are in all probability linked. After all, academics do not live in a social vacuum and are as much affected by contemporary currents of thought as the non-specialist, general public.

Prior to the 1960s, writing on the history of medicine was typically the preserve of physicians and surgeons, few of whom had experienced any formal historical training. They were largely concerned with discovering the roots of the modern scientific medicine that they practised, and as such, not surprisingly, tended to focus on the celebrated discoveries of past physicians. A case in point concerning the early modern period was the exceptional attention paid to medical innovators such as William Harvey, discoverer of the circulation of the blood, whose anatomical research was considered a major 'breakthrough' and, by implication, represented a rejection of the errors of the past (discussed in more detail in Chapter 7). In a similar vein, much history of science in this period focused on the remarkable achievements and insights of scientific 'geniuses' such as Nicholas Copernicus and Isaac Newton. This approach to the subject, which has been labelled by later generations of historians of science and medicine as the 'great man' approach, nonetheless shared something in common with mainstream historical writing at this time. Political history, for example, was dominated by the desire to produce an account of past politics that was largely a vindication of the present. In Britain, this gave rise to what Herbert Butterfield defined in 1931 as a 'whiggish' approach to history – that is, one that focused on the progressive evolution of Britain from its feudal, unrepresentative roots to a fully constitutional and democratic state in the twentieth century. (The term 'whig' derives from a key moment in this process when, in the Glorious Revolution of 1688, the Whigs overthrew the 'despot', James II, and instituted a constitutional monarchy in which the power of Parliament reigned supreme. This is largely seen as a historical 'myth' by modern-day historians.) At the heart of this kind of writing lay a deep-seated desire to explain the past in present-centred terms, or to produce a history, in Butterfield's words, that represented the 'ratification if not the glorification of the present' (Butterfield, 1951, p.v).

In the later decades of the twentieth century, this approach underwent a radical challenge. Now, the voice of those groups who hitherto had been marginalized in historical discourse was heard for the first time. The emergence of feminist history in the 1960s and 1970s, for example, challenged the privileged place of men in much historical writing. Other marginalized or neglected groups – the poor, working class, Jews, non-Europeans – attracted the attention of historians. The overall impact of much of this new 'history from below', which involved what E.P. Thompson eloquently described as an attempt to rescue such groups from the 'enormous condescension of posterity', has radically altered the way historians think about, and analyse, the past (Thompson, 1968, p.13). The past is now viewed from a variety of perspectives, and white, Eurocentric, male history no longer dominates the historical agenda. The emergence of the new social history of medicine was in large part shaped by these developments. The new feminist history, for example, forced a radical re-evaluation of the role of women in the medical sphere. It also led to a new interest in one of medicine's neglected sub-groups, patients. Much recent research, for example, has sought to shift the focus away from those responsible for dispensing medical wisdom and treatment on to the recipients of such advice and care, the patient (for a seminal essay in defence of this approach, see Porter, 1985). Previously seen as of little importance in the story of medicine's advance, there is now a vast and growing literature on the place and experience of the sick in medical history. As we shall see in a number of the chapters in this volume, this new interest in the patient has produced some fascinating insights, none more so than the realization that prior to 1800 the voice and opinion of the patient carried great weight. In a world in which learned medical practitioners had to vie for customers with a range of competitors, the relationship between healer and patient was less one-sided than is customarily the case today.

Such developments were undoubtedly linked to a growing disenchantment in both academic and popular circles from the 1960s onwards with conventional, scientific medicine and the privileged status of its practitioners. This growing mood of scepticism is best illustrated in the writings of academic critics such as Ivan Illich (1963), who launched a full-scale assault on the privileged status of modern, technocratic medicine. Physicians and psychiatrists were increasingly depicted as manipulative charlatans, many of whose 'remedies' consisted of little more than pills and placebos. Criticism of the medical profession was extended in particular to psychiatry, which some hostile observers stigmatized as a fraud. Thomas Szasz (1961, 1970), for example, went so far as to doubt the very existence of 'mental illness', preferring to see it as an example of the way in which bourgeois society labels and contains those who refuse to accept its dominion. Such criticisms were essentially founded on a fundamental critique of the political power wielded by the medical profession in the modern world. The elite status of physicians, and their privileged body of medical knowledge, which they alone understood, were widely seen as an obstacle to greater democracy in the medical field. The emergence of 'patient power', and the growing challenge to the authority of the physician, thus provided a powerful incentive for the historian to reinvestigate power relations in past medicine. One of the earliest and most influential critics to undertake such an approach was the French philosopher Michel Foucault (1926–84). Though much of his work is discredited by historians today, important elements of his legacy live on, most notably in relation to his understanding of medical knowledge as a form of power – an idea which he related to the growing medicalization of European society in the late seventeenth and eighteenth centuries (Foucault's legacy is discussed in a number of the essays in this volume).

Wider developments in western society at large have added to the growing chorus of disapproval. The emergence of 'alternative medicine' (more lately referred to as 'complementary medicine' in recognition of its growing acceptance in lay and specialist medical circles) clearly owes much to the growth of multiculturalism in western society, itself a product of the demise of western imperialism and the emergence of a post-colonial Europe after the Second World War. The 'discovery' in the west of Chinese and Indian medicine, and the alternative therapies associated with these two ancient cultures, has thus stimulated a radical rethink of the privileged place traditionally afforded to western, scientific medicine in the European past. In terms of the early modern period, interest in such 'alternative' cultures, and their related medical systems, has led to a renewed interest in the holistic nature of humoral medicine and has provided important clues to the remarkable longevity and popularity of this system. Like some eastern medical philosophies, it was predicated on principles that were accessible and intelligible to a wide, non-specialist audience. Unlike much current western medicine, herbal medicine and acupuncture appeals *because* it feels as though the patient understands, and is thus in control, of their own body and its treatment. Much the same argument has been made for the Galenic medical system, which dominated western medicine throughout our period (it was not superseded until the middle decades of the nineteenth century, a development that forms a central theme of the second volume in this series). Consequently, we are beginning to understand just why it was so long-lived and able to assimilate and fend off challenges to its supremacy (see, for example, Wear, 2000).

In April 2002, the *British Medical Journal* (*BMJ*) reported the results of a recent survey in which British doctors had been asked to identify popular 'diseases' or complaints that they would like to reclassify as 'non-diseases'. A total of 174 conditions were listed, many of which (such as baldness and bad breath) were non-controversial. However, there were a number of complaints whose appearance provoked much debate. These included chronic fatigue syndrome (CFS) and Gulf War syndrome, both of which display recognizable symptoms but do not have an agreed cause. The debate over the disease status of the latter clearly has political overtones, given the sensitivity of physicians to the authority of the military and its civilian paymasters. The former is particularly interesting since some practitioners have now given it a Latinate tag – myalgic encephalomyelitis – a sure sign of its need to be assimilated into the canon of recognized diseases. Others, however, have dismissed it as 'yuppie flu', an affliction of suspiciously recent origin which would appear to strike only those of a certain social background (predominantly middle class). The *BMJ* was keen to point out that the redesignation of an affliction such as CFS as a 'non-disease' did not mean that medical professionals would cease to take it seriously or to deny the genuine nature of the patient's experience. On the other hand, at a time when it is widely acknowledged that the resources to treat illness are a precious commodity, there can be little doubt that such attitudes must impact on the way in which individual medical practitioners treat those presenting with such symptoms. Disease, as the official *BMJ* website concludes, 'is a very slippery concept' – a tacit admission perhaps that those who have argued for a social constructivist approach to medicine in the past may have a valid point (*British Medical Journal*, 12 April 2002; *Guardian*, 10 April 2002).

A parallel case – this time in the field of mental health – concerns the extent to which some psychiatrists are beginning to question the existence of such widely accepted phenomena as stress and stress-related illnesses. The term 'stress', as used in a medical context, is in fact of recent coinage. It was first used in 1956 by the psychiatrist Hans Selye in his book *The Stress of Life*. Its recent invention and usage raises interesting questions, not least for the historian of early modern medicine concerned with diagnosing and charting the character and frequency of diseases in the period. As we shall see in Chapter 9, early modern medical practitioners employed a variety of terms to designate mental illness, some of which, such as melancholy, seem to have been specific to a particular social class. Other, more familiar conditions, such as hysteria, underwent radical redefinition in the period. The realization that medical understanding of the nature of disease might be shaped by specific historical and cultural conditions poses a number of problems for 'old-fashioned' medical history, much of which was concerned with tracing the 'history' of diseases, and the discovery of their biological causes, over the centuries. Nowadays, historians seek instead to understand how contemporaries thought about and understood disease *in their own time*, and to explore the various factors that impinged on such thinking.

One result of this new approach has been growing criticism in academic circles of those older studies that characteristically sought to apply the methodology of 'retrodiagnosis' to early modern patients. Retrodiagnosis – the ability to identify the illnesses of past sufferers through the application of modern medical knowledge – was once a popular pastime of those amateur medical historians who also subscribed to the 'great man' approach to medicine, and it remains popular among some general historians and the media. The field is, however, fraught with problems, not least those relating to the need for generally agreed definitions of recognizable diseases and complaints. If diseases are socially and culturally constructed, retrodiagnosis becomes little more than a game, with ill-defined rules and little academic credibility.

Debates of this kind alert the historian of medicine to the substantial problems inherent in assuming that diseases, like medicine itself, follow a straight path. Diseases mutate, according to local, contingent conditions in much the same way as medical knowledge and understanding is situated in and shaped by the wider world in which it is located. The job of the medical historian – as guided by the new social history of medicine – is to arrive at a better understanding of this process in all its myriad forms. The thirteen essays that follow attempt to do this while at the same time acknowledging the problems and pitfalls inherent in any attempt to recapture the medical world of past centuries. One danger lies in the present-centred concerns of modern historians. For example, there is a genuine possibility that the current preoccupation with the tribulations of patients, especially women, may produce a revised version of the past which paints an excessively nostalgic and upbeat view of what it was like either to be sick or to practise folk medicine in the past. A case in point is the history of early modern obstetrics, a field of medicine that was largely confined to women and excluded learned male physicians (discussed more fully in Chapter 8). The current interest in 'natural' birthing techniques, and the concomitant rejection of medical intervention (usually perceived as technological and male), should not obscure the fact that the experience of childbirth in early modern Europe was dangerous and frequently ended in death, for both the mother and the child. The dangers implicit in this approach are well summarized by Mary Lindemann:

> Instead of viewing previous medical practices as unscientific, irrational, superstitious, and simply bad [as many earlier generations of medical historians had done], these historians endow it with a preternatural wisdom and a coherence that it probably never possessed. It is possible, for instance, that the whole idea of a popular medicine conveyed by oral tradition through the centuries might be the figment of an overheated historical imagination.
>
> (Lindemann, 1999, p.4)

The task of the new social history of medicine is not a simple one. It needs to assimilate the best of the work of the past with the current fashion for a broader historical sweep. The work and thought of the great physicians of the past are part of this story and need to be incorporated (though the emphasis now should be on the wider social and cultural context in which they laboured, rather than on their 'heroic' status as pioneers). Above all, when encountering a world as radically different from our own as early modern Europe, we need to show far more sensitivity to the various forces, both medical and non-medical, that shaped the environment in which patients and healers functioned. Historians of medicine might disagree as to the extent to which it is either feasible or desirable to implement social constructivist approaches to the discipline. Few, however, would disagree with the positive overall impact that the new social history of medicine has had on our understanding of the medical past. In the essays that follow, we hope to provide a wide cross-section of much of the best of this new research, and the many debates it has spawned. At the same time, we appreciate that there is still much to be learned about the place of medicine in early modern Europe. Indeed, this volume, and the associated Open University course to which it relates, has been commissioned partly in the hope that it will stimulate further interest and research in the subject. We hope that you enjoy it as much as we have enjoyed its composition.

The essays that make up this volume have been specially commissioned and designed in order to appeal to as wide an audience as possible, both academic and non-specialist. Their chronological and geographical scope is large, and requires some justification. In terms of the period covered by the volume, the three centuries are, in medical terms, coherent and well defined. Despite medical innovation in both theory and practice, the general climate was one of continuity rather than change. In 1800, methods of cure and treatment were strikingly similar to those employed in 1500. In the field of learned medicine, the Galenic humoral system still held sway, and patients continued to choose their practitioner in much the same way as their ancestors had done three centuries earlier. Despite some regional variations, the same pattern prevailed over the whole of Europe. Indeed, as Europeans spread inexorably across the globe in this period so they took with them their own distinctive medical culture, which became transplanted in alien contexts (a central theme of Chapter 12).

The chronology and geography adopted here, however, is not altogether unproblematic. Some aspects of medical practice and theory did undergo change and challenge in the period. The most significant drawback, however, to a volume such as this lies in its European framework. This is problematic for two reasons. First, it accentuates the Eurocentric nature of early modern medicine at the expense of other, contemporary medical cultures elsewhere in the world. And second, it claims a European focus despite the fact that the new approaches pioneered by recent generations of medical historians have barely scratched the surface of large parts of Europe. As much as possible, we have tried to avoid both pitfalls. Any bias towards Britain, or English-speaking sources, is largely a product of the fact that so much of the new social history of medicine was first popularized in the English-speaking world. We thus know a great deal about how medicine, in all its various manifestations, flourished in the British Isles, especially in England, and rather less about other parts of the Continent. Slowly, this situation is changing. Italian and German scholars in particular are beginning to take a keen interest in the approaches pioneered by English-speaking historians of the subject, while many of the latter have begun to show much greater interest in developments on the other side of the Channel. Inevitability, much of this work has been slow to filter into the English-speaking world because of problems surrounding translations. In seeking to address these and related issues, the authors in this volume have sought, wherever possible, to paint as broad a picture as possible, while at the same time stressing regional and local variations in medical practices. In addition, Andrew Wear's chapter on colonial medicine addresses a growing concern with the clash between European and non-western medical cultures.

The essays in this volume do not constitute a comprehensive or chronological account of early modern European medicine. They do, however, seek to address some of the most important issues and debates that have arisen in historical circles in recent years. As a result, the chapters are arranged thematically, a format that precludes the approach of older histories of medicine that charted the triumphant march of medical progress from medieval superstition to the more enlightened modes of practice associated with the eighteenth century.

We begin our survey of early modern medicine in Europe by looking in Chapter 1 at the classical and medieval inheritance. Taking a rough starting date of 1500 – largely an arbitrary one – Sachiko Kusukawa describes the state of medical knowledge and practice in Rome. The choice of Rome is dictated partly because of its typicality (medical practice here was largely conducted along lines familiar to other cities in Europe at this time), but also because of its symbolic significance in early modern Europe as the centre of Christianity and the heir to a great, classical empire. The two themes – religion and the classical past – informed every aspect of medical culture in this period, in much the same way as they shaped the wider mental and cultural horizons of the age. In this chapter, the emphasis is on the nature of the classical legacy, in particular the medicine of the two great ancient physicians, Hippocrates and Galen, which informed early modern approaches to the diagnosis, prognosis and treatment of ill health. A key issue discussed here, and one to which we return in later essays, is that of the transmission of medical knowledge. Kusukawa thus asks how early modern Europeans acquired their understanding of this ancient source of wisdom. Integral to her answer is the idea of transmission as a process of mediation; in this case, she shows how classical medicine was interpreted selectively and partially by having been passed down through the hands of Arab and medieval translators and interpreters. Contemporaries around 1500 were becoming increasingly aware of this fact – so much so that some physicians, influenced by the vogue for Renaissance humanism, sought a return to the original sources in the belief that Galen and others had been 'corrupted' by such mediation.

A key development in this process was the utilization of the printing press by medical practitioners and writers, eager to use this new technology as a means of spreading the word and selling their wares. Printed books and pamphlets provided medical men, and sometimes women, with a multipurpose outlet. Both specialist and non-specialist markets created a huge demand for medical writings and provided a valuable opportunity for the propagation of new ideas and cures. By the eighteenth century, new forms of printed literature – newspapers, journals, novels, and so on – enabled medical ideas to circulate among all sections of society. Many contained illustrations, which complemented the written text and helped to reinforce the message of the author. This aspect of the social construction and dissemination of medical knowledge in early modern Europe forms a consistent theme of many subsequent essays. In Chapter 3, for example, Kusukawa analyses in detail the engravings that the celebrated anatomist Andreas Vesalius included in his groundbreaking work of 1543. Later chapters pick up on this theme and stress the vital importance of printing in the medical culture of the period.

Whereas the focus of Chapters 1 and 3 is on the acquisition and construction of medical knowledge, Chapter 2 is largely concerned with general issues surrounding the practice of medicine, particularly the variety of practitioners and the complex nature of the relationships that existed between them. In early modern Europe, medical assistance was sought and found in a variety of places. In recreating the vibrant and varied character of early modern medicine, Silvia De Renzi highlights a number of problems facing historians who wish to describe and account for such diversity. She notes, for example, that the professional status of medics – taken for granted in the modern world – was largely unclear in this period. Although learned physicians (usually defined as those who possessed an MD, or medical degree) invoked their privileged educational and social position in order to monopolize the field of medical practice, or at least to impose their control over it, their success remained patchy. The confusion is compounded by problems of definition and terminology. Contemporaries and historians have used a bewildering range of terms to describe those who offered their services in the medical sphere. Members of the three major medical occupations (physicians, surgeons and apothecaries), for example, routinely castigated those whom they saw as interlopers as quacks, empirics, charlatans or mountebanks. Historians, in seeking to come to terms with this diversity, have attempted to categorize these groups into various polarities: learned and unlearned; orthodox and unorthodox; elite and popular; professional and lay. The reality on the ground, however, defies the easy application of any or all of these terms. As De Renzi's case studies demonstrate, the boundaries between the various types of medical practitioner were much more 'fluid' and ill defined in early modern Europe than was previously thought.

Attempts to regulate medical practice and to impose some form of hierarchical organization were a feature of early modern medicine, but, more often than not, these attempts failed. There were several reasons for this. One reason was the inability of the nascent 'profession' to police 'illicit' practice. Another relates to the growing evidence for the 'empowerment' of patients in this period. In many respects, medical practitioners were at the mercy of their 'customers', though attempts to suggest that a lack of regulation combined with patient power created what some historians have referred to as a 'medical marketplace' in early modern Europe is now considered both anachronistic and wide of the mark (for recent trenchant criticism of the concept, and a call for its revision, see Pelling, 2003, pp.342–3). In choosing a medic, factors other than the purely commercial were often paramount. Moral and religious concerns, for example, played an important role in the choice of cure and the person responsible for its administration. It was not until the eighteenth century, and the growing secularization of the Enlightenment, that a fully fledged marketplace in medicine came into being, though as Laurence Brockliss demonstrates in Chapter 13, there were still marked variations in practice across Europe.

Knowledge of the dominant medical system of ideas – humoralism – was never exclusive to university-educated physicians. As both Kusukawa and De Renzi show, such knowledge, albeit modified, was regularly adapted and modified by those practitioners who lacked a medical qualification. Such ideas were also popular with patients. Not surprisingly, medical ideas and practice changed little in the three centuries between 1500 and 1800. Medicine, however, was not untouched by controversy and debate. The broad consensus sketched above was challenged, most notably in the sixteenth century by the iconoclastic figure of the Swiss physician Paracelsus. Paracelsus' medical ideas threatened the whole edifice of humoralism, which it sought to replace with a medical philosophy and practice based on the principles of the new science of 'chemistry'. Chapters 4 and 5 explore the contribution of Paracelsus and his followers to early modern medicine, focusing in particular on the way in which his works were accepted or rejected not just for their medical content but also because of their radical religious and political associations. As such, both chapters provide illuminating case studies in the social constructivist approach to medical knowledge and its dissemination. In particular, Ole Grell demonstrates in Chapter 4 how Paracelsus' medical worldview was profoundly shaped by the reformer's distinctive response to the social, intellectual and religious upheavals of the early sixteenth century. In the event, Paracelsianism succeeded only insofar as it was able to divest itself of its earlier, radical associations – a point reaffirmed in Chapter 5 where I discuss its reception in Europe, particularly in France and England.

Integral to both these chapters, and a theme explored throughout the book, is the extent to which religion informed medical knowledge and practice in this period. The religious upheavals of the sixteenth century, culminating in the Protestant Reformation and the Catholic response, the Counter-Reformation, impacted on all aspects of early modern life. It is hardly surprising, therefore, that historians have frequently stressed the impact of religion on medicine and healing. This is apparent, for example, in official attitudes to miraculous healing, madness and the curative properties of springs and wells – topics explored in Chapters 6, 9 and 11. It is particularly evident in the vital role played by hospitals in both the spiritual and the physical care of the poor and sick in early modern Europe. Even as official religion began to lose its grip on large sections of the population in the eighteenth century – especially in northern Europe – the ideals of Christian charity continued to inform many of the philanthropic and medical projects of that period. Consequently, it is impossible to deny a role for religion in any discussion of early modern medicine, though historians frequently fail to agree on its precise function in promoting or inhibiting medical innovation and change.

One of the more controversial historical issues raised by discussion of the place of religion in early modern Europe relates to its relationship to the state and to secular authority. Indeed, the concept of the 'state' is equally problematic in terms of the medical history of this period. Part of the problem lies in the difficulties attached to using this term in respect to the miscellaneous sovereign bodies or political authorities that existed in early modern Europe. Most of these were small, decentralized and impecunious. Moreover, few bore the hallmarks of the modern nation state. Often divided by language, culture and religion, the rulers of such 'states' rarely possessed either the manpower or resources to ensure uniform and effective government within their boundaries. Nonetheless, in an age when most people were unable to afford expensive health care, the state, however defined, was increasingly expected to address the medical needs of the poorest members of the community. In Chapter 6, De Renzi explores the role of the 'state' in formulating schemes of poor relief and health care in early modern Europe, and assesses its ability to carry these out. In so doing, she stresses the intricate web of political and administrative authorities, and the sheer variety of individuals and institutions, that were engaged in such schemes. Central governments, such as they existed in this period, had to operate through, and alongside, other agencies, which may or may not have shared their motivation or goals. There was, then, considerable overlap – and sometimes conflict – between the various bodies (central and local government, church and state, individual benefactors and charitable organizations) which addressed the needs of the poor and communities in times of medical crisis. This was particularly evident in the case of funding – a major issue then as now – since so many of the welfare schemes in this period were reliant on local sources of revenue.

These, and related issues, become most visible in this period when contemporaries were faced with the onset of infectious epidemics such as plague and smallpox, which were endemic to early modern Europe. As De Renzi's case study of contemporary responses to the plague illustrates, there was much that communities could do, despite the chronic administrative and financial shortcomings described above. Vital in this respect were early modern hospitals. For much of the period they constituted a social as well as a medical resource for the communities they served. However, as De Renzi shows, the cities of Renaissance Italy were increasingly focusing their attention on providing a range of medical services to the urban poor – a model which was gradually emulated throughout much of the rest of Europe in the centuries that followed. Health then, as now, was never divorced from political imperatives. In charting the evolution of the state's response to the health of its peoples, particularly the poor, De Renzi illustrates an omnipresent and underlying theme of the new social history of medicine – the political significance of medicine and the way in which medical and political concerns interacted in the wider world. These themes are taken up in later chapters, where, under the influence of Enlightenment ideals, the growing role of the state in the formulation of health care policies for its subjects is addressed. Once again, we are reminded here of Foucault's dictum that 'knowledge is power', as physicians increasingly lent their support to state initiatives designed to 'improve' the health and prosperity of their subjects (see, for example, Chapters 10, 11 and 13).

Another theme of much recent writing in the social history of medicine, as well as in related fields, is the general significance attached in early modern culture to the body (for a recent overview of work in this field, see Jenner, 1999). Chapters 7 and 8 in particular detail the changing way in which Europeans understood the function and operation of the body in the seventeenth and eighteenth centuries. In Chapter 7, the focus is on the exploration and discovery of new ways of understanding and conceptualizing the body, beginning with Harvey's discovery of the circulation of the blood. Successive case studies chart other approaches to modelling the body, many of which were indebted to a change in the climate of scientific investigation following the discovery of the microscope in the second half of the seventeenth century. Medicine and medical research was also profoundly affected by the demise of the Aristotelian world picture following the onset of the 'scientific revolution' (today, a controversial term among historians of science, many of whom now question both the revolutionary status of the event, and its scientific credentials; for a recent overview, see Osler, 2000; Shapin, 1996). The impact of these changes on medical thinking, particularly in terms of the body's structure and function, was profound. De Renzi is at pains to point out, however, that new theories of the body did not lead to a new therapeutics or more effective medical practice. On the contrary, humoralism demonstrated a remarkable ability to survive such changes and indeed to incorporate the new models of the body into the traditional canon of medical treatment.

In Chapter 8, De Renzi turns her attention to a particular type of body – that of women. Drawing on recent work in the field of women's history and gender studies, she focuses on the various ways in which medicine and women interacted in the early modern period. The chapter explores how medicine contributed to the understanding of sex differences and the nature of the female body, and how this in turn was used to establish and perpetuate gender roles in early modern society. Far from being uncontroversial, the nature of the female body, and in particular the role of women in procreation, was the subject of competing theories. The widely accepted assumption that women were physically inferior to men could on occasion be challenged in the medical arena. The chapter also looks at the recapturing of women's exclusive authority and competence in matters relating to pregnancy and childbirth in the period, and explores how these events were framed mainly in non-medical terms. During the course of the eighteenth century, however, the primacy of women's role in such matters underwent considerable challenge with the emergence of the man-midwife. De Renzi explores the origins of these developments (and the historical debates they have engendered), which led ultimately to a substantial redrawing of the boundaries of competence over the female body.

In Chapter 9, I discuss early modern medical understanding of mental illness and its wider place in society. Here, we touch again the complex and often controversial debate surrounding definitions of illness, and the unstable meanings that have been attached to madness in pre-industrial Europe. By focusing on the rural English medic-cum-clergyman Richard Napier, I discuss both popular and learned responses to mental illness in the seventeenth century. Napier's unique case notes clearly establish the historical and cultural specificity of early modern notions of madness, which were profoundly shaped by the dominant cultural assumptions of the age. This is most obviously apparent in the diagnosis of the condition known to contemporaries as melancholia, which became fashionable in educated circles from the late sixteenth century onwards. It is also evident in the way in which the mad were treated in this period. The growth of public and private asylums for the insane is subjected to historical scrutiny in the second half of this chapter, where recent arguments are presented to demonstrate that far from existing as dumping grounds, early modern hospitals for the insane were concerned with therapy and care.

In Chapter 10, we turn our attention to the relationship between war and medicine in the early modern period. In our own time, it is widely assumed that modern warfare has been 'good' for medicine. Here, Grell puts the case for an intimate connection between the two, emphasizing the significance of army and naval surgeons in particular in promoting innovation in surgical operations and implements. He also discusses the prominent role played by army hospitals and physicians in pioneering new approaches to the care and cure of sick soldiers, while acknowledging the fact that such changes were often only slowly adopted by civilian hospitals and authorities. Warfare, Grell concludes, was an important testing ground for medicine, a fact that was increasingly appreciated by the leaders of early modern states, who were eager to promote any reforms that might create fitter and healthier armies.

The growing intervention of the state is also evident in the way in which it encouraged the collection of medical statistics, and sponsored and encouraged a variety of medical initiatives. In Chapter 11, Mark Jenner explores these developments within the context of the wider early modern concern for environmental medicine – an issue that also figures prominently in much modern medical discourse. In particular, he traces the emergence of new responses to disease and its prevention, as epitomised in a case study concerned with the introduction of inoculation for smallpox. In addressing these issues, however, he once again stresses the importance of the wider social, economic, religious and political environment in the reception of medical innovation. Inoculation was not greeted with universal acclaim, and its implementation and acceptance required various strategies on the part of its supporters. Once again, the role of new forms of printed media such as newspapers and journals – themselves the products of the new consumerism of the eighteenth century – are identified as crucial in disseminating support for inoculation.

The importance of place and climate – an issue fundamental to environmental medicine – was particularly significant within the context of colonial medicine. In Chapter 12, we turn our attention from 'old world' Europe to investigate the relationship between colonialism and medicine. Andrew Wear's chapter starts by focusing on the impact of old world pathogens on the native populations of the Americas and Australasia. Here, he stresses the crucial role played by the 'importation' of such diseases in laying waste to the indigenous populations, and thus facilitating the successful colonization and conquest of new lands. Colonization, however, posed its own series of medical problems for the newcomers. Traditional medical theories routinely averred that individual constitutions were in part the product of native climates. Immigration to new lands, climates and environments thus posed a major medical dilemma. Early modern physicians found their way round the problem by either promoting the health-giving qualities of the new lands or, as was increasingly the case in hostile environments such as the Caribbean and the American South, advocating the virtues of acclimatization. Moreover, in some cases the health-enhancing qualities of native plants and drugs might be trumpeted. In such cases, however, as Wear's citation of the example of Spanish colonization in the Americas suggests, the native body of medical ideas associated with such drugs and herbal remedies was usually overlooked or denigrated. Once again, it is the ability of European practitioners to incorporate such novel cures into the traditional canon that speaks volumes for the durability and flexibility of the traditional Galenic system. Spanish hospitals in Mexico, for example, incorporated elements of native medicine and practice. And in his concluding section, Wear describes how aspects of black, African medicine survived, and in some cases competed with, white, colonial medicine on the slave plantations of the Caribbean and the American South.

In the final chapter, Laurence Brockliss focuses attention on the eighteenth century. This was a period dominated by the spread of 'enlightenment', which Brockliss defines as 'a movement of intellectual emancipation which ... preached the possibility of moral and material progress'. His chapter explores how medicine, like other areas of eighteenth-century life, was touched by these and associated developments in the economic, political and cultural organization of society. In particular, he traces changes in the nature and content of medical education and emphasizes the extent to which the old boundaries between physicians, surgeons and others were breaking down under the influence of market forces. The creation of a fully fledged 'medical marketplace' meant that medical transactions were now dominated by the purchasing power of the patient while learned physicians fought a losing battle in their struggle to undermine the pretensions of their unlearned competitors. To some extent, there was nothing novel about this situation. University-educated practitioners had struggled to establish their supremacy in earlier centuries (as suggested, for example, in Chapter 2). What made the situation different in the eighteenth century was the proliferation of new forms of training, allied to the expansion of literacy, which allowed a growing number of medical practitioners to compete on equal terms with the university-educated physicians.

References

Butterfield, H. [1931] (1951) *The Whig Interpretation of History*, London: G. Bell.

Illich, I. (1963) *Limits to Medicine: The Expropriation of Health*, Harmondsworth: Penguin.

Jenner, M. (1999) 'Body, image, text in early modern Europe', *Social History of Medicine*, vol.12, pp.143–54.

Lindemann, M. (1999) *Medicine and Society in Early Modern Europe*, Cambridge: Cambridge University Press.

Osler, M.J. (ed) (2000) *Rethinking the Scientific Revolution*, Cambridge: Cambridge University Press.

Pelling, M. (2003) *Medical Conflicts in Early Modern London: Patronage, Physicians and Irregular Practitioners 1550–1640*, Oxford: Clarendon Press.

Porter, R. (1985) 'The patient's view: doing medical history from below', *Theory and Society*, vol.14, pp.175–98.

Porter R. (2002) 'Disease and the historian' in P. Burke (ed.) *History and Historians in the Twentieth Century*, Oxford: Oxford University Press, pp.165–80.

Rosenberg, C.E. and Golden, R. (1992) *Framing Disease: Studies in Cultural History*, Brunswick, NJ: Rutgers University Press.

Selye, H. (1956) *The Stress of Life*, New York: McGraw-Hill.

Shapin, S. (1996) *The Scientific Revolution*, Chicago: University of Chicago Press.

Szasz, T. (1961) *The Myth of Mental Illness: Foundations of a Theory of Personal Conduct*, New York: Dell.

Szasz, T. (1970) *The Manufacture of Madness: A Comparative Study of the Inquisition and the Mental Health Movement*, New York: Harper & Row.

Thompson, E.P. (1968) *The Making of the English Working Class*, Harmondsworth: Penguin.

Wear, A. (2000) *Knowledge and Practice in English Medicine 1550–1680*, Cambridge: Cambridge University Press.

1

Medicine in Western Europe in 1500

Sachiko Kusukawa

Objectives

When you have completed this chapter you should be able to:

- describe the main characteristics of ancient Greek medicine;

- understand how ancient medicine was studied in western Europe in 1500;

- explain how ancient medical knowledge was used in western Europe.

1.1 Introduction

We have chosen to begin this study of the history of medicine in the year 1500, and my aim in this chapter is to give you a brief account of medical knowledge and practice in Europe at that time. Although the chapter covers a lot of ground, many features that I discuss will be examined in greater detail in later chapters. I shall focus in particular on the situation in Rome at the beginning of the sixteenth century. Rome has been chosen, not because it was a famous centre of medical learning (that reputation belonged to places such as Padua, Bologna and Montpellier), but because it reflected many of the most important features and trends in medical knowledge and practice that could be found across Europe at this time. Rome is also important for other reasons. As the heart of western Christianity for over a thousand years, Rome occupied a central point in the religious and cultural life of all Europeans. And as the ancient capital city of a vast and powerful empire, Rome was also increasingly the focus of scholars and others in the fifteenth and sixteenth centuries who were eager to recapture or revive its cultural and intellectual heritage. As you will see, this rich legacy was to play a vital role in reshaping the medical world of all sixteenth-century Europeans. It is therefore fitting to start the journey here, and to focus on the state of medical knowledge and practice in Rome at the dawn of the sixteenth century. You should then be in a good position to assess the extent to which medicine in 1500 was both characterized by continuity with its immediate medieval past and challenged by the new spirit of enquiry that typified the age of the **Renaissance**.

1.2 Rome and Europe in 1500

Let us begin by looking at Rome as it appeared in 1500. In many ways, the city was quite different from the Rome we know today: it had fewer bridges across the River Tiber, Michelangelo had not begun work on the ceiling of the Sistine Chapel, St Peter's Basilica had not yet been rebuilt, and there were fewer inhabitants. The Roman Empire had perished in the fifth century CE, but, as in today's Rome, the remains of the city's imperial past were everywhere to be seen. Unlike today, however, in 1500, these ancient structures were not kept as museums, but were put to different uses by the city's inhabitants. Thus, the Colosseum was used as a fortress, the Forum as a cattle market, and ancient temples were transformed into churches or civic buildings. One of them, the Temple of Antonino and Faustina, had been occupied by the pharmacists' guild since 1492 (Stinger, 1985, pp.14–46). Rome was also where St Peter, the leading disciple of Christ, worked and died. His successors as head of the Christian church, the bishops of Rome, thereafter claimed the title of pope. In time, a complex administrative system of ecclesiastical governance was created; termed the 'papacy', it oversaw the lives of all Christians in western Europe. Large numbers of pilgrims visited Rome every Easter, and the numbers swelled in 'jubilee' or 'holy years'. For such occasions, popes built new bridges and extended hostels to care for tired and sick pilgrims. In 1500, the Spanish Pope Alexander VI (1492–1503) celebrated the jubilee with much pomp and spectacle. Thus Rome, at this time, not only basked in its ancient imperial past, but also saw itself as the city of God and the heart of western Christendom. It was also in Rome, 1,300 years earlier, that Galen of Pergamum (now Bergama in present-day Turkey) practised Greek medicine and made his mark. He boasted that his achievement in medicine was equivalent to that of the Emperor Trajan (98–117 CE), who had extended the empire to Romania, Hungary, the Ukraine, Arabia and Armenia. Like Trajan's Column, too, very much in evidence in the Rome of 1500, Galen's heritage was monumental. You will be meeting Galen anon. What is important to note here is that this description of Rome in 1500 highlights two important features of medical knowledge in Europe at this time: a classical heritage and a Christian context.

Politically, Europe was very different in 1500 from the Europe of today (Plate 1). Instead of a country called 'Italy', for example, the Italian peninsula was composed of a conglomeration of semi-independent **city states**, such as the republics of Venice and Genoa. It also contained extensive territories belonging to the pope (the Papal States). Spain, which had been created out of the union of the kingdoms of Castile and Aragon in 1479, had other dependent European territories such as Sardinia, Sicily and Naples. During the early decades of the sixteenth century, Spain was to grow yet more powerful following the acquisition of vast territories in central and southern America, and the accession of the Spanish king to the **Habsburg** lands in central Europe, including Burgundy and the **Holy Roman Empire** in 1519. As the newly crowned emperor of vast dominions, Charles V (1519–56) revived memories of imperial Rome. He threatened briefly the peace of great powers like France, which now found itself surrounded by Spanish and Habsburg lands. In reality, however, Charles's real potential to recreate a unified empire on the model of ancient Rome was severely circumscribed. The Holy Roman Empire itself was little more than a loose confederation of semi-autonomous principalities and cities that covered much of present-day Germany, Switzerland, the Netherlands, Austria and Hungary. Each polity jealously guarded its independence and privileges and only reluctantly permitted imperial inter-ference in the day-to-day administration of government. There were in fact about 500 independent states and political entities in Europe in 1500. Politically, legally and economically, then, Europe was more fragmented in 1500 than in the twenty-first century. This in turn suggests that, from a medical perspective, we might expect similar diversity and fragmentation, reflecting the variety of local traditions and customs. This was not, however, the case. Despite regional variations, there was at this time a common body of medical practitioners operating throughout Europe who broadly shared a common approach to both the practice and the knowledge of medicine.

1.3   The organization of medical practice

Three distinct groups of medical practitioners can be identified in the Rome of 1500: physicians, barber-surgeons and apothecaries. These particular practitioners were those that had chosen to form collective bodies. Physicians had formed the College of Physicians, whose right to co-opt members and to fine unlicensed practitioners was confirmed by Pope Sixtus IV (1471–84) in 1471; barber-surgeons had similarly incorporated themselves in the Compagnia ed Università in the 1440s; and apothecaries had their own college by 1487. Generally speaking, physicians dealt with the inside of the body, treating diseases, fevers and inflammations, and they also prescribed and supervised any surgical or medicinal treatment. Barber-surgeons dealt with the outside of the body, treating external wounds and carrying out manual procedures such as bloodletting, **cautery** and bonesetting as well as offering more cosmetic services, such as shaving. Apothecaries prepared and sold medicines, usually on the instructions of physicians. During the **Middle Ages**, these practitioners had organized themselves into interest groups – guilds – just as other craftworkers and tradespeople had done. Outside this privileged triad, an amorphous collection of healers – tooth-drawers, bonesetters, eye surgeons, midwives, snake handlers (who sold cures for snakebites), wise-women and cunning-folk (who peddled herbal remedies, charms and love potions) – plied their trade, often in the face of official disapproval. Guilds represented and protected the economic, political and religious interests of their members: members alone were permitted to practise their craft or trade in the community; membership of a guild required proof of adequate training and proficiency in the craft; and guilds set the prices of goods and services and the conditions of labour and trade. Such guilds existed in most large towns and cities in western Europe at 1500, though there were some regional differences. In Florence, for instance, physicians and apothecaries had formed a single guild in 1236. Conflict between the three groups of practitioners was not uncommon. In Paris, for example, friction between the surgeon's college of St Cosmas (established in 1210) and the physicians of the medical faculty of the University of Paris was a constant feature of relations between the two bodies in the later medieval period (Porter, 1999, p.119).

Conflict was perhaps inevitable, given the fact that these three groups often worked side by side for the same clients, but cooperation was essential, too. Arrangements for working together varied. Some practitioners shared premises, or set up their shops close to each other (Plate 2). Apothecaries sometimes contracted physicians and surgeons to work at their shops for a fixed number of hours each week, to provide a sort of 'walk-in clinic' (Plate 3). It was cheaper for patients to consult a physician at an apothecary's shop than it was for them to arrange a visit to their home, and the arrangement also allowed physicians to treat more patients.

The three groups also worked alongside each other in the service of wealthier patrons. Popes and emperors typically had a retinue of six to eight physicians, a couple of surgeons and an apothecary in their main residence. These medical personnel catered for all the members of the household, which might include over a hundred retainers and servants. Some of these practitioners also fulfilled other functions within the court – for instance, the court apothecary sometimes doubled up as confectioner or grocer. Pope Alexander VI had seven physicians – one of them, Gaspar Torrella (whom we shall meet again later), was also the Vatican librarian. Those employed by the pope might also work for local hospitals or universities: an appointment at the medical faculty of 'La Sapienza' (that is, the University of Rome), for instance, may well have appealed to prospective papal physicians who were wary of the vagaries of court politics and the rapid succession of popes (Palmer, 1990).

The importance of water and the wider environment in **early modern** discussions of health is discussed in more detail in Chapter 11.

Rome also had a health board, whose officials looked after the community's interest as a whole by activities such as improving sanitation and implementing restrictions on movement during outbreaks of the plague. (In Rome, such officials were appointed by the pope, but elsewhere they were appointed by municipal governments.) From 1480, the three main streets of Rome that converged on Ponte Sant'Angelo were paved and subjected to regular cleaning, as were the public markets in the large piazzas. Health boards operated elsewhere in Europe, and several municipal governments contracted physicians and surgeons to serve their urban and rural inhabitants. Alexander VI also restored some of the ancient aqueducts, and helped drain marshy areas where the air was regarded as noxious. It should be noted, however, that these measures were often piecemeal: they did not constitute coordinated urban planning or public health policies. During the course of the sixteenth century, such developments grew apace, especially after the rebuilding of the city in the wake of the **Sack of Rome** in 1527.

Despite local variations in the organization of medical practice and official attitudes to health care, it is important to note that the threefold division of medical practitioners – physicians, barber-surgeons and apothecaries – could be found throughout western Europe in 1500.

1.4 The medical knowledge of the ancient Greeks

Anyone practising medicine in 1500 would almost certainly have been familiar with the names of Hippocrates and Galen, even if they had never read any of the texts written by these medical giants. One of the main features of western European medicine is that it was heir to an ancient body of knowledge that was Greek in origin. In order to understand the state of medical knowledge in 1500, it is therefore essential to familiarize yourself with some of the major concepts of ancient Greek medicine. I shall focus on two areas in particular: Greek ideas about the human body; and Greek ideas about diagnosis, prognosis and treatment.

Greek ideas about the human body

Galen (129–*c*.210 CE) was a Greek-speaking physician who worked in imperial Rome. He wrote a vast number of tracts on a great number of medical topics, and championed, systematized and developed Greek medicine as this had been passed down in the body of writings known as the 'Hippocratic corpus'. Though they bear his name, the sixty or so texts in the corpus were not all written by Hippocrates (*c*.460–377 BCE), about whom little is known (see Porter, 1999, pp.55–6). At the time Galen was practising medicine in Rome, individuals needed to obtain no standard educational requirement or qualification in order for them to become 'doctors', and sundry healers advertised wondrous cures. To distance himself from unlearned **empirics**, Galen wished to elevate the status of medicine so that it was regarded with the same degree of dignity afforded to other intellectual pursuits such as philosophy and science. In order to achieve this status, it was crucial for Galen's medicine to concern itself with the nature of causation in the human body since, for the Greeks, an understanding of how things worked was seen as integral to the pursuit of scientific wisdom. In this way, he was able to foster the idea that medicine constituted a unified and rational body of knowledge. Galen's ideal doctor was therefore both learned and methodical. Unlike empirics, who possessed no rational account for their cures, Galen and his followers were able to provide detailed explanations for their therapeutic methods. What is more, Galen also wrote in Greek, which in Rome was the language of the cultured person. He was quick to lampoon his non-philosophical competitors and trumpeted his own successes with the great and the good, including the emperor, Marcus Aurelius (Porter, 1999, pp.73–7). Galen's image of the ideal doctor, encapsulated in the title of his book *The Best Doctor is Also a Philosopher*, and found everywhere in his writings, was to endure and shape the image of the 'learned physician' in medieval and Renaissance Europe (Nutton, 1992).

Now let us look a little more closely at how Galen understood the structure and workings of the human body. (The study of the structure and organization of the body is called 'anatomy', and that of the body's functions is called 'physiology'.) In his learned treatises on medicine, Galen said that the skeleton was the fundamental structure of the body: he compared the function of the bones in the body to that performed by the walls of a house. In turn, this structure housed numerous vessels and organs that were linked by a series of channels – veins and nerves – that supplied the body with the fluids and **spirits** that gave it life, heat and sensation. By far the most important of these channels were the veins and the arteries, which Galen compared to the branches of a tree. Each was rooted in one of the principal organs of the body: the veins in the liver; the arteries in the heart. This reflected Galen's understanding that these two channels carried two different types of blood. For Galen, the **venous** blood was produced in the liver from digested food; its main function was to nourish each part of the body via the system of veins. Some of the venous blood also reached the left **ventricle** of the heart, where it mixed with the ***pneuma*** – life-giving spirits extracted from the air in the lungs – to produce the **arterial** blood. This gave heat and thus life to the body via the arteries – a system of vessels entirely independent from the veins. Both the venous and the arterial blood were 'used up' by the body and had to be constantly replenished, the former in the liver, the latter in the heart. Blood was attracted by and drawn to parts of the body where it had been consumed, and thus the movement of blood throughout the body was seen in terms of supply and demand, rather than of circulation.

Following earlier Greek ideas, especially those of Plato (427–347 BCE), Galen believed that every animal, including human beings, possessed a soul, and that this soul was responsible for overseeing every aspect of the animal's life – that is, it performed the three functions of respiration, nutrition and animation. It carried out these functions by means of the three medical spirits – vital, natural and animal. The 'vital spirits', which were conveyed to the rest of the body from the heart via the arterial blood, were so called because they endowed the body with life. The 'natural spirits', on the other hand, were the property of the liver and provided essential nourishment to the body via the venous system. The 'animal spirits' were so named from the Latin word *anima*, meaning 'life' or 'soul'. They represented the most refined form of arterial blood and were processed in the *rete mirabile*, a network of nerves and vessels that was thought to exist at the base of the human brain. They were transmitted to the rest of the body through the nerves, which Galen understood as hollow vessels, and were thus seen as the vehicle for thought, sensation and movement. In this way, the vital bodily functions came to be associated with three main areas of the body: the stomach and liver were associated with nutrition and growth; the lungs and heart with heat and vitality; and the brain with sensation and thought.

The soul as understood by Galen was clearly a very different entity from the Christian soul. For Galen, the soul was a material substance, albeit invisible to the naked eye, which lived and died with the body. This is very different from the Christian idea of the soul as something that exists apart from the physical body, and that lives on after the body's death. During the sixteenth and seventeenth centuries, Galen's materialistic view of the soul, and his rejection of Christianity (he lived two centuries after the death of Christ), would lead to accusations of atheism against some Galenic physicians. It certainly encouraged his critics to seek a new medical system, which was better able to accommodate key aspects of Christian dogma, including belief in a non-material and immortal human soul.

Another important concept for Galen was that of the 'humoral body'. This concept is an important one for medicine throughout the period covered by this book. It explained not only the causes of disease but also individual characteristics and mental habits, as well as general differences between men and women, the old and the young, and different races of people. For Galen, all mental operations and habits were ultimately reducible to natural or physical changes in the body. So how did the system work? Essentially, the belief was that all the organs, vessels and other parts of the body were ultimately reducible to four **qualities**: hot, cold, wet and dry. The proportion in which these qualities occurred differed from person to person, so that the amount of, say, heat and moisture that was natural for one individual was not necessarily natural for another. An individual's particular mixture of qualities was called their **complexion** or temperament. The complexion was an innate characteristic, acquired at the moment of conception and persisting through life, which might nonetheless vary according to external influences. Thus, there were some general patterns of complexion, according to age, sex and habitat: the young, for example, had more heat and moisture than the old; women were colder and moister than men (which, it was claimed, accounted for their timidity, their lesser intellect and their menstrual cycle); and those living in colder climates were colder and moister than those living in hot climates. The balance of these qualities was maintained through the interaction of the four **humours** that existed within an individual's body. These humours were bodily fluids essential to the physiological functioning of the organism. They were: yellow bile (also known as red bile or choler), black bile (also known as melancholy), phlegm and pure blood. Blood occupied a special place among the humours. The actual blood that flowed through the veins was made up of the pure humour, blood, mixed with a lesser proportion of the other humours, which were generated as part of the process of the manufacture of blood. The balance of these humours gave rise to different temperaments, with the predominant humour determining an individual's character. Thus a person who had yellow bile as their predominant humour was characterized as choleric (that is, hot-headed and quick to react); having black bile, or melancholy, as the predominant humour meant that he or she was sad and low-spirited; a phlegmatic person was lethargic and apathetic; and a sanguine person, in whom the humour blood was predominant, was warm and pleasant.

Humoral theory, as this way of looking at the body is often referred to, ultimately derived from classical Greek ideas about nature and natural causation. The most systematic expression of these ideas is to be found in the work of the Greek philosopher Aristotle (384–322 BCE). Aristotle had studied the natural world, including humans, in an attempt to understand why living beings functioned in the way they did. From his extensive observations, he concluded that all things in nature were composed of four **elements**: earth, air, fire and water, each of which was associated with a pair of qualities: dry–cold, hot–wet, dry–hot and cold–wet. All change in nature he saw as being caused by alterations in the balance of these four qualities. Humoral theory is thus a 'qualitative' explanation of change, as opposed to 'quantitative' or 'mechanical' explanations. Such mechanical explanations had been put forward by ancient philosophers such as Democritus (*fl*.420 BCE) and Epicurus (341–271 BCE), who based them on the idea that matter was composed of tiny particles, which were called 'atoms' (not to be confused with the modern, scientific meaning of the term). The theory was that atoms of different sizes, travelling at different speeds, randomly interacted with each other to cause physical change in nature. However, Aristotle – and indeed most other Greek philosophers – rejected mechanical explanations such as this, because in their seeming randomness, they failed to account for the order that could be observed in nature. The order and regularity of the natural world persuaded the philosophers that all things in nature – including all parts of the human body – had been created for a specific purpose: nature was believed to do nothing in vain. These purposes counted as causes for the Greeks and became the cornerstone of their philosophy. Greek medicine and Aristotelian philosophy therefore agreed in seeking to explain causation in the natural world in terms of qualitative change.

Although Galen's ideas may seem like a far cry from our modern understanding of how the human body works, they formed the basis of medical knowledge for centuries. In the following exercise, you will look at how Galen's ideas about the human body affected his understanding of health and disease. Galen defined medicine as 'the knowledge of what is healthy, what is morbid and what is neither'.

Note that he called this knowledge 'scientific' because it was based on a wide-ranging study of many cases, not just on unique or individual examples. This was an important point for Galen to make, as it distinguished his medicine from that of the empirics, who dealt with individual cases.

Exercise

Now read 'Galen's approach to health and disease: *The Art of Medicine*' (Source Book 1, Reading 1.1) and then answer the following questions:

1 How were the concepts of 'healthy', 'morbid' and 'neither' related?

2 According to Galen, what were the causes of change and therefore of illness? (Note that Galen used the word 'necessary' to describe these causes, to indicate that the body cannot escape them.)

Discussion

1 According to Galen, a healthy body had a good complexion – that is, a good balance of humours and arrangement of the parts of the body. A diseased body did not have a good balance – in fact, it had an imbalance caused by a deficiency in or an excess of one or more of the humours. In this view, disease was seen as some kind of disturbance to the internal balance of the human body, rather than as the result of external organisms invading it. Galen saw bodily health in terms of degree, with perfect health at one end of a spectrum and illness at the other. When an individual's body had the balance that was ideal for that particular person, then it was in a state of perfect health. When parts of the body fell short of that perfect balance, then the body was in a state of disease. In the middle of the spectrum was a state when the body was neither perfectly healthy nor diseased. Galenic medicine, then, was about restoring a disturbed balance of humours in the body.

2 Galen listed six major influences on the human body that might cause changes in the humoral balance and thus induce disease. He listed these as: contact with the ambient air; motion and rest; sleep and waking; substances taken; substances voided or retained; what happens to the soul. These became the important causes that Galen's philosopher-doctor had to master.

In the ninth century, Johannitius (809–73), a **Nestorian** Christian from southern Iraq who translated the *Art of Medicine*, called Galen's six causes the six '**non-naturals**' because they were not natural to the human body – that is, they did not form part of the body's internal workings. In his translation, Johannitius classified them as: surroundings (e.g. air); exercise (walks, riding, massages and sex); sleep (and waking); ingested substances (food, drink, medicine); those things that are eliminated or retained (secretions and excretions); the 'passions of the soul' (emotional states such as anger, grief and envy) (García-Ballester, 1993). These six factors, which are essential for health, could also affect an individual's innate complexion, and result in disease. Thus, by carefully managing the non-naturals, the physician could both restore a sick body to health and prevent a healthy body from becoming sick. As part of the course of treatment, or **regimen**, therefore, the physician would advise his patient on virtually all aspects of his or her daily life.

Diagnosis, prognosis and treatment

Galen and Hippocrates also wrote much about the practice of medicine – that is, about diagnosis, prognosis and treatment. Diagnosis involved taking note of a patient's appearance, and listening to his or her account of the course of their illness or pain. Since humoral theory was concerned with keeping the humours in the correct balance, anything that impeded the natural flow of fluids within the body was a possible cause of disease. Thus notions of stagnation, corruption and putrefaction assumed great importance. The body was believed to rid itself of accumulating pollutants and corrupt matter through bodily excretions such as urine, faeces, blood and sweat, which of course contained humours. Evidence about the patient's bodily state could thus be obtained by examining such excreted matter. Another important diagnostic technique for the Galenic physician was taking the patient's pulse. The pulse was regarded as a sign of vitality, and different types were thought to be indicative of different illnesses – Galen describes pulses as 'double-beating', 'hectic', 'gazelling', 'anting' and 'worming'. However, it is not clear whether all physicians were able to distinguish and identify the different types of pulse. In medieval Europe, the most common procedures used in diagnosis were inspecting the urine and taking the pulse (Figure 1.1).

Prognosis involved the ability to accurately forecast the course of a disease, based on the doctrine of 'crisis' or 'critical days'. All illnesses were believed to have 'turning points', whether for the worse or for the better, and the critical day represented this point. The calculation of these critical days depended on the phases of the moon, as set out in Galen's text *On Critical Days*. A sense of the limits of the healing arts made prognosis all the more important. Given that not all illnesses were curable, a physician needed to ensure that he was not blamed if his patient died. In such cases, the ability to predict that the patient had taken a turn for the worse helped to protect the physician's reputation; in more fortunate cases, a prognosis might enable him to find a cure, and thus engender confidence in the patient. Having confidence in the doctor was thought to relate to one of the six non-naturals, the passions of the soul, which in turn might have a beneficial effect on the humours. Accuracy in prognosis thus became the hallmark of a good physician.

Physicians prescribed treatments to help individuals maintain their health (such treatment is termed prophylaxis), as well as prescribing medication or surgery to restore sick or wounded bodies to health. The maintenance of health was usually achieved by adhering to a particular regimen, or course of treatment, designed to manage the six non-naturals. Medication in this period was based mainly on preparations made from herbs and some minerals. These natural products were collectively called *materia medica* and each was classified as having one of the four qualities (hot, cold, wet, dry) in different degrees ranging from one (imperceptible) to four (fatal). Because the function of medicine was to restore a balance that had been disturbed, the principle of medication rested on the idea of

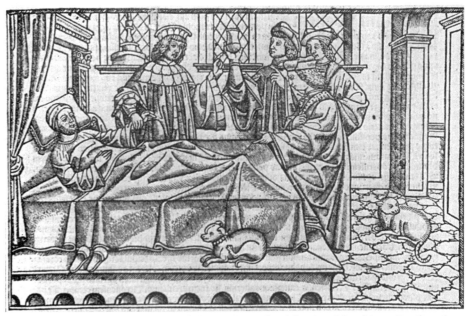

Figure 1.1   In this typical scene of diagnosis, a physician is taking his patient's pulse and examining his urine. Though they may possibly be household servants, the other men appear to be physicians too. The presence of more than one physician in attendance at his bedside would indicate that the patient is quite affluent. National Library of Medicine, Bethesda, Maryland

opposition. For instance, an illness that caused excessive heat was treated with a medicine that had a strong cold quality. The quantity of medicine was adjusted according to both the intensity of the illness and the extent to which the quality exceeded that which was normal for the patient. The *materia medica* could be used on their own, as **simples**, or could be mixed together to produce a compound. One of the most famous Greek compound medicines was 'theriac'. Originally an antidote to snakebite, and later believed to be an antidote to all poisons, its exact composition was a matter of great debate. Theriac was given as a general tonic well into the eighteenth century (Figure 1.2). Surgical operations that a physician might prescribe included the treatment of wounds, bonesetting, bloodletting (to rid the body of the noxious and excess humours) and cautery (to alter the flow and distribution of humours). Physicians might administer medicines to their patients themselves, but they preferred to leave the manual tasks involved in surgery to surgeons or barber-surgeons.

An important challenge faced by every doctor trained in Galenic medicine was that of applying this knowledge to individual cases. Individuals had different optimum complexions; they lived in different conditions and environments; they had different lifestyles and occupations; and they were affected by illnesses in various ways, depending on the critical days. To draw up his ***consilium***, the Galenic physician had to develop a means of applying his medical knowledge – which, as you have seen, aspired to being universal and scientific – to these individual patients. This difficult process led some physicians to question whether medicine was in fact an art rather than a science – the essential difference being that an 'art'

The debate as to whether medicine constituted an art or a science is discussed further in Chapter 2.

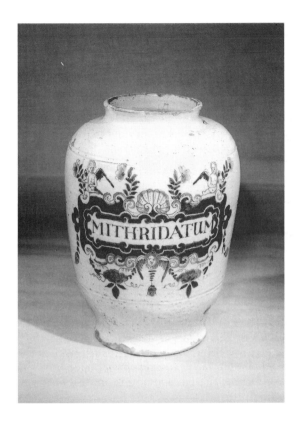

Figure 1.2   An eighteenth-century ceramic jar labelled 'Mithridatum'. Mithridatum was a version of theriac attributed to Mithridates VI, the king of Pontus (120–63 BCE). That it was still in use at this date attests to the persistence of the belief in this ancient and miraculous antidote to all poisons. Wellcome Library, London

remained conjectural and open to question, whereas a 'science' provided certitude. The difference between the two, as they were applied to medicine, was a continuing topic of debate in learned medicine. The following exercise will give you an idea of what was involved in a medieval medical consultation.

Exercise

Now read 'A medieval *consilium*: Ugo Benzi (1376–1439)' (Source Book 1, Reading 1.2). What aspects of classical Greek medicine were evident in the *consilium* of this medieval physician?

Discussion

In most respects, Benzi's *consilium* was faithful to ancient precedents. He described the case in terms of qualities and humours, and his regimen had instructions relating to six areas, which corresponded to the six non-naturals – those external conditions that affect the humours. The section on food and drink was the longest and most detailed, and reflected a long and unbroken interest, in medical circles, in the importance of diet in the preservation of health. Benzi was a university-educated physician who followed Galenic principles in all aspects of his medical practice.

1.5 The making of the learned doctor in medieval Europe

As we have already glimpsed in the case of Benzi, Greek medicine was studied and used in western Europe long after Galen's death, and it survived the political upheavals of the intervening centuries. To a large extent, it was kept alive by influential followers, such as Oribasius (325–97) and Paul of Aegina (*fl.*640), who compiled encyclopedias and compendia of his doctrines and remedies. Not all of Galen's works survived, and those that did were often preserved in translations, compilations and commentaries produced by Arab philosopher-physicians, such as Avicenna (980–1037), Averroës (1126–98), Rhazes (865–925), Haly Abbas (*fl.* late tenth century) and Albucasis (*fl. c.*940). As well as translating Galen's writings, such scholars also sought to develop and systematize Galenic medicine. (For a discussion of the Arabic translation movement, see Porter, 1999, pp.94–103.)

The key institution for medical learning in medieval Europe was the university. Around 1100, there developed in Salerno (already a renowned centre for medical practitioners) a tradition of medical instruction based on a canonical set of texts called the *Articella* [Little Art of Medicine]. From around 1200, groups of cathedral masters and students began to form corporations (similar to those of the craft guilds) called 'universities', to teach and confer qualifications in learning. By 1500, every university had a medical faculty, though some were more celebrated and better attended than others. In the thirteenth century, the universities of Paris and Montpellier superseded Salerno as the chief centres of medical teaching. They, in turn, were later eclipsed by Bologna in the fourteenth century and by Padua in the fifteenth century. But even Padua awarded only eight or nine medical degrees per year, at most, in its heyday. Medieval universities, then, were producing very small numbers of learned physicians. These university medical faculties were nothing like the large medical schools of today, which produce hundreds of medical professionals (Siraisi, 1990, p.64).

A student wishing to study medicine at university in 1500 would first have had to complete a course in the faculty of arts. Having mastered the seven **liberal arts**, the student would then have gone on to study philosophy, which encompassed logic (the discipline of thinking), **natural philosophy** (the science of nature) and moral philosophy (the science of action) before proceeding to the 'higher' faculties, of law, theology or medicine. Aristotelian logic provided the scaffolding for subsequent scientific and medical argument in antiquity and throughout the Middle Ages, and Aristotelian philosophy provided a theory of natural causation. Natural philosophy was a discipline based on the works of Aristotle, which encompassed what we might loosely describe today as science. It dealt, for example, with issues of causation in the heavens and on earth, as well as the relationship between the body and the soul, and was regarded as fundamental to prospective students of medicine. I mentioned above that Greek medicine and Aristotelian philosophy agreed in their aspiration to produce a body of 'scientific' knowledge as well as to explain the natural world in terms of qualitative change. An Aristotelian arts course and a Galenic medical education therefore offered a coherent outlook, and provided the foundation needed to be a 'learned doctor'.

Although some scholars, such as Pietro d'Abano (1257–*c*.1315), pointed to differences between Aristotelian and Galenic views of nature, the general affinity between them meant that they were linked within university walls well into the seventeenth century.

Throughout the Middle Ages, the teaching of the medical faculties continued to be based on the *Articella*, a collection of texts that included Galen's *Art of Medicine*, the Hippocratic *Prognostics*, the *Aphorisms*, and tracts on the urine and the pulse. You have already come across the *Art of Medicine*. The *Aphorisms*, attributed to Hippocrates, starts with the famous maxim *Ars longa, vita brevis* ('Art is long, life is short') and is a collection of rules of thumb covering diagnosis (for example, blood or pus in the urine indicates ulceration of the kidneys or the bladder), prognosis (jaundice occurring on the seventh, ninth, eleventh or fourteenth day of a fever is favourable unless the right **hypochondrium** is hard), medication (hellebore is a dangerous drug for healthy people since in these it induces convulsions) and reassuring truisms (desperate cases require desperate remedies).

From the thirteenth century, many more of Galen's works were translated into Latin from the Arabic. An important feature of medical education in medieval universities is that the Greek heritage was mediated by learned Arabic scholars and physicians. In the universities, instead of reading the numerous works of Galen and Hippocrates for themselves, students studied them by way of summaries and introductions that were written by Arabic commentators, and subsequently translated into Latin. Avicenna's *Canon* was particularly valued for its discussion of whether medicine was a science or an art, its synopsis of physiology, fevers, the principles of diseases and treatments and its listing of diseases from head to toe (Siraisi, 1987). Many compilations by other Arabic authors, such as Rhazes, Averroës and Haly Abbas, were also used and read in the universities, as they systematized, developed and clarified the teachings of their Greek predecessors. Thus, although based on the ideas and principles of Galen and Hippocrates, medieval university learning was by no means 'Galenic' in the strictest sense – it was learnt through the fruits of centuries of study by others, especially the Arabs. The learned physician therefore discussed philosophically and logically, not just the ideas of Galen and Hippocrates, but also the views of Arab commentators, such as Avicenna. Several medieval physicians, such as Benzi, in turn became noted for their scholarly commentaries on these canonical texts, using the logical and disputational skills they had learnt in the arts faculty (McVaugh, 1997b; Siraisi, 1990, pp.55–77).

There were further medieval developments of Greek medical thought in the area of astrology. In Galenic and Hippocratic medical texts, astrology and astronomy received little attention, apart from their use in the calculation of critical days. Though it was believed that the position of the planets exercised an influence on the health of individual human bodies, this was mainly in terms of the effects produced on the humours as a result of atmospheric and climatic changes. During the Middle Ages, however, medical students began to learn more developed theories of astrology from works that were attributed to Galen or Hippocrates but in fact were of **Byzantine** origin. The importance attached to astrology and astronomy in medieval universities can be seen in the medical curriculum at

Bologna in 1405, which stipulated that students attend four years of lectures on these subjects.

Astrology became the cornerstone of prognosis in the Middle Ages. In addition to knowing how to construct a horoscope, a budding medical student also had to learn such astrological information as: the division of the heavens into twelve sections, or 'houses', correlating to the signs of the zodiac, and how the moon's position in relation to these houses affected each part of the body; which zodiacal sign ruled which part of the body (for example, Pisces ruled the feet); the qualities of the planets (for example, the moon was cold and wet, the sun hot and dry); which planets were beneficent and which were maleficent (Jupiter, for example, was beneficent, whereas Saturn and Mars were maleficent); whether the relative positions of particular planets were favourable or unfavourable. Because the moon was the nearest planet to the earth it was thought to have the greatest influence on the body and to govern the 'critical' times of acute diseases. By constructing the patient's horoscope at the time the illness had set in, the physician was expected to predict the course of the illness and to suggest treatment, using astrological principles. Proficiency in astrology thus became another hallmark of the learned physician. In practice, however, most university-educated physicians found it difficult and time-consuming to work out from scratch the planetary positions on any given day or time. Instead, they relied on various astronomical tables and charts, which aided and simplified these onerous calculations. Many such charts and tables survive, which attests to their usefulness for physicians. There were some exceptions, of course: Paul of Middleburg (1446–1534), the physician to Francesco Maria della Rovere, the Duke of Urbino, was so accomplished at astronomical calculations that he was asked to help with the **calendar reform**.

Teaching anatomy by the **dissection** of human bodies was not standard practice in the medieval medical curriculum. Just as Galen had done, the earliest medical scholars dissected animals and used their findings to describe human anatomy. In the fourteenth century, however, a new tradition of public dissection was instituted at the University of Bologna by Mondino de' Liuzzi (d.1326). The universities of Montpellier and Padua quickly followed suit in stipulating attendance at a public dissection in their medical curriculum, but many other universities rarely conducted dissections. Mondino's anatomical demonstration, in which he dissected the bodies of hanged criminals, spanned three or more days. He divided the body into three parts – lower, middle and upper – which corresponded, respectively to the functions of nutrition, respiration and animation, as set out in the only two texts of Galenic anatomy known in the Middle Ages (*On the Treatment of Limbs* and the *On the Natural Faculties*). However, the aim of these dissections was to demonstrate what was already known, rather than to conduct original, observational research. Mondino's lessons are best understood as visual aids, to confirm the descriptions in Galen's texts. Thus, medical instruction at medieval universities remained predominantly book-based, though medical faculties did require students to gain experience of medical practice by accompanying the senior professor on visits to his patients, and to learn about medical cases by reading collections of *consilia* (Porter, 1999, pp.131–3; Siraisi, 1990, pp.73, 84–91).

Universities thus provided the institutional context through which Greek medicine, mediated via Arab translations and commentaries, was studied. University learning, and the possession of a medical degree, came to form and shape Galen's ideal doctor into the 'learned doctor' of medieval Europe. It enabled those physicians who had been educated at a university to claim expertise by virtue of the breadth of their knowledge of diseases and the depth of their understanding of causes, as well as their prowess in prognosis based on astrological training. This learning distinguished them from other practitioners and from empirics, who relied on experiential trial and error rather than on causal investigation. It therefore provided the basis for claiming authority over the whole practice of medicine. University-educated physicians and professors of medicine began to form colleges of physicians, which were authorized to examine and license those who wished to set up in practice. The role claimed by physicians, however, was often resented by other practitioners. The surgeon Henry of Mondeville (*c*.1260–*c*.1320) found the learning of university-educated physicians pernicious and controlling (McVaugh, 1997b, p.62). The important medical procedure of bloodletting was traditionally carried out by barbers or surgeons. Mondeville resented what he saw as the attempt by learned physicians to impose their authority over these practitioners by using their astrological and physiological knowledge to determine when, where and how much blood should be let.

The licensing of practitioners is discussed further in Chapters 2 and 13.

University learning was not, however, the exclusive privilege of physicians. Some Italian universities, such as Bologna, offered training and degrees in surgery, based on the study of a selection of Galenic and Arabic texts including those of Albucasis and Haly Abbas. Moreover, some surgeons wrote books on surgery in Latin, with learned references to academic authorities in medicine. One such surgeon was a Frenchman, Guy de Chauliac.

Exercise

Now read 'The history of surgery: Guy de Chauliac (1298–1368)' (Source Book 1, Reading 1.3). According to Chauliac, how and why was learning important for a surgeon?

Discussion

Chauliac places himself in the historical line of famous learned physicians, beginning with Hippocrates. He is not shy of exhibiting his knowledge of learned authorities in medicine, and makes frequent references to them. According to Chauliac, education was the hallmark of a surgeon: he had to know about health, illness and the non-naturals, the principles of medicine, geometry, astronomy and other branches of learning. For Chauliac, this learning was what distinguished a surgeon from other craftworkers such as leather workers, carpenters and smiths.

In some respects Chauliac was an exceptional member of his profession. His case does, however, reflect a growing trend in the Middle Ages towards greater differentiation in the practice of surgery. Learned surgeons possessed higher status

15

in their guilds and collegiate bodies. In the Parisian college of St Cosmas, for example, this distinction was manifest in the division between the more eminent 'long-robes' and their lesser brethren, the 'short-robes'. Increasingly, those surgeons with learning who claimed to understand the general principles of surgery began to argue that unlearned barbers should confine themselves to routine work such as bloodletting or cautery and avoid dangerous operations. Some even went so far as to claim parity with physicians, and most were proud to boast of their prowess in performing operations and using the complex instruments of their trade (Figure 1.3).

While experience and manual dexterity remained the identifying mark of a surgeon, learned or not, it is noteworthy that Chauliac also demands that a surgeon behaves in a manner appropriate to his privileged station. Knowledge of what was regarded as appropriate and seemly behaviour was important in the Middle Ages. Several surgeons intent on making surgery a literate, learned and respectable art, elaborated on this topic. They advised against drinking, philandering and social climbing; they recommended a clean and neat appearance, stipulating how long a surgeon's hair should be and what sort of clothing he should wear; and they advised on etiquette and sometimes on how to charge fees. These rules of

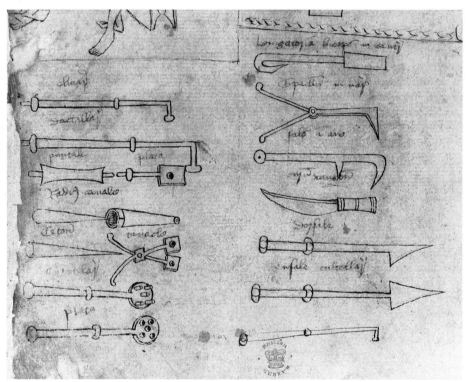

Figure 1.3 A table of surgical instruments, from an English manuscript of the fifteenth century. These drawings were copied from a manuscript of the works of Guy de Chauliac. To the left are various instruments for cautery, and to the right are tools for treating various **fistulae**. Courtesy British Library

comportment, governing the impression the surgeon made on his patients, were intended not only to raise his status, but also to help in effecting a cure. As I mentioned above, having confidence in the practitioner was thought to aid the patient's recovery. These discussions are often cited as early attempts to establish a science of professional ethics, but this was not their original purpose or intent. Their primary aim was to convince the patient that the learned practitioner in front of them was respectable and trustworthy (McVaugh, 1997a).

This preoccupation with comportment was by no means a medieval invention. Numerous Hippocratic and Galenic works discussed the conduct and etiquette that were appropriate to a physician. For example, they recommended that physicians should help those in need, should wear sober headgear and should not discuss their fee at the beginning of a consultation. Patients expected a good physician to be morally upright, as well as an expert in his field. By following such rules, a physician was likely to make a good impression on patients, and thus build up a good practice. These classical works were not recovered until the sixteenth century in Europe, but writings on the duties of physicians dating from the fifth and sixth centuries, but possibly based on earlier works, were known in the Middle Ages (Nutton, 1993).

University learning was not exclusive to physicians in yet another sense: academic books on medicine written in Latin could be translated into shorter and more practical forms. For instance, the *Treasury of the Poor*, ascribed to Peter of Spain (*c.*1210–77), was a compilation of diseases and their remedies aimed at practitioners without university training, which appeared widely in simple Latin and various **vernacular** translations. Likewise, certain herbals, extracted from the works of Galen and Dioscorides (*c.*40–*c.*90 CE), were compiled into reference works in which ailments were indexed in simple Latin or in the vernacular. These also listed indigenous herbs that might be substituted for ancient plants whose equivalent could not be found in medieval Europe. Apothecaries, who were normally trained by apprenticeship, required literacy and numeracy in order to read the prescriptions of physicians. In the sixteenth century, several of them could hold their own in debates with learned physicians over the names, effects and identities of herbs described by the ancient Greeks, while also cultivating and supplying new specimens from their own gardens. Even people who were unable to read at all could access medical information in the form of the calendars that were produced to provide details of the most favourable times for bloodletting, bathing, gathering herbs, and so on (Plate 4). Such activities were governed by astrologically auspicious and inauspicious days, the knowledge of which was calculated by university-trained scholars and made available to ordinary people in pictorial form. To use the calendars, people needed only to be able to recognize the attributes of the saints and the symbols used to denote days favourable for the various activities – knowledge that was in fact common to most people at this time.

These examples suggest the widespread diffusion of Galenic ideas across all levels of society. Doubtless, most people would have had, at best, only a shaky grasp of the medical knowledge behind these ideas. However, the great majority of people, who lacked formal medical training, were still able to share a common body of ideas about health and healing. These centred on the concept of a humoral body, which was affected by the surrounding air or by planetary conjunctions, and on the principle of treating diseases caused by particular qualities with their opposites.

In this section, I have described how Greek medical knowledge was transmitted to medieval Europe through the universities. 'Transmitted' is perhaps a misleading word to use in this context, as Greek medicine itself had undergone transformation at the hands of Arabic translators and commentators. Consequently, the medical knowledge taught in medieval universities was heavily mediated and did not represent a direct link with the classical past. Nonetheless, it was increasingly seen as the source of authority and respectability on which physicians and, to a lesser extent, surgeons could rest their own claims of superiority over rival practitioners.

1.6   Christianity and healing

There can be little doubt that the imperfect, but continuous, tradition of ancient medical learning provides one of the main contexts for an understanding of medicine in late medieval Europe. Equally important, however, in this respect is the role played by Christianity in both popular and learned conceptions of health and disease, and its successful management. Christian values were important in promoting aspects of Greek medicine that might otherwise have been overlooked. The Hippocratic oath (see Reading 1.4 in Source Book 1) is a case in point. Originally representing the interests of a small sect that followed the precepts of the geometer Pythagoras (c.530 BCE), it was not widely recognized in its own time as forming a basic covenant for the relationship between patient and doctor. It survived, in the west, however, because certain aspects of the oath, such as the sanctity of human life (including the embryo), struck a chord with Christian thinking on the same subject. (Suicide and abortion were both permissible in Greek society.)

During the Middle Ages, the Christian concept of an orderly and divinely inspired creation found the qualitative regularity of nature in Aristotle and Galen generally appealing. In particular, Christian scholars agreed with Aristotle's objections against the atomists, whose views seemed to imply chaos and thus deny God's providential hand in the day-to-day functioning of the universe. In addition, the stress laid by Aristotle and Galen on the purposiveness of nature – the idea that everything in the natural world, including human beings and the individual parts of the human body, was designed to perform a specific end – agreed well with the Christian view that God created the world with foresight. This is important to note when discussing medieval natural philosophy, since, although the books by Aristotle were read in the universities, they were read through the eyes of Christians. Nature was ultimately God's creation.

There were, however, some clear differences between the Christians and the ancient Greeks. One of them, as I mentioned above, was the concept of the soul. While Galen and Aristotle held that the soul was coterminous with the human body, Christians believed that it survived bodily death. The immortality of the soul, and its ultimate redemption, was central to Christian belief. Indeed, in many ways, the soul came before the body. Hence the laws of the church (canon law) stipulated that physicians should urge patients to confess their sins before treatment. The church also sought to license midwives, as they were expected to provide emergency baptism in cases of difficult deliveries, and professors of medicine paid for mass to be said for the souls of condemned criminals whose bodies were used in public dissections. Christians also believed that the immaterial Holy Spirit, as well as demonic spirits, could affect the physical world, including the human body. Illnesses caused by evil spirits required something more powerful than the natural cures of physicians. Epilepsy, for example, was widely held to be caused by demonic possession, and thus to require spiritual medicine. The surgeon Chauliac's prescription for epileptics was 'to write in their own blood on a piece of parchment the names of the Three Wise Men, and to recite three Pater Nosters and three Ave Marias daily for three months' (Porter, 1999, p.118). Today, matters of the soul are considered the preserve of religion, not medicine, but in the predominantly Christian culture of medieval Europe, in which it was believed that the soul's well-being could affect bodily health and vice versa, it is best to interpret these 'spiritual therapies' as an extension of 'healing'.

The widespread belief that bodily illness was ultimately the result of sin or divine displeasure meant that Christians also turned to God as the ultimate source of healing. Thus prayers to God, invocations to saints and pilgrimages were all recognized means of healing. The brothers Cosmas and Damian, early Christian martyrs who, among other things, were said to have miraculously replaced the gangrened leg of a white Christian with that of a dead Moor, became patron saints for physicians. The church of St Sebastian in Rome, a major pilgrimage site, not only promised visitors absolution from sins but also protection from pestilence. Other saints were called on to provide similar protection against specific diseases: St Christopher for epilepsy, St Apollonia for toothache, and so on. The sick flocked to the shrines of these saints, offering prayers and gifts in return for a cure. Christianity thus offered alternative and additional forms of healing, which complemented existing medical knowledge and procedures. In the early Middle Ages, monastic libraries contained medical books, some monks were trained as healers, and monasteries dispensed medical help to the public. Increasingly, the interests of the medieval church in the matter of healing paralleled those of elite physicians and surgeons, especially as they sought to eradicate empirics and wise-women who peddled charms, talismans and herbs together with a prayer or two. To the church, these quacks were falsely practising spiritual healing; to the elite physicians and surgeons, they lacked the proper training in medical knowledge.

Hospitals are discussed further in Chapters 4 and 6. The impact of sixteenth-century religious change on medicine is charted in more detail in Chapter 4.

Another form of medical care that evolved within a specifically Christian context was the institution of the medieval hospital. There had been hospitals in ancient Rome, in the form of army hospitals and the sickrooms that could be found in large rural households. Further impetus was given by the spread of Christianity, because Christians had a duty to provide charity – to care for strangers, the needy and the sick. Rome, the city of God, benefited from hospitals and hostels that were established and supported by popes and cardinals. (Although today we make a distinction, the terms 'hospital' and 'hostel' were used interchangeably in this period.) By 1500, the largest of these was the Santo Spirito, which was close to the Vatican. It was established in the early thirteenth century by Pope Innocent III (1198–1216) and was refurbished by Pope Sixtus IV in the 1470s. The Santo Spirito hospital housed nearly five hundred people, including the sick, the destitute, abandoned women and orphans, and regularly employed physicians, surgeons and apothecaries. Similar arrangements were evident in other famous large hospitals in Europe at this time, such as the Santa Maria Nuova in Florence and the **Hôtel-Dieu** [House of God] in Paris. By 1500, the Order of the Holy Ghost, whose centre was at Santo Spirito in Rome, provided medical care in infirmaries from Alsace to Poland. Rome boasted other medieval hospitals, such as San Salvatore and Santa Maria della Consolazione, which were smaller in size. Smaller hostels lacked resident medical assistance, but some of them cared for a specific group. In Rome, for instance, there were hospitals for pilgrims and invalids, reformed prostitutes and orphans. These institutions were supported by donations from Christians, who believed that such acts of charity facilitated their own salvation (Figure 1.4) (Partner, 1976, pp.102–10).

1.7 The old and the new

Let us return once more to the city of Rome in 1500. By that time, a new trend in learned circles could be discerned, which historians have called the 'Renaissance'. This trend, which began among the elite in the service of the pope, took the form of an increasing enthusiasm for the ancient world, the ruins of which were right on the doorstep of those who lived in Rome. For some, these ruins embodied a glorious, historical past, which was also accessible through the study of classical literature and history. The rediscovery of classical Rome thus gathered pace. Poggio Bracciolini (1380–1459), a papal secretary, discovered *On the Waters of the City of Rome*, a manuscript written by the Roman engineer Frontinus, which provided detailed descriptions of the names, locations and system of the aqueducts. He also discovered a manuscript of Vitruvius' *On Architecture*, which helped his friend Leon Battista Alberti (1404–72), a colleague in the papal secretariat, to understand the principles behind Rome's ancient buildings. Alberti, in turn, applied these principles to his architectural plans for the pope and other clients. Through the study of classical texts, yet another papal servant, Flavio Biondo (1392–1463), pinpointed the place where Julius Caesar had been assassinated and discovered the true function of the Colosseum. Hitherto it was thought to have been an ancient temple of the sun; now Biondo was able to explain that it was used to host the gladiatorial games. By discovering the original function and layout of classical buildings, these enthusiasts began to realize that centuries of misunderstanding and error lay between their world and that of ancient Rome. By 1500, recovering the culture of the ancient past, learning about it directly from original writings and emulating what was recommended in them, had become a fashion among the intellectual elites of Rome and the rest of Europe. The trend was most manifest, perhaps, in the increasing fondness for classically inspired art and architecture, represented in Rome by the recently completed suite of apartments in the Vatican palace that were commissioned by Pope Alexander VI.

This penchant for all things ancient, the 'Renaissance', affected all branches of learning. Scholars increasingly realized that many original works by earlier writers were lost, missing or corrupt. Their medieval commentators, both Latin and Arab, now seemed to *hinder* rather than to help in the understanding of the pristine knowledge of the ancients. The recently discovered technology of printing was put

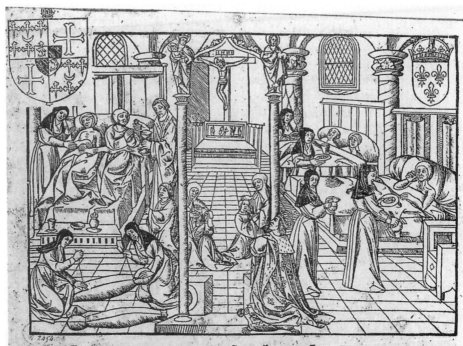

Figure 1.4   An appeal for donations from the Hôtel-Dieu, Paris. The text promises that those who make donations in the designated chests within the specified period will have their sins pardoned. This appeal aptly captures the importance of Christian charity. Bibliothèque Nationale de France, Paris

to use to rectify this defect by producing the works of classical authors in their original Greek or Latin. In this new style of learning – **humanism** – much greater emphasis was placed on retrieving the original message of classical authors through greater knowledge and understanding of the languages in which the ancients wrote, and this new perspective gradually affected the learned medicine of the universities. Around 1500, in the area of medicine, the printing press was still turning out staple traditional university texts such as the *Articella* and Avicenna's *Canon*, but some other works were beginning to appear in Greek. The full spate of recovery and printing of the Greek Galen – his *On the Use of the Parts*, *On the Opinions of Hippocrates and Plato*, and several other works either lost or unknown to the Middle Ages – was to come later in the sixteenth century.

The full impact of medical humanism is discussed in greater detail in Chapter 3.

Such efforts at recovering, editing, printing and reading the ancient authors in their original tongues led to a better grasp of a wider range of works, and showed up the differences, as well as the affinities, between the ancient world and that of the Renaissance. It had always been known, for example, that Galen and Aristotle denied the immortality of the soul, but Renaissance scholars now realized that there were other ancient authors whose views were more in accord with Christianity on this subject. For the Florentine humanist philosopher Marsilio Ficino (1433–99), the most important of these was Plato. Unlike Aristotle, Plato believed in a divine creation and an immortal 'soul'. His view of the physical body as but a shadow was more agreeable to Christians than Aristotle's materialism. Ficino was responsible for a new translation of Plato's works from Greek into Latin (printed 1484) and wrote at length on the religious dimension of Plato's thought in the *Theologica Platonica* (1482). Ficino's interest in Plato and in spiritual matters led him to develop a form of 'spiritual medicine' whereby the afflictions of the soul should be treated with music, astrology and magic. Struck by the affinity between Plato's religious philosophy and the central tenets of Christianity, Ficino went on to argue for the existence of an ancient tradition, the *prisca theologia* (pristine theology), which had been revealed by God to a chosen few, including Plato and Moses. Other **adepts** included Hermes Trismegistus, a contemporary of Moses, whose mystical writings on man and nature were also published by Ficino and his circle of **Neoplatonic** admirers in the late fifteenth century. During the sixteenth century, the **hermetic** texts inspired a new generation of scholars and physicians, including the medical iconoclast Paracelsus (*c.*1493–1541), to reject Galenism in favour of a radically different system of medicine that was more in accord with Christian principles.

Just as the attention of the scholarly world was being gripped by the rediscovery of its ancient past, news began to reach Europe of the discovery of a new world in the Americas. In 1492, Christopher Columbus (1451–1506), sailing under the auspices of Ferdinand and Isabella of Spain, alighted upon the 'new Indies'. Columbus opened up a new world: there were now new flora to be studied, cultivated and perhaps consumed; new fauna to be named, stuffed and exhibited in collections and museums; new peoples to be colonized and converted to Christianity. And, it was said, Columbus had returned to Europe with a new disease. This was commonly known as the 'French disease' (*morbus gallicus* in Latin), so called because its first appearance in Italy coincided with the invasion of

French troops in 1496. It was a horrible and painful disease, as described here by the German nobleman Ulrich von Hutten, who was afflicted by it:

> There were boils, sharp, and standing out, having the similitude and quantity of acorns, from which came so foul humours and so great stench, that whosoever once smelled it, thought himself to be infect. The colour of these pustules was dark green, and the sight thereof was more grievous unto the patient than the pain itself: and yet their pains were as though they had lain in the fire.
>
> (quoted in Cunningham and Grell, 2000, p.251)

This new disease began ravaging Europe during the pontificate of Alexander VI. Among those afflicted were the pope's own son Cesare and Cardinal Joan Borjia-Llançol, a relative of the pope, who had been suffering from it for over two years and was unable to appear in public. Another cardinal, Giuliano della Rovere, who succeeded Alexander Borgia as Pope Julius II (1503–13), was also afflicted by the disease. This new disease is better known by the name later given to it: syphilis. How did physicians react to this new challenge? Could the medical learning of the ancients provide a cure? Let us see how two of the pope's physicians tried to deal with it.

Exercise

Now read 'Reactions to the "French disease" at the papal court' (Source Book 1, Reading 1.5) and then answer the following questions:

1   What were the pressures facing Torrella and Pintor as university-trained physicians?

2   What was significant about the way in which the two men sought to define and treat the new disease?

3   Account for differences between Torrella and Pintor in the way they approached the disease. Were there any similarities between them?

Discussion

1   The French disease challenged the learned physicians intellectually. Because it was 'new', it appeared to have no ancient equivalent, and thus could not be tackled using the learned medicine at their disposal. Because this learned tradition, derived from the ancients, bestowed upon physicians their professional identity, any failure to act or to provide alleviation for the disease would threaten their professional status. In the eyes of their patients and the civil authorities, physicians would appear no better than empirics or unlicensed practitioners. Being papal physicians also raised the stakes. The French disease thus threatened the intellectual and professional survival of the university-educated physician.

2   Both Torrella and Pintor sought to incorporate the disease into the known canon of medical literature. Pintor named it *aluhumata*, and claimed that it was an obscure species of the *variola* disease discussed by the Arab physicians Avicenna

and Rhazes. Torrella, who was younger, was a little bolder. He coined a new name for the disease, *pudendagra*, and proceeded to classify it as a new species of what Avicenna had defined as scabies. Both exhibited boldness and confidence in their ability to tame the disease – attributes expected of a learned physician. Despite their differences, which were exacerbated by personal rivalry, it was clearly important to both men that they were able to demonstrate the proficiency of their learning and of their profession.

3   There were marked differences between Torrella and Pintor in the way they approached the French disease. Pintor was quite conservative; Torrella, however, was more open to new intellectual trends such as Neoplatonism, which seemed to offer grounds for optimism. Their differences can be seen as generational and educational, and it appears that these became more pronounced as a result of their professional rivalry. Yet there are some similarities between the two men: they both published in Latin, and neither doubted the importance of the learned medical tradition. They chose Latin names for the new disease in order to place it exclusively in the domain of the learned doctor. Significantly, both placed it in a pre-existing, learned classification of diseases based on the work of Avicenna. They developed treatments according to their understanding of the character of the disease. Both wished to use mercury, but felt the need to distinguish their usage from that of empirics and charlatans.

In the event, both men appear to have convinced their patron, the pope, that they were successful, and kept their jobs as papal physicians. What this episode illustrates is the remarkable flexibility of late medieval medicine in accommodating change and new challenges. Learning derived from ancient medicine continued to function as a way of maintaining status and authority over other practitioners, who were regarded as empirics, and it was subtle enough to be used to differentiate between the views of learned colleagues and rivals. Meanwhile, despite the claims of Torrella and Pintor, the number of those suffering from the French disease showed no sign of abating in Rome. In 1515, the medieval hospital of San Giacomo was rededicated to the care of the 'incurables', in particular those suffering from syphilis.

Ideas about a specifically Christian medicine are discussed in Chapters 4 and 5.

1.8   Conclusion

In this chapter, I have sketched out the state of medical knowledge around 1500, and its foundation in the Greek medicine of Hippocrates and Galen. I have shown how it provided the basis for the identity and authority of learned medical practitioners, as they tackled competition from their rivals and faced new challenges. This chapter has also anticipated some of the developments and transformations that were about to engulf medicine in the sixteenth century. War, population expansion, famine and religious upheaval represent just a sample. In the following chapters, you will explore these in greater detail. Before you can assess their impact on the healing arts, however, you need to look in more detail at medical practice on the ground, seeing it from the point of view of the patient, as opposed to that of the learned practitioner.

References

Cunningham, A.R. and Grell, O.P. (2000) *The Four Horsemen of the Apocalypse: Religion, War, Famine and Death in Reformation Europe*, Cambridge: Cambridge University Press.

García-Ballester, L. (1993) 'On the origins of the "Six non-natural things" in Galen' in J. Kollesch and D. Nickel (eds) *Galen und das hellenistische Erbe*, Stuttgart: Steiner, pp.105–15.

McVaugh, M.R. (1997a) 'Bedside manners in the Middle Ages', *Bulletin of the History of Medicine*, vol.71, pp.201–23.

McVaugh, M.R. (1997b) 'Medicine in the Latin Middle Ages' in I. Loudon (ed.) *Western Medicine: An Illustrated History*, Oxford: Oxford University Press, pp.54–65.

Nutton, V. (1992) 'Healers in the medical market place: towards a social history of Graeco-Roman medicine' in A. Wear (ed.) *Medicine in Society: Historical Essays*, Cambridge: Cambridge University Press, pp.15–58.

Nutton, V. (1993) 'Beyond the Hippocratic oath' in A. Wear, J. Geyer-Kordesch and R.K. French (eds) *Doctors and Ethics: The Earlier Historical Setting of Professional Ethics*, Amsterdam: Rodopi, pp.10–37.

Palmer, R. (1990) 'Medicine at the papal court in the 16th century' in V. Nutton (ed.) *Medicine at the Courts of Europe, 1500–1837*, London: Routledge, pp.49–78.

Partner, P. (1976) *Renaissance Rome 1500–1559: A Portrait of a Society*, Berkeley: University of California Press.

Porter, R. (1999) *The Greatest Benefit to Mankind: A Medical History of Humanity from Antiquity to the Present*, London: Fontana.

Siraisi, N.G. (1987) *Avicenna in Renaissance Italy: The Canon and Medical Teaching in Italian Universities after 1500*, Princeton: Princeton University Press.

Siraisi, N.G. (1990) *Medieval and Early Renaissance Medicine: An Introduction to Knowledge and Practice*, Chicago: University of Chicago Press.

Stinger, C.L. (1985) *The Renaissance in Rome*, Bloomington: Indiana University Press.

Source Book readings

Galen, *The Art of Medicine* in Galen, *Selected Works*, ed. by P.N. Singer, Oxford: Oxford University Press, 1997, pp.345–8, 374–6 (Reading 1.1).

D.P. Lockwood, *Ugo Benzi: Medieval Philosopher and Physician 1376–1439*, Chicago: University of Chicago Press, 1951, pp.54–6 (Reading 1.2).

G. de Chauliac, *Great Surgery* in J.B. Ross and M.M. McLaughlin (eds) *The Portable Medieval Reader*, Harmondsworth: Penguin, 1977, pp.640–9 (Reading 1.3).

The Hippocratic Oath in O. Temkin and C.L. Temkin (eds) *Ancient Medicine: Selected Papers of Ludwig Edelstein*, Baltimore: Johns Hopkins Press, 1967, p.6 (Reading 1.4).

J. Arrizabalaga, J. Henderson and R. French, *The Great Pox: The French Disease in Renaissance Europe*, New Haven and London: Yale University Press, 1997, pp.113–19, 131–42 (Reading 1.5).

2

The Sick and their Healers

Silvia De Renzi

Objectives

When you have completed this chapter you should be able to:

- explain the notion of medical pluralism and its implications for the relationship between the sick and their medical practitioners;

- discuss the relationship between lay and expert medical knowledge;

- identify various types of early modern medical practitioners and explain how they built their knowledge, established their expertise and organized their activities;

- describe how practitioners related to each other;

- compare the ways in which different practitioners understood diseases and treated the sick.

2.1 Introduction

Within mainstream western culture, a clear distinction is now made between the relative certainty of scientific treatment and the less easily quantifiable benefits of complementary medicine. The state is acknowledged as responsible for testing the efficacy of medical procedures and drugs according to precise scientific standards, set by university-trained professionals, who play a major role in the provision of health care. In some western countries, the state is also the main provider of care via a national health service. All this is recent, much of it dating from the twentieth century. In this chapter, I explore what happened before any of this was in place.

My focus here is on the period between 1500 and 1700, which falls within what historians call the early modern period. A major feature of early modern medical practice is the range of medical services on offer – much wider than was previously thought. Chapter 1 introduced you to three important types of medical practitioner: physicians, surgeons and apothecaries. In this chapter, I look in more detail at these practitioners, and place them within the broader context of the many other healers, all competing for custom. The order in which I discuss these practitioners largely follows the path most people would have taken when they fell sick – though, as you will discover, early modern people had no qualms about consulting more than one healer at the same time. I begin by exploring ideas about how to keep healthy, and then look at examples of some of these various healers: noblewomen and wise-women; itinerant sellers of remedies; surgeons and apothecaries; and physicians. At this period, physicians were usually the only practitioners to receive their medical training at a university. As you saw in Chapter 1, this had a great effect on how they viewed themselves and other healers. The fact that I have left them till last does not mean that physicians were the main providers of medical care. On the contrary, although they struggled hard to impose a monopoly over healing – and eventually succeeded – for a long time they were simply one provider among many.

The reason why we should look at the wide range of providers of medical care rather than focus on the activities of learned physicians has been clearly explained by Margaret Pelling and Charles Webster, who carried out seminal research on the great variety of healers active in early modern England:

> Any balanced view of medicine in the early modern period, or in non-western societies, must take into account all practitioners involved in dispensing medical care ... The entire body of individuals identified as healers by the community should be regarded as eligible for inclusion in a study of medical practitioners.
>
> (1979, pp.166, 232)

Drawing on the approach used by anthropologists to investigate non-western cultures of sickness and healing, historians of medicine are now trying to view past medical knowledge and practice from the vantage point of contemporary sufferers and healers. An important part of this is the reconstruction of how past people behaved when illness struck, including what kind of care they sought and who they trusted. To assess the efficacy of the treatment offered by past practitioners on the basis of modern medical knowledge, or to look for 'forerunners' of what modern practitioners believe is 'good medicine' (as medical historians have traditionally done), is now regarded as anachronistic, and of little use in understanding the past.

2.2   Medical care: its economy and control

In early modern Europe, the bulk of medical care was provided by practitioners who had no formal medical training. It was not unusual for people to seek medical help from within their circle of family and friends, as well as from the wide range of healers on offer, of whom physicians were a minority. Furthermore, early modern patients played an active role in their treatment. While the word 'patient' was already in use to mean a sick person undergoing treatment, it did not carry the sense of passivity that is sometimes associated with the role of the patient today – especially in relation to the authority of the doctor. It was also quite normal for people to seek a cure from several different sources simultaneously – from wise-women, nuns or priests renowned for their healing powers, and from friends knowledgeable in health matters, as well as from physicians. Economics, of course, played a part: physicians were usually more expensive than other healers, and therefore not everyone could afford their help. However, economic factors were not the only consideration. As the historian Mary Lindemann writes:

> expense has often been evoked to explain the antipathy many people felt towards physicians. Whether such crude kinds of cost-accounting drove people's choice of healers is doubtful. Medical decision making was complex. People often paid what might (objectively) seem like exorbitant sums for medicine and advice, and a simple correlation comparing, for

example, the amount of a day's wage to the cost of a drug or a treatment misses the point. Most important, early modern people were medically promiscuous. They often, perhaps usually, consulted several practitioners, serially or consecutively. Medical promiscuity was by no means limited to the lower elements of society; a monarch, a lord, or a wealthy patrician was just as liable to seek advice from a range of practitioners as was an artisan or a cowherd. It is simply not true that the well-to-do patronised 'legitimate' practitioners, and especially surgeons and physicians, while the less well-off (or less knowledgeable) frequented the lower ranks of medical practitioners or visited 'quacks'.

(1999, pp.198–9)

So, by and large, patients perceived no social or cultural barrier between different medical practitioners, and behaved accordingly. Historians term this feature 'medical pluralism'. That they are increasingly keen to investigate it reveals a fundamental change that has taken place in medical history. Following a broader trend to write history 'from below' – that is, from the perspective of those who did not have political power – the focus of much research is now on reconstructing patients' experience of health and sickness. Pluralism, however, does not mean anarchy. The economic and political forces at work in the early modern period were crucial in shaping the organization and provision of medical care.

The impact of the Reformation and Counter-Reformation is discussed in Chapter 4.

Between 1500 and 1700, the countries of Europe were extremely diverse politically, ranging from large monarchies to small republics ruled by merchants. However, there were some common features. These included the existence of an intricate web of overlapping political and administrative institutions, the relative independence of bodies such as town authorities, and the continuing power exerted by influential families and individuals, not to mention that of the various religious institutions, the power of which in Catholic countries had been strengthened following the upheavals of the sixteenth century. Early modern societies were therefore made up of juxtaposed bodies, each one claiming authority, and this had far-reaching consequences for people's social conduct and expectations. For example, it is difficult to overestimate the role played by personal relationships and patronage in early modern society. Only very gradually did these features disappear, as a state bureaucracy with its impersonal relations, and an economy ostensibly based on the principle of freedom, particularly freedom of trade, slowly gained sway. In the pre-industrial world, economic activity was structured by, and organized around, corporations that represented the interests of a particular trade or craft. Wool merchants, tanners, grocers – each would have their own guild or company. Those who wished to take up a particular trade had to be accepted as members of the appropriate body, usually by examination after a period of apprenticeship. In return, guilds protected their members' interests, and guaranteed them a wide range of privileges. As you saw in Chapter 1, in most parts of Europe, physicians, surgeons and apothecaries also organized themselves into such bodies, which set rules for their respective area of expertise, policed practice and issued licences to practitioners.

In theory, all those providing medical care were required to have a licence. For practitioners such as apothecaries and surgeons, the licensing authority was their respective guild. The licence was issued after the applicant had completed an apprenticeship at the shop of a senior member of the guild and, at the same time, the applicant became a guild member himself. Physicians, too, had to obtain a licence. Before a newly graduated physician could practise, he had to apply to receive authorization from the local college of physicians. These colleges sometimes, but not always, had connections with a university medical faculty, and were also responsible for the medical teaching carried out in it. Since the Middle Ages, colleges of physicians had changed dramatically: they had lost their identity as 'professional guilds', and instead had become rather closed and elitist institutions. To obtain a licence from a medical college, therefore, did not mean that a physician automatically became a member of the college. Membership was reserved for those who were regarded as worthy of a place among the elite.

Not all healers had an associated trade guild or professional body. Some, such as midwives, were simply barred from doing so because of their sex (guilds made up solely of female members were disallowed); others, such as bonesetters or **lithotomists**, did not have a clear 'professional' profile or a 'trade' with which they could identify. They learnt their skills informally and usually complemented their healing practice with other activities. However, they still had to have an official licence. To obtain one they could apply to a bishop (midwives especially followed this route), or to a municipal authority, or to the crown. That medical practitioners were licensed by such a variety of bodies is an important feature of the early modern period and stands in stark contrast to the system of modern medicine. In the seventeenth century, the licensing procedure attracted increasing controversy, as colleges of physicians claimed unique authority to license all kinds of practitioners. This caused friction with the surgeons' and apothecaries' guilds, and only slowly did colleges of physicians manage to impose their control.

The licence established what kinds of treatment a practitioner was allowed to perform – helping women in childbirth, setting bones or treating eye diseases, for example. It also set down the geographical limits within which the licence was valid. Proof of the applicant's ability was usually in the form of testimonials provided by people of authority or accounts of the healer's successful treatments. If practitioners relocated, the licence would not necessarily be recognized by the governing authority of the new area; if they continued to practise without obtaining a new licence, or if they breached in any way the limits set for their activities, they could face prosecution, followed by either a ban or a fine.

That was the theory. But historians have shown that most medical practice across Europe, especially in England, was in fact carried out by unlicensed practitioners. In 1518, following the example of earlier colleges established in Italy, the London College of Physicians was founded. The physicians' aim was to have formal jurisdiction over all medical practitioners within a 7-mile (11 kilometre) radius of the city, which meant that no one was allowed to practise any form of healing without a licence from the college. Their attempts to impose control varied greatly during the period we are considering but, overall, they failed, and unlicensed practitioners, or practitioners licensed by other authorities, proliferated in London. In the rest of the country, particularly in rural areas, medical practice was largely unregulated.

Exercise

Now read 'Medicine: trade or profession?' (Source Book 1, Reading 2.1) and answer the following questions:

1   In the extract, Margaret Pelling discusses the two main features of the early modern medical economy. Can you identify these?

2   How did these features make early modern practice different from the way in which medicine is organized today?

Discussion

1   The two main features Pelling discusses are the abundance of medical care on offer and 'diversification' on the part of its practitioners. She suggests that medical practice was rarely the healer's only source of income or their only specialization. It was quite common for barbers, surgeons, apothecaries and even physicians to be involved in a variety of more or less related occupations, trades and pursuits, including the food trade and distilling. Medical care could also be provided on a part-time basis by people in a variety of social positions, for example poor women, priests and schoolmasters.

2   This overlap of activities, which was characteristic of economic activity in other occupational groups at this time, is one of the most obvious differences from the way in which medical practice is organized today: that is, as a full-time, autonomous activity carried out by a well-defined category of qualified professionals.

Can we apply Pelling's conclusions about England to the rest of Europe in the sixteenth and the seventeenth centuries? Overall the answer is a tentative 'yes' – medical practice did not remain impervious to transformation in this period, but by and large continuity prevailed. Moreover, medical pluralism was certainly common to all European countries, as was the organization of trades in guilds and the overlap of administrative and political bodies. But there are good reasons to look at geographic differences.

Two countries that tackled medical care in markedly different ways were England and Italy, and interesting comparisons can be made between them. (For convenience, though I refer here to 'Italy', historically it is more accurate to speak of the 'Italian states', into which the Italian peninsula was divided politically at this time; see Plate 5.) From the late Middle Ages onward, Italy had developed a highly complex political structure. It had also established numerous renowned medical faculties, which had resulted in the existence of a large body of university-trained physicians. Taken together, these factors contributed to the establishment of a sophisticated and, in theory, strictly regulated medical system. At its centre were powerful institutions such as medical colleges, which were responsible for the licensing of physicians, the *protomedicato*, a powerful medical office linked to the college or to the political authority and in charge of policing all the other practitioners, and health boards. The latter were particularly active during epidemics. Italy was a highly 'medicalized' society, where it was not uncommon for town authorities to hire physicians to treat the poor and needy inhabitants. Although even in Italy rules were flouted, and in reality unlicensed medical practitioners flourished there as they did in the rest of Europe, many countries – in particular England – looked to emulate the Italian model. Compared with medicine in Italy, English medical practice was largely unregulated. Its physicians' corporate bodies, both medical faculties and colleges, were weak; unlicensed practitioners proliferated; and the political authorities displayed only a minimal interest in public health care. England and Italy are therefore interestingly different. In the rest of the chapter, I examine the activities carried out by some early modern medical practitioners in both countries.

2.3 The maintenance of health

Let us start by looking at a passage from a work by Leonardo Fioravanti (1517–c.1584), a successful healer, whose frequent travels and confrontational attitudes towards the authorities made him well known throughout Italy. In his book *Capricci Medicinali* [Medical Caprices] (1561), Fioravanti described asking a very old man for the secret of his longevity. Here is what the old man reportedly said:

> My rule has always been to get up early and eat early in the morning. I always make sure that the first glass of wine I drink in the morning is the best I can get hold of, and I never eat more than twice a day. I always go to bed early and I never go out at night ... I never take any medicine, though once every spring I take some soldanella [a sort of bindweed], which is very common here. Each time I take it, it makes me vomit violently, and this leaves my stomach so clean that I do not get sick for the rest of the year. And every year, in May, I take three sprigs of rue, three of sage, three of wormwood, and three of rosemary and infuse them in a glass of good wine until the following morning. I drink the infusion before eating, and I do this for fifteen or twenty mornings, every year.
>
> (quoted in Camporesi, 1997, p.54; my translation)

So what are the old man's secrets? The passage contains several important points.

- The old man was confident that he knew how to maintain his own health. He said he never took any medicine, by which he meant that he took no prescribed remedies. By extension, we can assume that he never sought the advice of an 'expert'.

- He regarded his lifestyle (going to bed and getting up early, drinking good wine, eating only a small amount of food) as an important factor in maintaining his health.

- He routinely dosed himself with specific herbs and plants, and knew when and how to prepare the **infusions**. The way he did this resembled a sort of yearly ritual.

- Overall, the old man seemed to think of his body as a vessel to be kept clean; the most important procedure in his self-medication was vomiting.

Rather than being 'secrets', these were, on the contrary, popular and widely known precepts. The old man's system may have reminded you of what you read in Chapter 1 about Galenic medicine. Learned medicine had long instructed people in how to live a regular and thus a healthy life, and much of the advice was centred on diet and regimen – for example, what things to eat or not to eat according to the season and the individual's **constitution**. The old man's confidence that he could take care of his own health by following similar rules indicates that, in the early modern period, boundaries between lay and expert medical knowledge were more fluid than they are today.

Both learned and popular medicine taught that the main way to avoid illness was to keep the body in balance – that is, to have an appropriate mixture of the humours that was just right for each person. Because illness was believed to result from an imbalance caused by the defect or excess of one or more of the humours, close attention was paid to what went into the body and what came out of it. Problems might occur when the digestive tract became blocked, when superfluous matter was not properly evacuated, when foods containing qualities not suitable for the person's complexion had been ingested, and so on. Those who could afford it, therefore, took preventive measures, such as following a diet appropriate to their constitution, eating fresh food to avoid sources of putrefaction, having their blood let regularly to prevent the build-up of noxious humours, and, at the first sign of discomfort, taking **purgatives** to remove putrid matter. To keep the body's passages open and its fluids flowing was essential for good health. The widespread belief that illness was the result of sin or of divine disapproval also meant that it was important to live a morally irreproachable life.

So what did people do when their preventive measures failed and they became sick? Contemporary accounts in letters and diaries reveal that **lay people** were quite knowledgeable about health matters. They would often treat themselves, or seek a cure from a family member or a neighbour, before they would contemplate resorting to a paid expert. This was the case even for educated people from the upper social strata, who would have been able to afford the services of a physician. Some people, despite having no formal medical qualifications, were considered particularly knowledgeable in health matters and their remedies were trusted. But where did they get their knowledge from? Much popular medical wisdom came from family and friends, perhaps handed down through the generations by word of mouth or in handwritten recipe-books. Other sources of medical knowledge were the innumerable vernacular medical books that were being published at this time. These books, written not in Latin (the language of the learned), but in the language people spoke everyday, dealt with a variety of health issues. Mainly practical, such volumes included collections of recipes for drugs, almanacs containing astrological information about the best times for bloodletting and purging, and publications presenting various kinds of regimen. Their popularity demonstrates the existence of large numbers of people who were interested in matters to do with health, who had some education, but no official medical training, and who were keen to acquire medical knowledge (Slack, 1979). I will return later in the chapter to the relationship between the 'learned' and the 'popular', or lay, medical traditions – in particular, to what extent they borrowed from each other.

2.4   Women as healers

The sick were mostly cared for and treated at home. At a time when local communities were close-knit and a great source of support, remedies and advice were freely provided by visiting neighbours and relatives. While we have visual and written evidence of how the sickroom was organized in a rich household (Plate 6), it is very difficult to say what happened in the homes of the much more numerous families of modest or little means. It is likely that the close proximity that was usually necessary within poorer households simply continued, and that the sick person would have continued to share a bed with other family members.

Given women's importance in the domestic sphere, it is no surprise that they played a particularly active role in looking after the sick. Yet, until recently, women's medical activities have received little attention in historical accounts. Now, however, they have begun to attract interest, and a range of sources has been successfully tapped. The two examples I shall focus on here are particularly illuminating because they come from the opposite ends of the social spectrum: the activities of Lady Mildmay, an English aristocrat, and the healing practices of poor women in London.

Lady Mildmay: a charitable noblewoman

Lady Grace Mildmay (1552–1620), who belonged to the landed elite and lived a sheltered life in rural Northamptonshire, left a vast number of papers, including autobiographical and medical notes. Although she did not receive a formal medical education – women were not allowed to go to university – from the hundreds of recipes she collected and her observations about causes of diseases and treatments, it is clear that she provided medical services on an impressive scale. Her house was fully equipped for the production of a variety of drugs, based on both plants and minerals, and she supervised the complex processes of boiling, infusing, distilling, straining and storing medicines. Patients also came to her for a medical consultation: she was therefore responsible for diagnosing their ailments, suggesting a course of treatment and preparing the medicines (Pollock, 1993). Her patients were usually poor people, for whom she provided her services and medicines free, as an act of Christian charity. It is possible that in certain cases she consulted physicians and surgeons, but she clearly had deep and wide medical knowledge.

Exercise

Now read the extract from Lady Mildmay's notes in 'Women practitioners: the prescriptions of Lady Grace Mildmay' (Source Book 1, Reading 2.2). What do they suggest about the theoretical framework within which she practised medicine? Don't worry about trying to understand the terminology used in the passage. Just try to identify the general area of medical knowledge on which she based her treatment.

The presence of technical and unusual terms such as 'cephalgia', 'cephalia' and 'apoplexy' shows her familiarity with the learned tradition, which at this time was based on the works of Galen. There are several other clues to indicate that Lady Mildmay was conversant with the main tenets of Galenic medical knowledge and practice: her classification of bodily signs and their interpretation – for example, the meaning of the colours of the face and eyes in relation to different kinds of headaches; her reference to phlegm (one of the humours) and her use of remedies to 'mitigate' the imbalance of the humours.

Paracelsianism is discussed in Chapters 4 and 5.

The Galenic framework within which Lady Mildmay practised medicine, however, coexisted with her knowledge and wide use of chemical remedies, which belonged to the new Paracelsian medicine. This suggests that Lady Mildmay was abreast of the most innovative medical theories of her time. What were the sources of her up-to-date knowledge? She recalls that a governess introduced her to medicine, and this suggests the existence of informal channels through which knowledge circulated among women (Hellwarth, 1999). At the same time, we know from her notes that Lady Mildmay kept herself informed by collecting and reading a great variety of books. Caring for one's sick neighbours, especially if they were poor, was a traditional charitable activity for noblewomen. However, wealthy ladies were by no means the only female healers.

Female healers in early modern London

Evidence that female medical practice was widespread can be found in the papers of the London College of Physicians, which allow us to glimpse activities that otherwise have left scanty traces. Among those healers prosecuted by the college for practising without a licence were women who prescribed purging herbs, ointments and pills. The records show that most of them belonged to the lowest social strata, and that providing medical services was a way for them to support their households. However ignorant, and even dangerous, these women were in the eyes of learned physicians, they catered for a broad clientele. Unlike noblewomen such as Lady Mildmay, they charged for their services, but they were usually well integrated in their community and much sought after, possibly because they were cheaper than licensed practitioners. They usually practised at home, as extant bills and advertisements show (Pelling, 1997).

Such women normally prescribed simple herbal remedies for common conditions, though they sometimes specialized in the treatment of a particular ailment. Knowledge of the healing powers of various herbs circulated by word of mouth among those who could not read, but it remains difficult to say how, precisely, these urban female practitioners acquired their skills. Their activities show how widespread medical knowledge and practice were, and this prompts reflection as to how we should describe and understand the relationship between these practitioners and their more learned rivals.

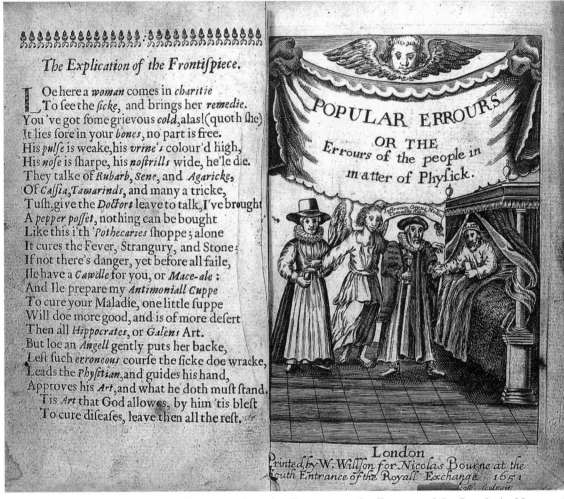

The Explication of the Frontispiece.

Loe here a *woman* comes in *charitie*
To fee the *ficke*, and brings her *remedie*.
You 've got fome grievous *cold*, alas! (quoth fhe)
It lies fore in your *bones*, no part is free.
His *pulfe* is weake, his *vrine's* colour'd high,
His *nofe* is fharpe, his *noftrills* wide, he'le die.
They talke of *Rubarb*, *Sene*, and *Agaricke*,
Of *Caffia*, *Tamarinds*, and many a tricke,
Tufh, give the *Doctors* leave to talk, I've brought
A *pepper poffet*, nothing can be bought
Like this i'th *Pothecaries* fhoppe ; alone
It cures the Fever, Strangury, and Stone :
If not there's danger, yet before all faile,
Ile have a *Cawdle* for you, or *Mace-ale* :
And Ile prepare my *Antimoniall Cuppe*
To cure your Maladie, one little fuppe
Will doe more good, and is of more defert
Then all *Hippocrates*, or *Galens* Art.
But loe an *Angell* gently puts her backe,
Left fuch *erroneous* courfe the ficke doe wracke,
Leads the *Phyfitian*, and guides his hand,
Approves his *Art*, and what he doth muft ftand.
Tis *Art* that God allowes, by him 'tis bleft
To cure difeafes, leave then all the reft.

POPULAR ERROURS

OR THE
Errours of the people in
matter of Phyfick.

London
Printed by W. Willfon for Nicolas Bourne at the
South Entrance of the Royall Exchange 1651

Figure 2.1   Frontispiece to James Primrose, *Popular Errours or the Errours of the People in Matter of Physick*, 1651. Wellcome Library, London

First, look at Figure 2.1, the frontispiece of *Popular Errours*, a book by the seventeenth-century physician James Primrose, and read the accompanying verses. Now read 'The place of women in learned medicine: James Primrose's *Popular Errours* (1651)' (Source Book 1, Reading 2.3). How would you describe Primrose's attitude towards female healers?

Primrose thought that women did not possess the knowledge required to provide effective medical treatment. He admitted that they were capable of tending the sick, and that they also had knowledge of various remedies, but he criticized them for attempting to carry out surgical procedures and to treat serious illnesses. His main point was that they lacked the methodical and well-grounded knowledge of learned physicians, which was the only basis on which treatments tailored to the needs of particular individuals could be provided. Notice his disdain for what he saw as the two sources of women's knowledge: English books, as opposed to learned medical literature in Latin, and the informal communications of others. In the picture in the frontispiece, an angel is shown keeping a woman away from the bed of a sick man, while allowing a physician (note the hat and robe) to step forward. The verses further explain how the woman refutes Galen and Hippocrates and boasts that her remedies cannot be found at the apothecary's shop. Primrose was keen to stress a complete separation between learned practice and female healing; he portrayed female healers as being antithetical to learned physicians and as drawing on their own, and in his opinion dangerous, therapeutical recipes.

It is never a good idea to rely on just one source, however; historians always try to combine a variety of sources to get a more balanced view. This is what the author of the next reading has done.

Exercise

Now read 'Lay and learned medicine in early modern England' (Source Book 1, Reading 2.4). In what sense does Doreen Evenden Nagy think that learned and popular practice were part of an interdependent system?

Discussion

By exploring a variety of sources, Evenden Nagy shows how, well into the late seventeenth century, learned physicians borrowed remedies and treatments from a popular tradition of healing. She takes this as evidence of the strength of popular practice and also argues for the interdependency between learned and popular medical knowledge and the fluidity of their boundaries. Learned physicians claimed that their treatments were based on entirely different principles from popular cures, in order to eliminate competition. The reading shows that this was far from true.

It is now widely accepted that learned and popular practitioners shared much more medical knowledge than the former were prepared to acknowledge. However, Laurence Brockliss and Colin Jones have called into question the existence of an autonomous tradition of popular medicine, arguing instead that popular medicine fundamentally derived from the tradition of learned medicine. To explain how medical knowledge trickled down from the elite to the lower strata of society, they have drawn attention to the activities of literate, though non-university-trained, medical practitioners, who travelled around, selling their services. Brockliss and Jones claim that such practitioners 'acted as cultural intermediaries facilitating the diffusion of orthodox medical ideas' (1997, p.279). One such was our old friend Leonardo Fioravanti.

2.5 Leonardo Fioravanti: a sixteenth-century itinerant healer

Historians have long portrayed Leonardo Fioravanti as the epitome of the cunning and dishonest charlatan. However, recent research on the activities of informally trained and itinerant practitioners has shown how little we still know about such people, and how limiting it is simply to label them as 'charlatans' or 'quacks': doing so still does not explain who they were, why they were so successful and what they did. In the early modern period, several different terms were used to describe itinerant healers such as Fioravanti. In Italy, for example, a healer might be called a *ciurmatore* (from the Tuscan word *ciurmare*, 'to charm' or 'to bewitch'), a *ciarlatano* ('charlatan', from *ciarlare*, 'to chatter'), a *saltimbanco* ('mountebank', because they usually mounted a stage to sell their remedies) or a *circulatore* (from the Latin *circulator*, 'peddler' or 'stroller'). These terms were ambiguous even in their own day. Learned physicians might use a word such as 'mountebank' in a derogatory way, to denigrate the activities of these practitioners. However, in ordinary conversation, most people probably used 'mountebank' in a more neutral way. Until recently, the writings of elite physicians formed the main historical source for scholars, and so for the most part itinerant healers have been portrayed as confidence tricksters, who, after they had bamboozled simple people by staging faked cures, sold them useless syrups and ointments. Today, however, historians are keen to look beyond such stereotypes, to discover what these healers actually did and how they were regarded by ordinary people (Gentilcore, 1995). Although Fioravanti had much in common with itinerant healers, he was not typical of the majority of them, not least because he was literate: it is rare, for example, to find in the work of others such an articulate attack as he launched against learned medicine. He also portrayed himself in a markedly different way from how he was seen by the medical establishment (Figure 2.2). In his eventful life, he moved between popular and elite cultures, and this mobility makes him an interesting and important witness to the practice of early modern medicine. Our main source for Fioravanti's career is his autobiography, *Il Tesoro della Vita Humana* [The Treasury of Human Life] (1570). His bombastic style may sometimes make it necessary to read between the lines, but Fioravanti's writings are now recognized as a valuable historical source (Camporesi, 1997).

His life and medical ideas

Fioravanti was born in Bologna, Italy. In the early sixteenth century, Bologna was the site of an illustrious faculty of medicine, but Fioravanti did not attend the lectures there. Rather, his autobiography suggests that he may have started his medical career as an apprentice to a surgeon. However, as you will discover, he practised a variety of medical skills. Constantly in search of patronage and new clients, we know from his writings that he travelled the length and breadth of Italy, from Palermo and Naples to Milan and Venice. Fioravanti lived in Venice – a major centre of printing – for many years, and most of his works were published there. At

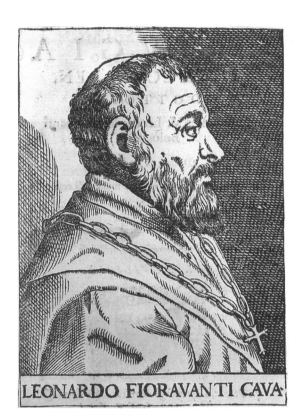

LEONARDO FIORAVANTI CAVA·

Figure 2.2   Portrait of Leonardo Fioravanti, from his book *La Cirugia* [Surgery], 1582. Note that the truncated word *cava* means *cavaliere* ('knight' or 'gentleman'). Fioravanti clearly wanted to emphasize his respectable status. This message was also conveyed by certain contemporary pictorial conventions: note the cross and chain around Fioravanti's neck, his decorous garb and his stern expression. Wellcome Library, London

some point, he joined the Spanish navy, where he learned new surgical techniques; he also spent time in Madrid, at the court of Philip II, and even practised at the papal court in Rome. Fioravanti regarded travelling as an essential means of acquiring knowledge, and believed that his wide experience and variety of medical skills made him equal, if not superior, to most university-trained physicians. In his autobiography, Fioravanti included letters showing that sick people had consulted him about various ailments, for which he would prescribe a remedy – often without seeing the patient. This form of written medical consultation was not unusual at the time, but might be seen by learned physicians as straying into their territory. Other letters were from learned medical practitioners, who had expressed an interest in the recipes for his potent drugs. Fioravanti was a skilful businessman, with a network of clients extending well beyond Italy, and he built good relations with the various apothecaries who made up his prescriptions.

Fioravanti maintained that his successful career rested on his skill in two major areas: performing daring surgical operations, which he described in great detail, and prescribing powerful drugs. He claimed always to have been willing to learn about new treatments, regardless of their source. Indeed, the less medically educated were his informants, the more valuable he thought them. In Fioravanti's view, women, peasants, soldiers, priests and even animals all knew how to cure themselves and so were invaluable sources of information. Unlike learned physicians, whose knowledge was bookish and dry, these untutored healers had put their remedies to the test many times. It was this direct experience that made their knowledge so useful.

To boost sales, Fioravanti gave his drugs attractive names, such as 'angelic **electuary**' and 'magistral syrup', but they appear to have been extremely violent in their effects. Believing that disease was the result of putrid matter accumulating in the stomach and then affecting other parts of the body, he took an aggressive approach to its cure. He seems to have been obsessed with purging his patients, and his drugs made people sweat, vomit and evacuate excessively. These extreme measures contrasted with the gentler and slower treatments of traditional Galenic medicine, which involved subtle changes to the patient's regimen. Although Fioravanti's treatments ultimately fell within a traditional framework, his emphasis on corruption and on purging the body violently and thoroughly did not form part of learned medical practice. Indeed, it has been argued that Fioravanti's obsession with purging owed more to the religious practice of exorcism than it did to medical theory (Eamon, 1993). Whatever the reason for the violence of his treatments, his patients certainly seem to have liked the fact that they had such visible effects.

Facing prosecution

Fioravanti's success infuriated the medical establishment. University-trained physicians felt aggrieved because he prescribed remedies without consulting them, and his overweening confidence in his own abilities exacerbated the situation. In Rome, for example, a group of physicians openly denounced Fioravanti to the authorities and demanded that his licence to practise surgery and to prescribe some medicines be withdrawn. To make his position more secure, in 1568 he applied for and obtained a degree in medicine from the University of Bologna – a process that involved being examined on a medical topic of which he was notified at short notice, and the payment of a conspicuously large fee to the college of physicians. However, when he was establishing himself in Milan, just a few years later, in 1573, his medical degree was no protection against the accusations brought against him by the local college of physicians. Arguing that he was not following the proper rules of medicine, and that too many of his patients had died, the physicians had him arrested and imprisoned.

Recent research has established that in addition to licensing physicians and policing other medical practitioners, colleges of physicians functioned as tribunals to which patients could turn when they thought they had been victims of medical malpractice; of course, their complaints were one of the best weapons that physicians had in their fight against other practitioners (Pomata, 1998). Fioravanti's defence against the Milanese physicians was defiant and well argued. He claimed that some of his patients were bound to die whatever the treatment; if physicians were asked to account for the patients who had died while in their care, they would all be in prison. Furthermore, Fioravanti challenged the physicians to put their knowledge to the test, asking that twenty-five patients be put under his care and another twenty-five, who suffered from the same illnesses, be treated by the physicians. He stated that if he did not succeed in healing his patients more quickly and effectively than the physicians, he would leave the city (Camporesi, 1997, pp.290–1).

This episode vividly illustrates three key points. First, it shows the strict control that physicians tried to establish over those whom they regarded as unsuitable practitioners. Colleges of physicians had the power to have an individual imprisoned, though more often than not they were happy to levy a fee and issue a licence limiting the practitioner's future activities, or to impose a short ban on their practising. The fact that Fioravanti was not a native of Milan amplified his problems. The colleges treated 'foreigners' particularly harshly in order to protect the trade of local healers. On the other hand, itinerant practitioners constantly defied geographical boundaries in search of business. Second, it illustrates Fioravanti's great confidence in his own experience and practice. Demonstrable success in curing the sick was to him the benchmark by which medical ability should be assessed, and in this he believed that he could outdo the physicians. Fioravanti was not alone in his scorn for the bookish quality of learned medicine: numerous satires were produced at this time, which portrayed physicians as pompous and ineffective. Third, although it is unlikely that there was an actual competition, Fioravanti's challenge to the medical establishment reveals a competitive attitude, which might best be summarized as 'Let the best man win'.

Where had Fioravanti learned this approach to medical practice? He was accused by his enemies of being a *circulatore*, a word usually denoting a peddler of drugs and remedies, but he refused to be grouped with such individuals, and made much of his credentials as a 'proper' medical practitioner. However, he clearly drew part of his identity from the culture and activities of itinerant healers.

Medicine on the stage

Contemporary visual sources usually present itinerant healers as standing on a stage, like actors – in the act of charming their open-mouthed and naive audience, but ready to cut short the performance and start the sale (Figure 2.3). However rich in detail they may be, these visual sources belong to a 'genre', a stereotypical representation, which cannot be taken at face value.

In his work on Italian itinerant healers, David Gentilcore has studied the records of the colleges of physicians to which they applied for a licence. The records reveal that these healers were not a homogenous group. Most of them were selling simple remedies, which most people regarded as useful and effective against various minor ailments: powders for cleaning the teeth and for treating toothache, waters for sore eyes, ointments for burns. Some of them also advertised their remedies as effective against more serious diseases. Often a family would run the main business from a shop, but would also have someone who travelled around, selling their treatments further afield. Dynasties were established, and skills and recipes were transmitted from generation to generation. Some of these healers were far from uneducated: they had access to books and skilfully used the new print culture to promote their goods. Like Brockliss and Jones (1997), Gentilcore sees these itinerant healers as 'intermediaries between learned and popular forms of healing' (Gentilcore, 1995, p.300). Their theatrical performances, and the various props they used, including the stage and its banners – to which colourful costumes, exotic animals and mysterious boxes could be added – were advertisements, designed to attract people rather than to con them. It is true that secrecy was part of their

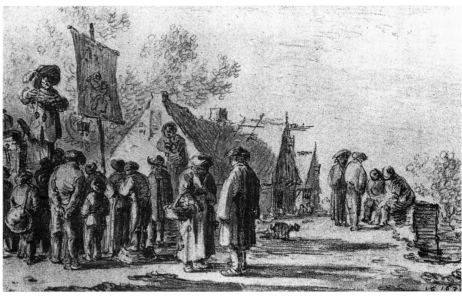

Figure 2.3   Jan van Goyen, *Village Scene with a Charlatan*, drawing, 1631. Here an itinerant healer (left) is shown addressing a small gathering of people. Notice that he is standing on a stage and to attract the attention of his audience has hoisted a standard. He is clearly in the middle of a performance and is displaying his wares. Wellcome Library, London

business, but in this they were by no means unique. The desire to protect particular 'trade secrets' from outsiders was a common feature of contemporary trades and crafts, which were themselves often known as 'mysteries'.

In challenging the physicians of Milan to a competition, in which they might all put their skills and medicines to the test, and let the general public judge who was the more successful healer, Fioravanti was looking at medicine from the perspective of someone engaged in trade rather than that of a learned academic. However, unlike most itinerant healers, Fioravanti was not content simply to make a profit: he also vigorously attacked learned medicine and challenged the authority of physicians. Fervently believing that medicine was a business like any other, and that no one should be immune from the risks of competition, he maintained that fame and respectability should rest only on demonstrable success in curing the sick. This was the reason for his bold challenge, but it was also the reason why the physicians of Milan could not accept it. One of the learned physicians' strongest beliefs was that their knowledge was not for sale in the way other goods were. To the medical elite, medicine was most certainly *not* a business like any other. Throughout the early modern period, physicians constantly maintained that the money they were paid for their services was not the same thing as the price customers paid craftspeople and traders: the physician's fee had the special status of an honorarium, or voluntary payment. Their insistence on this practice was an oblique reference to the unbridgeable gap between practical or manual skills and intellectual pursuits. It was thus unthinkable for a physician to pit his abilities against those of his fellows, as though they were practising a common craft or trade. Fioravanti's life vividly reveals the complex relationships between learned and popular practitioners in both their medical and their social roles. It also allows us to glimpse the entrepreneurial world of healers who had no academic education, but who were determined to build up a successful business. On the other hand, his desire not to be grouped with what he regarded as lower status charlatans and mountebanks shows how varied and complex such a world was.

Fioravanti began his career as a surgeon, and claimed that his success partly depended on his innovative surgical procedures. In the next section, I explore the training and the status of surgeons, as well as the kinds of treatment they usually provided. To do so, I move from sixteenth-century Italy to seventeenth-century London, and discuss the activities of Joseph Binns, a very successful surgeon, whose casebook has been the object of intensive study. I also look briefly at the work of apothecaries.

2.6   Barber-surgeons, surgeons and apothecaries

Barber-surgeons and surgeons in early modern London

Although there had been some innovations in techniques, surgery at the beginning of the early modern period was very little different from surgery in the Middle Ages. Surgeons had close occupational links with barbers, and often the two trades were carried out by the same practitioner: the barber-surgeon. Barber-surgeons and surgeons considerably outnumbered physicians and played an important role in medical care, particularly in urban areas. Written sources, such as surgeons' casebooks, provide useful evidence about what they did. In this section, I have drawn on Lucinda McCray Beier's (1987) study of the casebook of Joseph Binns (d.1665). Binns completed his apprenticeship to a London surgeon in 1637, and immediately started his own private practice. After ten years, he also took up a position at St Bartholomew's Hospital. A member of the Barber-Surgeons' Company, Binns later became one of its wardens.

A surgeon's apprenticeship could last up to seven years. During this time, the apprentice not only received a practical training in surgical techniques, but also gained some theoretical knowledge about the structure of the body, especially the arrangement of blood vessels, bones and muscles. At the end of a surgeon's apprenticeship, he was examined to test whether he was 'well exercised in the curing of infirmities belonging to surgery of the parts of man's body commonly called the anatomy' (quoted in Pelling and Webster, 1979, p.175).

Binns visited his patients at their homes, and from his descriptions we know that most of them were from middling or lower social groups – although he did have a few wealthy patients and he also treated the very poor at the hospital. Usually, however, surgeons and barber-surgeons carried out their practice from a shop. Research on the geographical distribution of barber-surgeons in early modern London has shown that they tended to concentrate in the most populous areas of the city, where all sorts of trades were carried out, including entertainment and prostitution (Pelling, 1986). The following exercise reveals the range of activities that might take place in a barber's shop.

Exercise

Now read 'Physical appearance and the role of the barber-surgeon in early modern London' (Source Book 1, Reading 2.5). What were the main services provided in a barber-surgeon's shop, and how did these fit in with contemporary perceptions of hygiene and fashion?

Discussion

In early modern London, barber-surgeons' shops offered a range of services for the male body that are best understood within the context of contemporary perceptions of bodily care. Appearance was very important: although clothing hid most of the body, the areas that could be seen (hair, hands and face) received particular attention. Cosmetics and perfumes were widespread, and washing was probably more common than was previously thought. By looking after their customers' skin, hair and teeth, barber-surgeons offered an essential service, in which the boundaries between beauty care and health care were blurred. They treated all sorts of skin problems, including minor blemishes, as well as permanent disfigurement caused by diseases; they also carried out bloodletting, which was universally regarded as a preventive and therapeutic measure to restore the balance of the humours. But their shops could also be places of entertainment, including, at times, sexual activities.

To make sense of Margaret Pelling's findings we need to understand the significance of the distinction made in this period between the body's surface and its interior. Medical practitioners today can use a range of instruments and techniques to see inside the body, but in the early modern period the interior of the body was hidden. To determine what was happening internally, practitioners were dependent on outward signs, the interpretation of which was a complex and difficult skill. Physicians used the distinction between the inner and the outer body to claim yet again their superiority – this time over surgeons. It was one thing to apply ointments, dress wounds, let blood, deal with bone dislocations, and so on (Figure 2.4), but an altogether different matter to diagnose a disease by understanding the causes of humoral imbalance, which had their origin inside the body. The mouth was the main access to the inner body: this is why the prescription of remedies to be taken by mouth was regarded by doctors as their prerogative. The skin, as the main boundary between the outside and the inside, was treated by practitioners of a lower status. The importance of the distinction between the inner body and its surface also explains why amputations were the surgeons' turf: cutting off a limb did not affect the inside of the body (the realm of the humours), but merely repaired damage to its outer surface. Bloodletting was an important medical intervention, and physicians tried to exercise a degree of control over it by retaining the right to prescribe it as a treatment. However, the

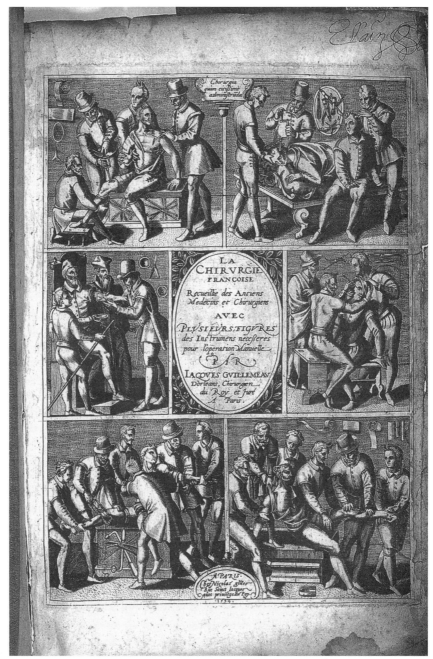

Figure 2.4   Title page of J. Guillemeau, *La Chirurgie françoise* [The French Surgery], 1594, showing the range of operations performed by surgeons. Clockwise from top left: dressing wounds (keeping a wound open was thought to help the evacuation of putrid matter); carrying out **trepanation**; treating eye ailments; treating dislocated limbs; carrying out amputations; bloodletting. Notice that in each vignette, the instruments used in the various procedures are also displayed. Wellcome Library, London

actual procedure was a manual, and therefore a menial, task, and one that physicians were happy to delegate to barbers and surgeons.

In reality, the easier accessibility of barbers and surgeons meant that patients consulted them about all sorts of illnesses and expected to receive a wide range of treatments from them. Binns's casebook confirms this. He routinely treated common ailments relating to the surface of the body – wounds, fractures, infected swellings, tumours. The majority of his cases related to syphilis or other venereal diseases. Venereal diseases were usually treated by surgeons, because they gave rise to skin problems. In the course of his treatment, however, Binns often prescribed medicines to be taken internally, even though prescribing was in theory the province of the physician. Likewise, patients also asked Binns's advice about illnesses such as epilepsy and stomach ache, for which, strictly speaking, they should have consulted a physician. From his casebook, therefore, we can conclude that Binns and his patients routinely breached the boundaries that physicians sought to impose on surgeons. Yet Binns's casebook contains frequent references to certain physicians with whom he cooperated and, unlike his son, who was also a surgeon, Binns was never prosecuted by the London College of Physicians for his activities.

Bear in mind that the lower social status of surgeons and barber-surgeons when compared with physicians is something of a generalization. In fact, the status and earnings of a surgeon could vary enormously: while some made a meagre living, others, like Binns, became wealthy and highly respected. Furthermore, a 'learned' tradition of surgery was also alive, especially in southern Europe, where university-trained surgeons taught and published books, just like physicians. Claiming that surgery had as venerable a tradition as medicine, and that its practice was every bit as important and respectable, educated surgeons were keen to distinguish themselves from the mass of barbers and barber-surgeons (Nutton, 1985). Even in England, surgeons and barber-surgeons constituted a varied community; for example, starting from the late sixteenth century, the Company of Barber-Surgeons included a group of learned and dynamic members who, in addition to teaching, published books, kept abreast of medical novelties, and felt equal to physicians. The relationship and the social dynamics between physicians and surgeons changed over time and became increasingly complex. For example, as anatomical practice expanded in the seventeenth century, and experience and observation became highly regarded sources of knowledge, physicians began to hold surgeons in higher regard, and to emulate their techniques. In the eighteenth century, the boundaries between the training and practice of a physician and those of a surgeon were redrawn.

The erosion of the traditional distinction between physicians and surgeons is discussed in Chapter 13.

Apothecaries

Another group of practitioners with whom physicians had to compete, and over whom they tried to exert control, were apothecaries. Originally wholesale merchants and importers of spices, during the early modern period apothecaries organized themselves into guilds that were independent from those of grocers, and claimed a monopoly over the production of and trade in drugs. New plants were being imported from America and other recently discovered lands, and apothecaries took a keen economic interest in them. Their familiarity with centuries-old techniques of distillation made apothecaries among the most active investigators of the expanding *materia medica*. They experimented, prepared and sold drugs, and, despite the physicians' monopoly over the prescription of remedies, were often consulted by patients on all sorts of medical issues. Inevitably, this triggered a response by the physicians. In Italy, for example, they insisted on their right to scrutinize both the ingredients kept in apothecaries' shops and the procedures by which their drugs were made. Should these be different from those officially approved by physicians, or should it emerge that apothecaries were prescribing remedies without consulting a physician, the *protomedicato* had the right to impose a fine. This, however, did not affect the popularity of apothecaries with patients.

In this survey of the various avenues open to sick people in the early modern period, you have come across several instances which reveal that university-trained physicians saw themselves as very different from other practitioners. Although in practice they were in constant competition with hundreds of other healers, they claimed for themselves a privileged role, and tried to impose a medical system in which they exercised complete control. It was not that physicians disliked the plurality of healers; on the contrary, they recognized the necessity for having a large number of less exalted practitioners to do all the work that needed to be done. Physicians had no desire to dress wounds, prepare ointments or supervise childbirths. As long as they retained their rights of diagnosis and prescription, they happily left such activities to other practitioners. However, the learned medical establishment saw it as imperative that other healers kept within the proper boundaries, and did not trespass into areas that physicians regarded as their own. Even though the efforts of physicians to impose such order and control were frequently thwarted, we should not underestimate their determination to succeed. Let us now explore what made a good physician.

2.7 The skills and career of a physician: Girolamo Cardano

Girolamo Cardano (1501–76) was a prolific and original writer on a range of subjects, including mathematics, astrology, natural history and medicine. Eccentric and idiosyncratic, Cardano's views on nature brought him to the attention of the **Inquisition**, and he spent some time in prison. By profession he was a physician, very influential and much respected, who, despite early difficulties, won fame throughout Europe (Figure 2.5). Such was his international reputation that one wealthy patient called him to Scotland for a consultation, and his numerous books were widely read and commented on. His successful, but less than smooth, career makes him a valuable witness to the world of learned medicine in early modern Europe (Siraisi, 1997). As I mentioned earlier, the way in which learned physicians organized their education and practice in Italy became the model that was followed in most other European countries, so it is useful to look at this in some detail.

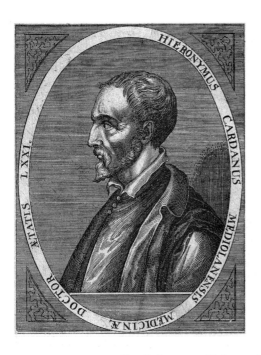

Figure 2.5   Engraving of Girolamo Cardano by C. Ammon the younger, 1652. This is a copy of an earlier portrait of Cardano as an elderly man. The Latin caption running around the image reads: 'Hieronymus Cardanus, doctor of medicine from Milan, at the age of seventy-one.' Notice that no other signs or symbols of his medical activities are shown; he is simply presented as an austere and serious man. Wellcome Library, London

Studying medicine: the university curriculum

The son of a respected teacher of mathematics, Cardano was born out of wedlock – a circumstance that could greatly affect one's future prospects, as he was to discover. He obtained his medical degree at the University of Padua, in Italy, in 1526. At that time, the university's medical faculty was one of the most famous in Europe, attracting dozens of students, including foreigners, every year (Figure 2.6).

The medical curriculum of an early modern university retained many features of its medieval predecessor. Although there was some new content – for example, in the second half of the sixteenth century, new courses in anatomy and *materia medica* were provided – most changes were simply additions to the established curriculum. Italian universities had a high reputation. Before pursuing their medical studies, students spent two years studying logic and natural philosophy. These subjects were seen as providing the ideal foundation for understanding health and sickness, and were taught mainly by the student reading and commenting on the texts of Aristotle. Logic trained students in how to analyse an argument, an essential skill for understanding the canon of ancient texts on which a medical education was based; a knowledge of natural philosophy gave them an explanation of the natural world. After this, students could start their medical education, which usually lasted three years. Lectures were divided between medical theory (for example the Galenic theory of the four humours) and medical practice, where students learned about particular diseases and their remedies. Professors taught both theory and practice in the same way – that is, by the exposition and clarification of the works of the standard ancient and medieval authorities: Hippocrates, Galen and Avicenna. Printed commentaries and abridged versions were also available to help readers navigate these texts. Students were required to attend just one

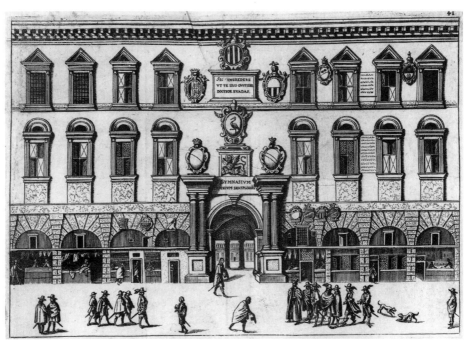

Figure 2.6   Main entrance of the medical faculty, University of Padua. Bodleian Library

anatomical dissection, during which they were shown the structure of the body. In general, therefore, they would complete their medical training without having had much experience of sick people.

Shortly after Cardano had graduated, a university professor in Padua, Giambattista da Monte (1498–1552), started to teach practice by taking students into a hospital and talking about the medical conditions of actual patients. This innovation seems to have been well received, but it is not clear to what extent it was taken up by other professors in Padua, or elsewhere. Although Italian universities were renowned for their emphasis on practical training, it was not until the end of the eighteenth century that 'bedside teaching' became central to medical education. Throughout the sixteenth and most of the seventeenth centuries, students learned medicine largely by listening to and taking notes on the expositions of learned professors, by reading books, and by identifying and memorizing the pros and cons of opposing arguments within the established medical tradition.

The controversial status of medical knowledge

Because of its venerable tradition, medicine had always been one of the most highly regarded disciplines, and this bestowed authority and prestige on physicians. Yet, roughly at the time Cardano was studying in Padua, medicine became the target of strong attacks by famous men of letters such as the Italian Gianfrancesco Pico della Mirandola (1469–1533) and the German Henricus Cornelius Agrippa (1486–1535).

Now read 'Renaissance critiques of medicine: Pico and Agrippa' (Source Book 1, Reading 2.6). What aspects of medicine were Pico and Agrippa attacking?

Pico was disconcerted by the fact that the array of authorities which constituted the venerable medical tradition were constantly contradicting each other. Fundamental questions about the physiology of the body – for instance how semen was formed – had been disputed for centuries but had never been resolved. Physicians were also divided as to the status of medicine. The problem was whether medicine was a science, and therefore able to provide certain knowledge and universal truths, or an art, which, although capable of achieving practical goals, dealt with individual cases and could never rise above this level. By Aristotelian standards, this was the mark of second-rate knowledge. In some respects, medicine seemed to be a science, as it was grounded on Aristotelian philosophy, but the practical and empirical nature of medical practice made it more like an art. Agrippa also criticized the quality of medical knowledge. In addition, he cited the allegedly poor results of medical practice and attacked physicians for their greed and cruelty. He infused an unprecedented hostility into centuries-old stereotypes. Interestingly, one of his polemical weapons was a reference to illiterate women's knowledge of plants and remedies, which made physicians' learning look inadequate.

Such attacks were mainly directed against medieval medicine and the physicians who devoted their time to learned hair-splitting. Despite their very radical slant, the polemics of Pico and Agrippa are best understood as part of the more general discontent with medieval philosophy and medicine expressed by the humanists. One of the final outcomes of this discontent was a fundamental change in the traditional distinction between 'art' and 'science' and about the overall classification of disciplines. However, the status of medical knowledge, especially when compared with disciplines such as mathematics, was an issue that could not be easily solved; it remained controversial even when anatomy seemed to provide a firmer basis for understanding the body and its functions.

Becoming a physician: an elitist profession

After graduation, which consisted of an oral disputation on a medical topic, a new physician had to do two things: obtain a licence to practise and learn how to deal with real patients. Gaining experience with patients was a relatively simple matter: new medical graduates usually associated themselves with senior practitioners and followed them while they visited their clients. We have seen above that to obtain a licence, a graduate had to apply to the college of the city in which he wanted to practise and take an examination. Cardano decided to settle in Milan, but it took many years before he got his licence: the college was suspicious of the conditions surrounding his birth – and his growing disdain for Milanese doctors did not help matters. As you see, it was not only healers such as Fioravanti who ran into trouble with the college in Milan. Even university-educated physicians like Cardano sometimes found it difficult to deal with the extraordinarily elitist inner circle of the medical establishment.

Although only a tiny minority of the population could afford a university education, learned physicians were by no means a socially homogenous group. At one end of the spectrum there were doctors practising in the country or in small towns, who dealt mainly with poor people or people of modest means; at the other end, there were physicians from wealthy and well-connected families, who were in the service of prestigious clients (Cipolla, 1976). Rivalry between individual physicians was intense. In addition to guaranteeing a good income, acquiring wealthy or powerful clients could help a physician to gain a position at a university. Teaching might lead to the publication of a book, which in turn would further enhance a physician's reputation. To become a member of a college (which, you will recall, was different from receiving a licence) was regarded as the pinnacle of a physician's medical career. However, colleges were very closed institutions and, as with many other bodies in the early modern period, membership was often the result of family connections or patronage, rather than merit.

In Italy, one way for a newly qualified physician to begin his practice was for him to be appointed to look after the health of a particular community – a village, say, or a convent. This type of appointment was called a *condotta*. In return for his work, the physician received a fixed salary. A *condotta* was regarded as a secure, but not particularly prestigious office, which could be complemented by private practice. Cardano started his medical career by working in small towns but soon moved to Milan, where he was appointed as physician to a convent. No doubt he hoped his name would soon start to circulate in the big city.

Building up a private clientele could take a lot of effort and networking. Cardano's longest practice was carried out in Milan and Pavia between the mid-1530s and the late 1550s. We know from his writings that word of his successful treatments spread among the friends and relatives of his patients, and he quickly won the trust of several wealthy families. His reputation grew, until eventually he numbered among his clients some extremely powerful people. It was probably thanks to their patronage that Cardano managed to break the resistance of the college of physicians and become a member in 1539. In 1543, he was appointed as a professor of medicine at the University of Pavia. But when in 1562 he moved to Bologna to take up another university position, the civic and university authorities that appointed him did so reluctantly, and later argued that, given his high salary, he should have cured more patients. The fluctuations in Cardano's career show just how dependent a physician was on the support of powerful institutions and patrons. What attracted clients to a physician was his reputation for successful treatments: physicians mostly relied on informal recommendations, but some also published books detailing their successes. In his book *On the Method of Curing* (1565), Cardano included a section entitled 'Remarkable cures and predictions of diseases'. The title emphasizes not only Cardano's success rate at curing diseases – most of the cases he presented were common disorders, but persistent and difficult to eradicate – but also his skills in prognosis. He also scattered accounts of his cures in his other works – a typical practice among all learned physicians. But what exactly might a learned physician offer to his patients? And how did his knowledge shape and direct his practice?

The medical practice of a learned physician: diagnosis, prognosis and treatment

Before reading further, you may find it useful to reread Section 1.4 of Chapter 1, where a number of key theoretical concepts of the Galenic tradition are explained.

Cardano is famous for his astrological works and audacious horoscopes of influential people (including Christ), which brought him into conflict with the religious authorities. Yet, as a physician Cardano differed little from most of his colleagues in the use he made of astrology in his medical practice. In the remainder of the chapter, you will study one of Cardano's own medical cases to see how a Renaissance physician might approach a patient, formulate a diagnosis and attempt a cure.

Exercise

Now read 'Cardano's description of the death of a patient' (Source Book I, Reading 2.7). To explore this rich source in detail, it is helpful to divide it into four main sequences. First, read the whole extract through from beginning to end, and then reread the sequences indicated below in conjunction with my commentary.

Commentary on sequence 1

From 'Vicenzo Cospo ...' to '... no other symptoms'

Cardano's description of his patient included the colour and structure of his body, and his psychological state; these signs indicated the patient's complexion – that is, the ratio of the qualities of hot, wet, cold and dry, and of the humours, with which he was born. Information about Cospo's age and social status would have helped Cardano make sense of how his original complexion might have changed in the course of his life. You can see that Cardano also took into account Cospo's habits, how he exercised and rested, what he ate: these factors were the non-naturals – aspects of everyday living that the physician could adjust as part of the treatment. Notice the emphasis on diet, and the reference to unhealthy food such as cheese and watermelons. All food had its own mixture of the four qualities and thus might affect the humoral balance of the individual. Because the patient's body was likely to demonstrate the current state of sickness, the physician had to identify the patient's innate complexion. This task required careful observation and skilful interrogation. Cardano had been called following a fever which had tormented Cospo. Notice the symptoms Cardano listed: the 'rigor' (rigidity) in the limbs, vomiting, the unusual colour of the faeces, the lack of perspiration. Because they were thought to contain the noxious humours produced by the sick body, excretions were the main signs by which a diagnosis could be made. Medical textbooks discussed the meaning of the particular colour and consistency of the excretions, and colour charts for the inspection of urine were widely used. As you read earlier, consultations were often carried out in writing, with the physician interpreting the accounts submitted to him by the patient or by another doctor. In such cases, careful verbal descriptions of the signs and symptoms were extremely important.

Commentary on sequence 2

From 'In the morning ...' to '... egg yolk'

Before you read my commentary on this sequence, try to answer the following questions.

Exercise

1 What was the main medical procedure that Cardano carried out?

2 Why was this procedure so important within the Galenic framework?

3 What does the presence of another physician at Cospo's bedside suggest?

Discussion

1 Cardano's main procedure was taking Cospo's pulse.

2 The pulse-beat was one of the major signs a learned physician used to make a diagnosis, and to take a patient's pulse was his quintessential act: it would allow him to 'feel' the power of the vital spirits that moved in the arterial blood. The various kinds of pulse-beat were analysed at length in medical textbooks. Notice the richness of the adjectives Cardano used to describe Cospo's pulse-beat: 'very languid, small, not very fast but rather frequent'.

3 Consulting more than one practitioner at a time was common practice: learned physicians might discuss – and vie with each other over – the patient's condition at his or her bedside. In this case, Cardano, who was also a university professor, was confident of his status – he said that he 'warned' his colleague, a word that suggests he felt some superiority over him.

Cardano was by now sure of his diagnosis – double tertian fever – but how had he arrived at this conclusion? Fever, which to us is a symptom of a disease, was at the time thought to be a disease in its own right. It could be one of several types, depending on a number of characteristics, including the frequency and timing of its appearance. Galen had argued that fever was caused by an excess of one or more of the humours, which might accumulate in a particular part of the body, causing putrefaction and excessive heat. In general, to reach a diagnosis, the physician observed the patient's bodily signs, then checked them against lists of the signs and causes of various diseases. Different diseases might manifest themselves through similar signs and it was the physician's task, by a process of elimination, to arrive at the correct diagnosis. To pinpoint the causes of a disease was also difficult because, given the interconnectedness of the body, symptoms might show in one organ but be caused by putrefied humour or blockage and stagnation in a completely different part. In a section of his account not reported here, Cardano goes through all the possible diseases that were consistent with the signs shown by Cospo: poisoning, the plague, a tumour. One by one he rules them out. It is on the basis of this mental procedure that Cardano comes up with his diagnosis and makes his dietary prescription of a light supper of wine and egg, both supposed to have therapeutic effects.

Commentary on sequence 3

From 'The following morning ...' to '... were applied'

The patient's bodily signs were reassessed at each visit and, following a diagnosis, physicians usually made a prognosis – that is, they would predict the outcome of the disease. Not surprisingly, prognosis was a highly valued medical skill. It included knowledge of the usual course of the disease, and of its critical days – those days on which important changes were expected to occur. The seventh day after the onset of the disease was seen as one such critical day. Whether the physician made a favourable or unfavourable prediction depended largely on what happened and when. Reams of paper were written by physicians – including Cardano – on the critical days, and medical textbooks always included a discussion of them. We do not know whether Cardano had ventured a prognosis, but he expressed his concerns about the seventh day having passed, possibly because no clear sign of recovery had appeared. As part of his task, Cardano recommended a therapy, which, after the wine and egg, included an ointment and theriac, a drug widely regarded as a sort of panacea and made up from dozens of ingredients. You may notice that bloodletting, one of the most common medical procedures, is not mentioned.

Commentary on sequence 4

From 'When I came about the sixteenth hour ...' to '... he died'

This account does not end happily. Yet Cardano clearly did not feel that the patient's death tainted his reputation, otherwise he would not have selected the case for publication. Cardano's confidence in recounting even his failure to cure a patient shows what it was that university-educated physicians valued most in their practice: the fact that it was based on rational thinking. The account of Cospo's disease exemplifies Cardano's ability to read signs, make a diagnosis and provide a treatment. Their mastery of a venerable literature crammed with disputes about symptoms, qualities, humours and treatments meant that, unlike the empirics, physicians could justify what they were doing by referring to an authoritative and coherent, theoretical framework. Throughout the seventeenth and eighteenth centuries, what bestowed authority on physicians' practice was their highly individualized approach to patients. They prescribed treatments, including dietary advice and carefully chosen drugs, that were tailored to the patient's complexion, and to the specific causes of his or her condition (Cook, 1994). It was the ability to appreciate what made each case unique and to intervene accordingly that distinguished learned physicians from mere empirics. In the physicians' eyes, nothing was further from their rational practice than the charlatan's cure-all or a herbal concoction prescribed by a woman who had no understanding of the principles that made it work. Physicians saw the preservation and restoration of health as a long and complex procedure and not the result of a quick fix.

2.8 Conclusion

The early modern period was characterized by the great variety of medical practitioners to whom patients could turn. Furthermore, patients felt free to seek the help of many healers at the same time. This 'medical pluralism', meant that, despite their continuous attempts to impose a monopoly, learned physicians were regarded by ordinary people as simply one among many providers of medical services. The variety of medical care on offer also included lay medical knowledge, which remained strong and vital well into the nineteenth century. To appreciate how widespread medical knowledge was at this time, we need to understand the variety of channels, both written and oral, formal and informal, through which it circulated.

The economics of early modern medical care was based on the specific organization of contemporary trades and crafts, and on the competition which all the healers, including learned physicians, experienced. This competition was a direct result of the existence of so many sources of medical care, and the fact that sick people appear not to have differentiated between them to any great extent, although financial constraints of course would have limited their choice. On the other hand, medicine need not always have an economic basis. The case of Lady Mildmay shows that it was also perceived as one of the activities by which wealthy patrons or physicians could express their charity to the poor. So, the relationship between the sick and their healers in early modern Europe was variable: for many people the provision of health care was a business; for others it retained the nature of a spiritual pursuit.

University-trained physicians were willing to acknowledge the necessity for other practitioners, provided they limited themselves to very specific ailments, and preferably dealt with the outside of the body. While trying hard to exert control over other healers, physicians regarded their own ability to 'read the body' and its signs, and to tailor their intervention to the unique complexion and history of a patient, as the trademark of rational medicine and firmly played it against what they perceived as ill-founded and dangerous popular practice. On the other hand, part of the appeal of the aggressive drugs advertised by some of the empirics, with their visible effects, lay in the fact that they differed from the mild remedies and the regulation of diet and regimen advocated by traditional learned medicine. You will see in the following chapters, especially Chapter 5, how the debate over traditional therapeutics developed as new remedies were introduced, and how the medical establishment reacted to them.

References

Beier, L.M. (1987) *Sufferers and Healers: The Experience of Illness in Seventeenth-Century England*, London: Routledge & Kegan Paul.

Brockliss, L. and Jones, C. (1997) *The Medical World of Early Modern France*, Oxford: Clarendon Press.

Camporesi, P. (1997) *Camminare il mondo: vita e avventure di Leonardo Fioravanti medico del cinquecento*, Milan: Garzanti.

Cipolla, C. (1976) *Public Health and the Medical Profession in the Renaissance*, Cambridge: Cambridge University Press.

Cook, H.J. (1994) 'Good advice and little medicine: the professional authority of early modern English physicians', *Journal of British Studies*, vol.33, pp.1–31.

Eamon, W. (1993) '"With the rules of life and an enema": Leonardo Fioravanti's medical primitivism' in J.V. Field and F.A.J.L. James (eds) *Renaissance and Revolution: Humanists, Scholars, Craftsmen and Natural Philosophers in Early Modern Europe*, Cambridge: Cambridge University Press, pp.29–44.

Gentilcore, D. (1995) '"Charlatans, mountebanks and other similar people": the regulation and role of itinerant practitioners in early modern Italy', *Social History*, vol.20, pp.297–314.

Hellwarth, J.W. (1999) '"Be unto me as a precious ointment": Lady Grace Mildmay, sixteenth-century female practitioner', *Dynamis*, vol.19, pp.95–117.

Lindemann, M. (1999) *Medicine and Society in Early Modern Europe*, Cambridge: Cambridge University Press.

Nutton, V. (1985) 'Humanist surgery' in A. Wear, R.K. French and I.M. Lonie (eds) *The Medical Renaissance of the Sixteenth Century*, Cambridge: Cambridge University Press, pp.75–99.

Pelling, M. (1986) 'Appearance and reality: barber-surgeons, the body and disease' in A.L. Beier and R. Finlay (eds) *London 1500–1700: The Making of the Metropolis*, London: Longman, pp.82–112.

Pelling, M. (1997) 'Thoroughly resented? Older women and the medical role in early modern London' in L. Hunter and S. Hutton (eds) *Women, Science and Medicine 1500–1700: Mothers and Sisters of the Royal Society*, Stroud: Alan Sutton, pp.63–88.

Pelling, M. and Webster, C. (1979) 'Medical practitioners' in C. Webster (ed.) *Health, Medicine and Mortality in the Sixteenth Century*, Cambridge: Cambridge University Press, pp.165–235.

Pollock, L. (1993) *With Faith and Physic: The Life of a Tudor Gentlewoman, Lady Grace Mildmay 1552–1620*, London: Collins & Brown.

Pomata, G. (1998) *Contracting a Cure: Patients, Healers, and the Law in Early Modern Bologna*, Baltimore and London: Johns Hopkins University Press.

Siraisi, N.G. (1997) *The Clock and the Mirror: Girolamo Cardano and Renaissance Medicine*, Princeton: Princeton University Press.

Slack, P. (1979) 'Mirrors of health and treasures of poor men: the uses of the vernacular medical literature in Tudor England' in C. Webster (ed.) *Health, Medicine and Mortality of the Sixteenth Century*, Cambridge: Cambridge University Press, pp.237–73.

Source Book readings

M. Pelling, 'Trade or profession? Medical practice in early modern England' in M. Pelling (ed.) *The Common Lot: Sickness, Medical Occupation and the Urban Poor in Early Modern England*, London: Longman, 1998, pp.240–5 (Reading 2.1).

L. Pollock, *With Faith and Physic: The Life of a Tudor Gentlewoman, Lady Grace Mildmay 1552–1620*, London: Collins & Brown, 1993, pp.123–4 (Reading 2.2).

J. Primrose, *Popular Errours; Or the Errours of the People in Matter of Physick, First Written in Latine ... Translated into English by Robert Wittie Doctor in Physick*, London: W. Willson, 1651, pp.19–21 (Reading 2.3).

D. Evenden Nagy, *Popular Medicine in Seventeenth-Century England*, Bowling Green, OH: Bowling Green State University Press, 1988, pp.43–53 (Reading 2.4).

M. Pelling, 'Appearance and reality: barber-surgeons, the body and disease' in A.L. Beier and R. Finlay (eds) *London 1500–1700: The Making of the Metropolis*, London: Longman, 1986, pp.89–95 (Reading 2.5).

N.G. Siraisi, *Medicine and the Italian Universities 1250–1600*, Leiden: Brill, 2001, pp.184–202 (Reading 2.6).

G. Cardano, *Opera Omnia* (Lyons, 1663), translated by N.G. Siraisi, *The Clock and the Mirror: Girolamo Cardano and Renaissance Medicine*, Princeton: Princeton University Press, 1997, p.210 (Reading 2.7).

3

The Medical Renaissance of the Sixteenth Century

Vesalius, medical humanism and bloodletting

Sachiko Kusukawa

Objectives

When you have completed this chapter you should be able to:

*   appreciate the importance of humanist methods and techniques as applied to the study and practice of medicine in the sixteenth century;

*   comprehend how visual sources and printed books encouraged new ways of understanding the body in the Renaissance.

3.1   Introduction

In Chapter 1, you encountered the terms 'Renaissance' and 'humanism', which characterized new trends in western Europe after 1500. This chapter examines the impact of these new trends on medical learning. As an example, I shall be focusing on the physician Andreas Vesalius (1514–64), who published a major new work on anatomy in 1543. Vesalius' *De Humani Corporis Fabrica* [On the Structure of the Human Body] contained no shattering discoveries, but it laid the groundwork for observation-led anatomy (Porter, 1999, pp.179–81). What is fascinating about Vesalius is that he appears to be conservative and innovative at the same time. Vesalius embraced fully the ideals of Renaissance humanism, and took Galen as his model; his aim was to revive the pristine anatomy of Galen in sixteenth-century Europe. All this may appear rather conservative, and backward-looking. In the process, however, Vesalius also realized that Galen had never dissected humans and had thus made mistakes in his descriptions of anatomical structures. Vesalius sought to restore a dissection-based anatomy to what he saw as its rightful place at the heart of medical learning, and he used beautifully drawn illustrations to convey this message. These features make him appear more forward-looking. As we shall see, these aspects were not contradictory. Vesalius is an excellent example of how looking back to the ancients could produce innovation.

In order to understand how Vesalius developed his original ideas on the structure of the human body, it will be necessary to look in more detail at specific debates in medical circles at this time, in particular that relating to the most common therapeutic practice of the age: bloodletting. In the process, you should be better placed to appreciate and assess the significance of Vesalius' work from the perspective of the man himself and of those colleagues with whom he clashed.

3.2   The Renaissance and medical humanism

'The Renaissance' is a name used by historians today to denote both a period of European history (roughly from 1400 to 1600) and a distinctive set of values and beliefs. Its defining feature was the emphasis contemporary scholars placed on the rediscovery or revival of all aspects of classical Greek and Roman culture – hence the term 'Renaissance' or 'rebirth'. The term has long been used by art historians, for example, in discussing the work of such famous artists as Michelangelo (1475–1564) and Leonardo da Vinci (1452–1519). Since the nineteenth century, historians have extended its use to cover all areas of cultural and intellectual activity in the period, including science and medicine. Those who conveyed the ideals of the Renaissance are widely referred to as 'humanists': scholars and learned men who sought in one way or another to revive all or part of the cultures of ancient Greece and Rome. Typically, Renaissance humanists saw these classical civilizations as representing the pinnacle of human achievement, and sought to emulate them by recovering the legacy of this past golden age. Crucial to this project was the rediscovery of the literary legacy of the ancients. Humanists were eager collectors of ancient manuscripts and classical works, many of which had disappeared from circulation in the interim period, the Middle Ages, and it was through the intensive study of such writings that they hoped to recreate a new golden age in learning and the arts.

'Humanism' is a difficult term to define with any precision. Today, historians use it in a broad sense to denote a reverential attitude to classical culture rather than as a rigid set of ideals and values that were shared by everyone. Those who subscribed to the humanist projects of the Renaissance, however, shared above all else a passion for the literary traditions of the ancient Greeks and Romans. Humanists believed that writing in elegant Latin after the style of Roman orators such as Cicero or Quintilian was the mark of a cultured person. Many also read – or aspired to read – ancient Greek, a language that was largely unknown in the Christian west before the fifteenth century. An elite few, such as the German scholar Johannes Reuchlin (1454/5–1522), wished to master Hebrew, though excessive devotion to Hebrew was often regarded with suspicion because of its connection with the Jewish religion. Desiderius Erasmus (c.1466–1536), probably the most renowned humanist scholar of the Renaissance, spoke of a 'trilingual' man – that is, one fluent in Latin, Greek and Hebrew. On Erasmus' recommendation, a college was established at Louvain in Brabant (in modern-day Belgium) that specialized in the teaching of these three ancient languages, and which henceforth became known as the 'trilingual college'. One of its earliest graduates was the young Vesalius.

Humanists believed that ancient learning – especially that of the Greeks – constituted the most important repository of true knowledge and wisdom about man and the natural world. Consequently, philological study – that is, the study of words, languages and texts – was widely believed to hold the key to recovering the ancient verities in the works of Greek and Roman writers. Humanists were particularly critical of the way in which many ancient manuscripts had been preserved in faulty copies or translations during the Middle Ages, and they were scathing of the role played by Arab scholars in both preserving and perverting this rich heritage of ancient wisdom. The desire to recover the writings of ancient authors made humanists avid manuscript hunters and book collectors. They collated manuscripts, resolved variant readings, corrected erroneous transcriptions, removed extraneous interpolations, established clear definitions and authentic terminology, and sought to 'fix' the correct version of an ancient work by recourse to the new technology of the printing press. In short, humanist culture was essentially 'bookish', though many humanists were aware of the double-edged nature of the multiplying power of the printing press – it could perpetuate errors as well as disseminate correct readings. The humanist Niccolò Perotti (1429/30–80) even felt duty bound to call for active censorship of the presses in order to stop a rival (and, in his view, incompetent) humanist scholar from publishing a newly edited classical text.

Above all, in preface after preface to the newly printed editions of classical authors, humanists enthusiastically extolled the virtues of recovering pristine knowledge by returning to the original source (they used the Latin phrase *ad fontem*, meaning literally 'to the source or spring'). They chastised their predecessors' efforts at Latin translations (often via Arabic intermediaries) as 'barbaric' and consistently preferred to cite the original Greek and Latin sources rather than their Arabic commentators. The humanist enthusiasm for 'pure knowledge' extended to all branches of human understanding and activity: literature, history, politics, philosophy, religion, mathematics, medicine and the natural sciences. The scope of humanist scholars reflected this universal desire to recreate in its entirety the wisdom of the ancients. Erasmus, for example, produced editions of the works of Roman writers such as Cicero, Lucian, Terence and Seneca, as well as new editions of **patristic** authors, including St Ambrose, St Basil and St Jerome. In addition, he compiled a very popular booklet of classical sayings or adages, wrote manuals on rhetoric and produced new Latin and Greek translations of the New Testament. To accompany these translations, he provided commentaries in which he explained the corrections he had made to earlier Latin and Greek translations of the Scriptures, many of which had been used in the Christian church since antiquity.

Humanist methods and techniques such as these were equally applicable to medicine and were eagerly taken up by a growing number of physicians who had been trained in the humanist academies of Europe. Inspired by Erasmus, the famous humanist printing firm of Aldus Manutius in Venice printed the Greek text of Galen's complete works in five large volumes in 1525, followed a year later by the Greek version of the works of Hippocrates. New Latin translations, based on these Greek editions, soon became available to the learned medical profession throughout Europe. Anatomy, too, benefited from these humanist endeavours, culminating in the publication in 1531 of Galen's *On Anatomical Procedures* by the Parisian medical humanist Johann Guinther von Andernach (1487–1574). This text by Galen, which laid down the procedures for carrying out dissections, had, like his other works on anatomy and surgery, remained in obscurity in the Middle Ages.

From the late 1520s, Paris became the leading centre for the publication of medical humanism. In 1536, Guinther published an important guide to his translation of Galen's *On Anatomical Procedures*. His colleague in the Parisian medical faculty, Jacobus Sylvius (1478–1555), was responsible for numerous new

Latin editions and translations of the works of Galen and Hippocrates, and compiled new introductory textbooks for medical students. Both men were committed to restoring medicine to its original, Greek-inspired, purity. Both, too, sought to establish a new terminology for anatomy, which they reaffirmed in the regular public and private dissections that they performed in Paris at this time. Nicolò Leoniceno (1428–1524) was in many ways the godfather of medical humanism, and his pioneering research laid the foundations for the later achievements of men such as Guinther and Sylvius.

Exercise

Now read 'Leoniceno and medical humanism at Ferrara' (Source Book 1, Reading 3.1). What aspects of Leoniceno's life and career exemplify his commitment to the cause of medical humanism?

Discussion

Leoniceno had an excellent knowledge of ancient Greek and was an expert in philology. He stocked his library with Greek manuscripts, sought to replace Roman and Arabic authorities in medicine with Greek ones (Galen, Dioscorides and Hippocrates), called for a return to the original sources and dedicated his long life to editing the texts of Greek authors and teaching Greek medicine. His work was entirely orientated towards books, in that he concentrated on textual emendations and the search for perfect translations, often at the expense of practical experience.

3.3 Bloodletting

While men such as Leoniceno, Guinther and Sylvius concentrated their energies on largely literary pursuits, some of their students were more concerned with the impact of these new studies on the day-to-day business of medical practice. Galen himself had advocated numerous therapeutic techniques that were still in wide use in the sixteenth century, none more so than the practice of bloodletting. People from all walks of life had their blood let, the healthy as well as the sick. The practice itself was based on the Galenic view of the humoral body. Blood (containing all four humours) was understood to be a product of food. Food was first liquefied in the stomach and delivered to the liver. In the liver this liquefied food, called 'chyle', was turned into blood. This blood was then distributed throughout the body for nourishment through the veins. Galen had described the veins as being like the branches of a tree, which had its roots in the liver (the arteries were similarly rooted in the heart). The trunk of this 'tree' was a large vein called the **vena cava**. From the liver, blood passed through the inferior, or lower, vena cava to the lower part of the body, and through the superior, or upper, vena cava, via the right ventricle of the heart to the upper part of the body (Figure 3.1).

See Chapter 1 for an explanation of the humoral body and Galen's understanding of blood flow.

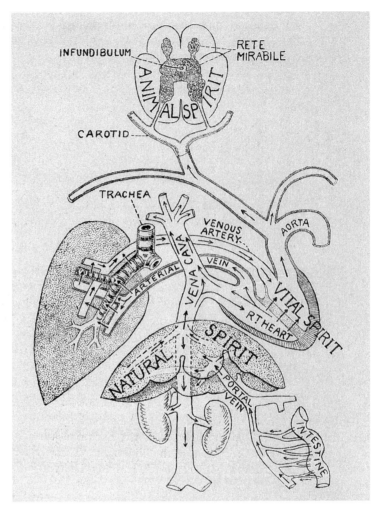

Figure 3.1   The Galenic system of blood flow. Wellcome Library, London

It was widely believed by Galen and his successors that the body sometimes produced more blood than it could use up. This excess of blood was known as **plethora**, and when it occurred there was a danger that the blood could stagnate and putrefy, causing humours to turn noxious, and thus cause a variety of ailments. A general excess of 'corrupt' blood in the whole body might cause fevers. Alternatively, if the noxious humours in the blood became localized they might cause inflammation or tumours in a particular part of the body. The important task of preventing or remedying the condition was largely based on the principles of evacuation or dietetic intervention. Physicians might tell their patients to reduce their food intake, to take emetic drugs or laxatives, to take medicines to induce perspiration or to have their blood let. The practice of bloodletting is also commonly referred to as **phlebotomy** or **venesection**, though to be precise, both these terms refer to the operation of letting blood from the veins – the most common form of treatment. Letting blood from the arteries – arteriotomy – was also possible, but this procedure demanded great care and skill and was consequently performed less frequently. Galen himself considered bloodletting to be a safer and more reliable method than drugs to rid the body of noxious humours. By the Middle Ages, it was considered effective for a whole host of ailments, as is suggested by the following extract from the manual of a medieval physician:

> Phlebotomy clears the mind, strengthens the memory, cleanses the stomach, dries up the brain, warms the marrow, sharpens the hearing, stops tears, encourages discrimination, develops the senses, promotes digestions, produces a musical voice, dispels torpor, drives away anxiety, feeds the blood, rids it of poisonous matter, and brings long life. It eliminates rheumatic ailments, gets rid of pestilent diseases, cures pains, fevers and various sicknesses and makes the urine clean and clear.
>
> (quoted in Talbot, 1967, p.131)

Having one's blood let was widely seen as beneficial for everyone, with the exception of children under a certain age, the elderly and pregnant women. But special care had to be taken in the performance of the surgical operation and various rules were developed and widely applied. It was generally agreed, for example, that noxious blood should not be drawn through vital organs such as the heart. In addition, elaborate charts were devised to indicate the most favourable times and conditions for bloodletting. It was usually carried out, for example, as part of a normal, healthy regimen, in the spring or autumn, when seasonal changes in the weather were thought more likely to upset the balance of the humours. Another important principle governing the timing of the activity was based on the astrological belief that the position of the planets exercised an influence on the health of individual human bodies. The moon, for example, was thought to exert a particularly powerful effect on the flow of liquids, such as blood; it was considered to be at its most powerful when it was full, and at its weakest when it was new. The fate and health of individuals was largely dependent on the sign of the zodiac under which they were born. In addition, each sign was linked to a specific part of the body, an idea frequently illustrated in the figure of the 'zodiac man' (Figure 3.2). This showed that Aries ruled the head, Gemini the shoulders, arms and hands, Pisces the feet, and so on. The moon's position in relation to the signs of the zodiac was believed to affect a particular part of the body. Charts featuring a 'zodiac man' could thus be used as a reminder not to let blood from the head when the moon was in Aries, or from the shoulders when it was in Gemini, and so on. Other charts gave guidance on the veins from which to let blood in the case of specific ailments (Figure 3.3). Not surprisingly, astrological medicine constituted an important part of the education of a learned physician in Renaissance Europe.

Various methods of letting blood were available to the physician. Venesection was the most common. It involved binding a ligature around the patient's limb in order to tie off the blood vessels and make the vein visible so that the barber-surgeon could make an incision with a small double-edged knife called a lancet. The patient was often given a stick to grasp, to help swell the vein, and the blood was caught in a bowl. The physician would then examine the colour and texture of the blood to gauge the patient's state of health. Blood could also be let, however, by other

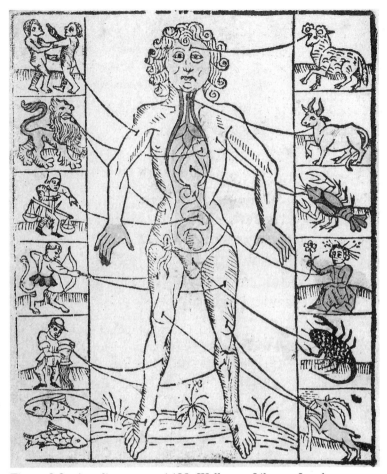

Figure 3.2   A zodiac man, *c*.1483. Wellcome Library, London

methods. Scarification, for example, involved the creation of numerous tiny incisions in the surface of the skin and the application of a heated glass vessel, or cup, to create a vacuum which drew blood to the surface. (This procedure is also known as cupping.) The application of leeches, which sucked out the blood, was another popular method.

Various manuals depicting the correct procedures for bloodletting survive from the Middle Ages. Many were learned tracts, written in Latin and produced by university-educated physicians. However, knowledge about the technicalities of bloodletting was not the exclusive preserve of the medical elite. Latin tracts on phlebotomy were frequently translated into the vernacular, and simple calendars and manuals known as girdle books made such information available to a wide range of practitioners, often in the form of easily understood summaries and rules (Figure 3.4). Much to the annoyance of learned physicians, bloodletting was frequently performed in the Middle Ages and Renaissance by a whole host of unsupervised practitioners, including barbers, monks, quacks and Jewish doctors. As the university-educated physicians became increasingly concerned with

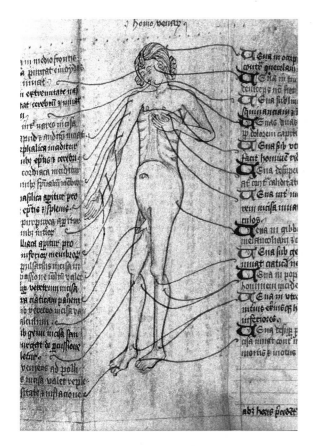

Figure 3.3   Diagram showing bloodletting points, 1463. Lines link sites on the body suitable for bloodletting with a textual explanation in the margin. For example, in the left-hand margin, the sixth caption from the top says that the **basilic vein** in the arm should be opened for ailments of the liver and spleen. A line links this text to a position on the inner arm, above the elbow. Wellcome Library, London

maintaining their status and authority over rival practitioners from the sixteenth century onward, they made greater efforts to bring the ubiquitous practice of bloodletting under their control. The normal practice throughout Europe at this time was therefore for the physician to prescribe and supervise bloodletting, which was then carried out by the barber-surgeon. This was certainly the case in those towns and cities where physicians and barber-surgeons were contracted and paid by the municipal authorities.

Exercise

Now read 'Bloodletting in Renaissance medicine' (Source Book 1, Reading 3.2). What factors does Nancy Siraisi suggest to account for the continuing popularity of bloodletting in the Renaissance?

Discussion

Bloodletting was less painful and dangerous than many other forms of medical intervention, and it had a long and respected history, knowledge of which was preserved throughout the Middle Ages in the learned commentaries of medieval and Arab scholars. These in turn were readily systematized and simplified in a variety of popular manuals that provided detailed advice and specific rules, which

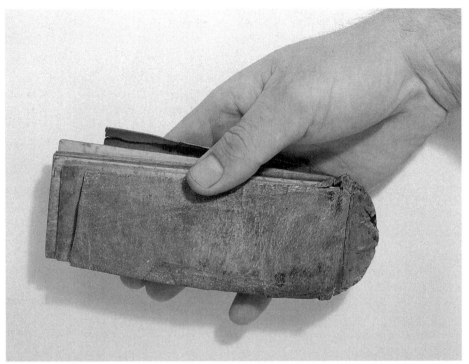

Figure 3.4 A girdle book, which might contain such information as a calendar, a picture of a zodiac man, a diagram showing bloodletting points and charts for determining planetary positions. Wellcome Library, London

could be followed by a range of practitioners. As a result, bloodletting was widely available and proved a highly popular form of therapy throughout the Renaissance – a period in which further debates arose as to specific aspects of the procedure.

3.4   Humanism, bloodletting and a new medical controversy

In Reading 3.2, Siraisi refers to the fact that there were two recognized ways of drawing noxious blood away from an affected part, such as the site of an inflammation: by taking blood either from the side of the body furthest away from the affected part, or from that nearest to it. These two methods had been used since antiquity, and were known, respectively, as revulsion and derivation. In revulsion, the blood was diverted away from the affected part before being drawn off. This method was considered useful in the early stages of an illness. Derivation was employed when the noxious humours had localized around the affected part, which was usually the case once the illness had become established. In such cases, the noxious blood was drawn off from a point much closer to the affected part. Medieval physicians normally interpreted the difference between revulsion and derivation as a matter of distance, and so understood revulsion as a method

whereby blood should be let from the point furthest away from the affected part –
that is, on the opposite side of the body. In practice, this meant that if an
inflammation occurred on the left-hand side of the body, blood was revulsed from
the right-hand side of the body, and vice versa.

In the first two decades of the sixteenth century, the practice of revulsion came
under close scrutiny from humanist physicians in their desire to recover the
correct meaning of the original Greek medical terms for this practice. In particular,
Pierre Brissot (1478–1522), an admirer of Erasmus who taught at the University of
Paris, condemned the received definition of revulsion as the spurious invention of
Arab physicians. He argued that in the true method of revulsion, as described by
Hippocrates and Galen, blood should not be let from the opposite side of the body,
but rather from a point much closer to the affected part. Brissot claimed to have
achieved spectacular success with this method during epidemics in Paris and Evora
(in present-day Portugal) of an ailment he referred to as 'pain in the side'. (The
Latin term used is *dolor lateralis* or *pleuritis*, which means 'pain in the side'; this
should not be confused, however, with the modern disease of pleurisy.) To back up
his argument, he quoted extensively from the texts of Galen and Hippocrates,
sometimes citing the original Greek. He also pointed out that pain in the side
occurred in the **thoracic** region, where blood flowed through the vena cava. Figure
3.5 shows the diagram that Brissot drew to indicate that, anatomically speaking,

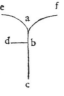

æquale.vt sit in diagrāmate vena caua a b c.lo-
cus pleuritidis sit d in latere dextro . vena quæ
costas alit sit b d . Diuidatur autem vena caua
a b c,in a e venā brachij dextri, & in a f venam
brachij sinistri:iam æquales sunt venæ e a,f a,&
communis est vena a b d. Igitur à loco d,ad loca e & f,per cōmunē a b, quæ vnica est, par est
distātia,id est à pleuritide dextri lateris ad vtrū-
que cubitū.Ergo vt detur quicquid petis, quid
tibi cū hac distātia, ex qua vides nihil posse col-
ligi , quod tuas partes foueat , potius q̄ meas?
Hanc ob causam præstantissimi ex recētioribus,
vt Nicolus Florentinus,putant id nō posse vlla
ratione probari,sed sola experientia.cōferre etiā
inter initia vnius brachij venæ sectiōnē in pleuritide potius,q̄ alterius. Galenus etiam ipse li-
bro de venarū sectione, siue de flobothomia, &
naturæ imitatiōnē, & suam experiētiam addu-
cit,cum alioqui semper soleat rationem reddere
etiā in minimis rebus: quasi ea res sola experiē-
tia cōfirmari possit.sed id postea accuratius scru
tabimur,huic rei dicato libello,vbi ostendemus
& tractū & pulsum humorum à natura optime
ac expedite fieri eo modo quo venarū stamina
procedūt siue filamēta siue villi,& hāc appella-
ri rectitudinē ab Hippocrate & Galeno.Hanc
enim ob causam,ab eo latere quod dolore affectū
est,sanguine detrahunt retractionis gratia.For-
b·j.

Figure 3.5 A page from Pierre Brissot,
*Apologetica Disceptatio, Qua Docetur Per
Quae Loca Santuis Mitti Debeat In
Viscerum Inflammationibus, Praesertim In
Pleuritide* [An Apologetic Debate, in which It
Is Taught from which Place Blood Should Be
Let in Visceral Inflammations, Especially for
Pain in the Side], 1525. In the marginal
diagram, the line *abc* represents the vena
cava, *af* the veins of the left arm, *ae* the veins
of the right arm; *d* represents the affected
part, and *db* the vein that takes blood from
the vena cava to the affected side of the
thorax. The diagram shows that there is no
difference in distance between *dbae* and *dbaf*.
Wellcome Library, London

there was little difference in terms of distance between selecting the right or the left side of the body for the purposes of bleeding. Brissot's arguments were typically humanist. Note his disdain for Arabic commentators and the use of extensive citations from the original Greek authorities to bolster his position. In addition, he pointed to the anatomical structure of the thoracic veins to support what he considered to be the correct and pristine method of the ancient Greeks.

After his death, Brissot's claims split the learned medical world into two camps, for and against. In an attempt to restore peace, the medical faculty of the University of Salamanca was asked to adjudicate on the controversy. Its decision to support the new method, however, only prompted Brissot's opponents to appeal to an even higher jurisdiction, that of the emperor, Charles V (he was also king of Spain). In the event, Brissot secured Charles's support (in all probability because a noble acquaintance and friend of the emperor had died after having had his blood let in the traditional way), as well as that of some of the most prestigious figures in contemporary medicine, including Giovanni Manardus (1462–1532), a student of Leoniceno at Ferrara, Matthaeus Curtius (*c*.1475–*c*.1532), a professor of theoretical medicine at Bologna, and Leonhart Fuchs (1501–66), a professor of medicine at the German university of Tübingen. Fuchs in particular was an inveterate opponent of the Arabs and their medieval successors, whom he termed 'barbarians', and campaigned tirelessly for a return to the original medical sources. The escalating temperature of the controversy can also be gauged from the accusation hurled at Brissot's supporters that they were acting like 'Lutherans' – that is, causing a schism in the medical world in much the same way that the religious reformer Martin Luther (1483–1546) had split the Catholic church in Europe.

Lutheranism in relation to medicine is discussed further in Chapter 4.

3.5 Andreas Vesalius

Born into a medical family in Brussels, Vesalius first attended the trilingual college in Louvain before travelling to Paris in 1533 where he began his medical studies. As you have seen, Paris was then a centre of medical humanism. The physicians Sylvius and Guinther were at this time enthusiastically reviving Galenic medicine, especially anatomy, in print and in their teaching. The precocious student seems to have found his niche quickly. In his textbook on Galenic anatomy, published in 1536, Guinther acknowledged Vesalius' help with anatomical matters. In the same year, Guinther translated two Galenic texts on bloodletting as the controversy surrounding it that had been initiated by Brissot continued to reverberate through the medical faculties of Europe.

In 1537, Vesalius left Paris for Padua, where he was appointed as demonstrator and lecturer in surgery at the city's prestigious university. Here, he confirmed his reputation in anatomy and received his doctorate in medicine. In the following year, he published a series of anatomical illustrations that reflected the humanist culture he had imbibed in Paris. These illustrations, now known as the *Tabulae Anatomicae Sex* [Six Anatomical Tables], depict the anatomical structure of the human body – in particular the veins, arteries and bones, which, in a break with tradition, he labelled alphabetically (Figure 3.6). He also supplied in the margins the name of each part in Latin and Greek, as well as in Hebrew and Arabic. Many of

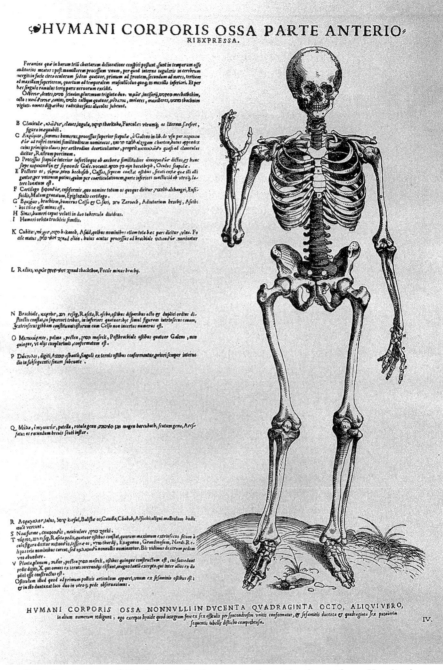

Figure 3.6   The bones of the human body as seen from the front; from Vesalius'
Tabulae Anatomicae Sex, 1538. For the bone of the forearm (labelled *K*), for
example, Vesalius gives the Latin *cubitus*, the Greek *pechys*, the Hebrew *hakaneh*
and the Arabic *asaid*. Wellcome Library, London

the Latin and Greek terms he used, such as '**azygos** vein', had only recently been established by his teachers, Guinther and Sylvius. These anatomical illustrations thus functioned as a pictorial concordance of anatomical terms for the purpose of establishing pristine medical terminology.

Another important feature of this series was the emphasis which Vesalius placed on the bones: three of the six illustrations depicted the human skeleton, as drawn by Jan Stephanus Calcar (d. *c*.1546) from a skeleton Vesalius had assembled himself (the remaining three illustrations were drawn by Vesalius). Galen had regarded the bones as the fundamental structure of the body – he compared them to the walls of a house. This message was strongly reinforced in the newly discovered and translated *On Anatomical Procedures*, in which Galen had recommended that the bones should be studied and dissected first, followed by the muscles, nerves, veins and arteries, and finally the internal organs and the brain. Traditionally, anatomists had begun by dissecting the internal organs located in the body cavities, because these were the first to putrefy.

Vesalius' *Tabulae Anatomicae Sex*, then, represented cutting-edge humanist scholarship on human anatomy, allied to a fundamentally new way of depicting the human body that utilized some of the latest techniques in Renaissance art and printing. In the following extract, Vesalius explains what had led him to produce this innovative series of drawings:

> Not so long ago ... having been chosen for the lecture of surgical medicine at Padua, I was dealing with the treatment of inflammation; and while I was about to explain the opinion of the divine Hippocrates and of Galen on revulsion and derivation, I incidentally drew the veins on paper, reckoning that what Hippocrates understood by the expression *kat' ixin* [Greek for 'in line with'] could readily be demonstrated. For you know these days how much expression of disagreement and contention has arisen among the learned over venesection, since some affirm that Hippocrates had indicated the agreement and straightness of the fibres, and others I know not what else. Indeed, that drawing of the veins so pleased the professors of medicine and all the students that they strenuously sought from me the description of the arteries and also of the nerves. Since the administration of Anatomy pertains to my profession, I could not fail them, especially as I knew that a drawing of this kind would bring no ordinary profit to those who might attend dissections.

> (Vesalius, preface to *Tabulae Anatomicae Sex*; my translation)

The specific context for Vesalius' publication of his groundbreaking illustrations was, therefore, a lecture on dissection in which the young anatomist was trying to explain the meaning of the Greek phrase *kat' ixin*. He regarded the correct definition as fundamental to the true understanding of revulsion, and to help his students understand its meaning, he drew the arrangement of the veins. The favourable reaction of his students and colleagues showed him how useful drawings could be in the teaching of anatomy. The *Tabulae Anatomicae Sex* thus arose as a result of Vesalius' engagement with the most hotly debated medical issue of the day: bloodletting.

Figure 3.7 shows Vesalius' drawing of the veins of the human body. Let us now consider in a little more detail how Vesalius' pictorial description, combined with his thirst for humanistic learning, enabled him to come down on the side of the Brissot camp in the war of words over bloodletting in cases of pain in the side. Central to Vesalius' explanation was the role that he accorded to the azygos vein, which he observed to issue from the right side of the vena cava at a point above the heart, whence it nourished the eight lower ribs – the source of *pleuritis*. In order to avoid drawing blood through the right **auricle** of this vital organ, he thus concluded that it was far safer to let blood from a point above that where the two veins met. Moreover, because the azygos vein issued from the right side of the vena cava, it made more sense for blood to be let from the right arm, which was considered more 'in line with' the affected area. This was directly opposed to the traditional idea that revulsion should be performed from a point on the body opposite to the site of pain. Putting to one side the technicalities of Vesalius' argument, the important point to note is the way in which Vesalius used his observations of the anatomical structure of the veins in general, and the azygos vein in particular, to support his contention about the best point from which to let blood.

Vesalius considered his finding to be so important in the ongoing controversy over bloodletting that in 1539 he published his thoughts on the subject. In his *Epistola, Docens Venam Axillarem Dextri Cubiti In Dolore Laterali Secandam* [Letter, Teaching That in Cases of Pain in the Side, the Axillary Vein in the Right Elbow Be Cut], Vesalius repeated Brissot's original argument that the essential difference between revulsion and derivation was not simply a matter of distance, and cited his own anatomical observations to prove the point. He also quoted fragmentary comments on the matter from both Hippocrates and Galen to show how Arab and medieval commentators may have erred in their earlier translations – the hallmark of a humanist scholar. And, once again, he clarified his point by drawing a diagram (Figure 3.8).

It is clear from this diagram that the structure and position of the azygos vein, which could be established only through direct anatomical observation, was fundamental to Vesalius' understanding. Significantly, Vesalius' description of the function and location of the azygos vein diverged from that of Galen. Vesalius was so convinced that his own observations revealed the vein's true structure that when he came to edit a new translation of Galen's *On the Dissection of Veins and Arteries* (1542), he corrected Galen's text to accord with his own description.

Exercise

Look again at Figures 3.7 and 3.8. Do you think these illustrations are realistic representations of what they were seeking to depict? What role did these illustrations fulfil for Vesalius?

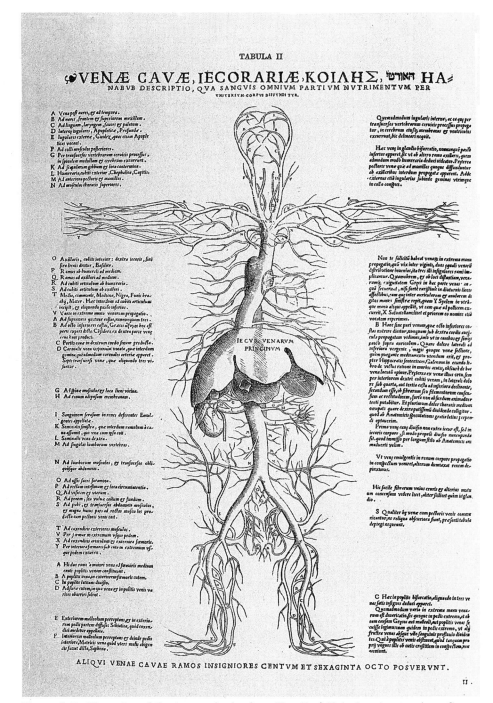

Figure 3.7   The veins of the human body, from Vesalius' *Tabulae Anatomicae Sex*.
This is a Galenic picture of the veins, with the liver in the centre, and the veins
extending from it, like the branches of a tree – an expression that Galen himself had
used. The azygos vein is shown as a bulge issuing from the 'trunk' of this tree (to the
left of it as you look at the diagram), just below the origin of the blood vessels feeding
the arm. Wellcome Library, London

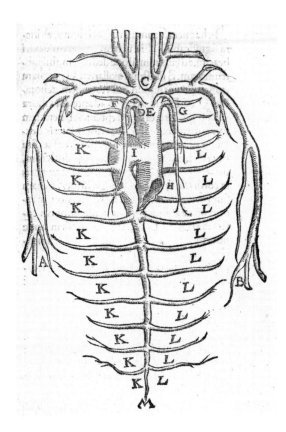

Figure 3.8   Vesalius' diagram of the thoracic veins, from his *Epistola, Docens Venam Axillarem Dextri Cubiti In Dolore Laterali Secandam*, 1539, p.41. The azygos vein (labelled *I*) nourishes all the ribs (labelled *K* and *L*) apart from the three that lie above the point at which it issues from the right side of the vena cava. These three ribs are thus exceptions to the rule that, for most cases of pain in the side, blood should be let from the right-hand side only (i.e. because the vena cava is more 'in line with' the affected area). For pain in the side that occurs in the area of these three ribs (labelled *F* and *G*), blood should be let from whichever side

Discussion

These illustrations are not realistic representations of the veins in an actual dissected human body, where the blood vessels would be intermingled with other matter, such as muscles, fat, cartilages and nerves. In fact, they are highly artificial images, in which Vesalius picked out only those details he needed in order to prove that, in most cases of pain in the side, blood should always be let from the right side of the body. For Vesalius, the drawings were a way of presenting to others the structures he observed, by selecting only those parts of the body that he considered important – in this case, the position and arrangement of the veins.

How influential was Vesalius' interpretation of bodily structures? In the following exercise, you will discover what effect drawings such as these had on a student who was present at one of Vesalius' anatomy lessons. Note that Vesalius was using illustrations even in a dissection class, when a human body lay before his students' eyes. Again, he used these illustrations to draw their attention to specific anatomical features.

Now read 'Attending a public dissection by Vesalius, Bologna, 1540' (Source Book 1, Reading 3.3). What was Heseler's reaction to Vesalius' drawings?

In his diary, Heseler noted his conviction that what was depicted in Vesalius' drawings corresponded with what he saw in the body 'completely': 'I saw this with my own eyes, as I stood quite near.' Clearly, the drawings were very effective as a tool of learning.

It is perhaps worth noting that in the human body the azygos vein does not in fact issue from above the heart, and that it is not as large as Vesalius described it, nor does it extend as far to the right. What Heseler 'saw' in the dissected human body, then, was Vesalius' way of seeing the body (in this case, the azygos vein) mediated via pictorial representations; these pictures were so convincing that Heseler was persuaded to accept Vesalius' interpretation. Henceforth, anatomical drawings were to become an important vehicle whereby Vesalius was able to establish a new understanding of the structure of the human body – one that owed much to Greek precedent while at the same time breaking new ground in anatomical research.

3.6 The *Fabrica*

In the summer of 1543, Vesalius' *De Humani Corporis Fabrica* [On the Structure of the Human Body] was published at Basel by the celebrated printer Johannes Oporinus. It was a lavish pictorial project. In the printer's preface, Oporinus makes it clear that he went to great pains to follow Vesalius' instructions with regard to the illustrations. The book itself contains full-size drawings of the dissected human body – the skeleton and muscles, nervous system, blood vessels and organs – in lifelike poses and set against landscape backgrounds. Also included are pictures of partial anatomical sections embedded in famous ancient sculptures, such as the **Belvedere torso**, and large initial capitals in which are depicted anatomical themes. Clearly, pictures were important to Vesalius, the humanist, in illustrating how the knowledge of the ancients should be read and, if necessary, corrected. But what exactly was he seeking to achieve in resurrecting the work of ancient physicians and anatomists such as Galen? One way of interpreting Vesalius' anatomical research and publications is to envisage his work as part of a wider project that entailed the revival and completion of the work begun by his revered master, Galen, in imperial Rome 1,400 years earlier.

The title page of *De Humani Corporis Fabrica* (Figure 3.9) can be read as a pictorial manifesto of Vesalius' project. The scene is a public dissection, which is taking place in the august surroundings of a classical anatomical theatre. At this period, these were mostly temporary structures that were often modelled on ancient theatres, the ruins of which could still be seen in Rome or Verona. Here, the theatre is teeming with spectators eager to see what is going on. In the centre,

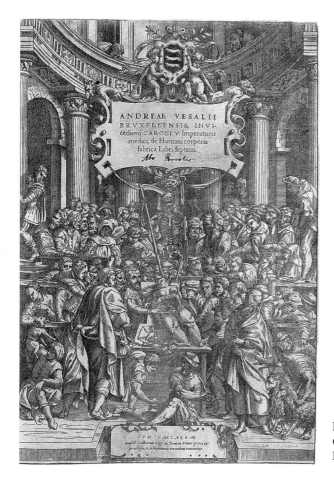

Figure 3.9   Title page of Vesalius' *De Humani Corporis Fabrica*, 1555 edition. Wellcome Library, London

Vesalius stands beside the body of a woman that he has just opened up; with one hand he points to the cadaver, and with the other to heaven. Above him is a human skeleton, representing the all-important structure of the Galenic body. Standing near to Vesalius are three larger-than-life figures in classical attire. It has been suggested that the man to the right of Vesalius, being distracted by a dog, is Aristotle. To the left, with a physician's pouch, stands Galen, and between Vesalius and Galen, and partly obscured, one can just make out the figure of Hippocrates. Vesalius is thus depicted as the focal point of this illustrious quartet, with the ancients looking on, in admiration or even in awe. In terms of Vesalius' wider project, it is easy to see why he has chosen to depict himself in this way. He is seeking both the approval of the ancients for his innovative anatomical research while at the same time daring to go beyond the established bounds of knowledge, as represented by the three great men of ancient medicine and science, Aristotle, Hippocrates and Galen. This is a bold strategy, but an essential one for Vesalius if he wishes to succeed in gaining the approval of his humanist audience.

The significance of this fictional scene may be set into sharper relief by comparing it with an earlier representation of a public dissection (Figure 3.10), in which the body is used to confirm what is described in Galen's text. Vesalius' title page presents us with a dramatically different image and message. Vesalius, the lecturer, also performs the dissection: he cuts open the body, points to what he sees, and uses his observations to understand the body as Galen had enjoined others to do. He is seeing with his own eyes – the literal meaning of the Greek word 'autopsy'. But how, we might ask, is this the action of a typical 'humanist'?

Exercise

Now read 'Vesalius and the anatomical renaissance' (Source Book 1, Reading 3.4). How did Curtius and Vesalius, both humanists, differ in their approach to Galen and his legacy?

Discussion

For the senior figure, Curtius, Galen was the master, whose descriptions of the body were always true. In addition, though his humanist ideals spurred him to rediscover and translate Galen's works, his teaching methods were highly traditional: he expected his lectures on the text of Galen to be confirmed in the dissections, rather than using the dissections as a means of uncovering new truths. The pristine text of Galen retained its primacy. For Vesalius, in contrast, the body was the book – the non-lying book, as he calls it elsewhere – that he desires to read and understand. Vesalius dissected the body, while at the same time commenting on and correcting Galen, much to the annoyance of the traditionalist, Curtius. The important difference between the two men is that Curtius sought to revive Galen through reason, logic and philological study, while Vesalius sought to revive Galen's *practice* of anatomy – that is, the personal experience of cutting open the body with his own hands and seeing with his own eyes.

As the title page of the *Fabrica* so powerfully illustrates, the book is about the body as presented in a public dissection. Vesalius made an important distinction between private and public dissections. In the former, it was sufficient for anatomists to use whatever corpses they might come by in order to practise the requisite skills of dissection and to learn about the diseased body. By contrast, in public dissections, Vesalius argued that it was important that the body chosen for dissection was that of a man or woman of middle age, who in life had a temperate complexion. Physical abnormalities were shunned and ignored. In other words, in public dissections and the *Fabrica*, Vesalius sought to present the viewer/reader with an ideal version of the human body, against which all other bodies might be compared. In this, he was again following the ancients, who regarded the statue of Doryphorus, by the famous sculptor Polycleitus (*fl.* fifth century BCE), as displaying the perfect proportions of the human body. The statue was well known to classical authors, including Galen, and was called the 'canon' or the 'mean' by which all sculptors and artists were to judge beauty.

So how did Vesalius attempt to establish a 'canon' of the human body? Typically, he based it on his own personal anatomical observations, which he compared with Galen's descriptions. Then, by comparing and pointing out differences between the

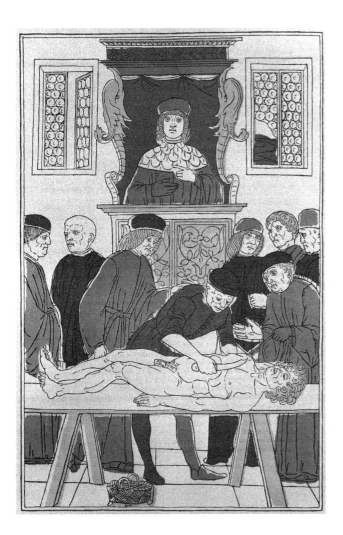

Figure 3.10   A traditional dissection scene from Johannes de Ketham, *Fasciculus Medicinae*, 1495. A university professor reads aloud from a prescribed anatomical text, quite literally *ex cathedra* ('from the chair'), while a barber-surgeon cuts open the body, and an *ostensor*, or demonstrator, points to the parts referred to in the text. Wellcome Library, London

muscles of humans and of animals, Vesalius defined what belonged to the human body and what did not. In the process, his increasing knowledge of human anatomy led him to realize that Galen had erred in basing his knowledge of the human body on the dissection of animals. Nonetheless, Vesalius was at great pains to stress that he did not wish anyone to construe such conclusions as amounting to a criticism of his ancient master. Though he was able to argue that his view of human anatomy was more accurate than that of Galen, he by no means envisaged his work as being anti-Galenic. By documenting Galen's errors (in all, he noted about 300), Vesalius was consciously seeking to revive the practice of Galenic anatomy, which for him meant subjecting Galen's text to the scrutiny of anatomical inspection. Anatomy was akin to seeing for oneself; Galen's authority had to be confirmed by 'autopsy'.

Another way in which Vesalius constructed his view of the canonical body was by defining variations from the norm, or abnormality. He maintained that human anatomy could be learnt only by studying human bodies – as many as possible. To discover what was normal or abnormal in bodily structures, he recommended students to examine samples of bones in a cemetery to establish which structures occurred most frequently. If few or no examples of a particular structure were found, their occurrence might be said to be rare or impossible. For example, Galen, relying on animals, had stated that the human lower jaw consisted of two parts. Vesalius refuted this by stating that 'although I have seen a very large number of lower jaws ... both elsewhere and especially in the Cemetery of the Innocents in Paris, I have never ever found one in two parts' (Vesalius, 1999, vol.I, p.107). Another way of confirming what was normal was to take the opportunity to examine the bones of any animal that was served up as food. Vesalius suggested, for example, that to understand the structure of the **ossicles** in the ear, students should dissect the head of a calf or a lamb; to understand the workings of the **scapula**, they should dissect those of a sheep, goat or hare; and to understand the ligament of the neck they should slice through that of a calf, piglet, kid or ox. Such exhortations were designed to have an immediate didactic effect, as Vesalius' dissection lectures took place both before and after meals.

Vesalius was not yet 28 years old when he finished *De Humani Corporis Fabrica*. Despite his studies at Louvain, Paris and Padua, his job as a demonstrator and lecturer in surgery at Padua was poorly paid and afforded lowly status in contrast to that of a professor of theoretical medicine. He was well aware that he lacked the authority or reputation to be taken seriously by the learned medical community, and so he dedicated his book to the emperor, Charles V, in the hope that such an august association would lend him the desired respectability and authority. This was a common strategy in the period for budding academicians, who sought the endorsement of powerful patrons in order to enhance their own personal status as well as that of their discipline. The successful French surgeon Ambroise Paré (1510–90), for example, boasted in print of his medical successes not only on the battlefield but also at the French court. A related strategy, designed specifically to enhance the academic credibility of 'lesser' or 'practical' disciplines such as anatomy, was to adopt the literary style and conventions of higher status academic pursuits. The Italian anatomist Jacopo Berengario da Carpi (d.1530) pursued this approach in a number of his published works on anatomy that were written in the style of scholarly commentaries on theoretical and philosophical subjects. Vesalius himself had embraced the principles of humanist scholarship that were so fashionable among the learned elite and noble patrons, and had been a knowledgeable and outspoken participant in one of the most hotly debated medical issues of the time. To further enhance his credibility, he adopted a variety of tactics in the *Fabrica*, many of which bore little relation to medicine.

Exercise

Now read 'Vesalius, *On the Fabric of the Human Body* (1543)' (Source Book 1, Reading 3.5). How did Vesalius seek to enhance his authority?

Discussion

Vesalius named the eminent people who have supported him. He vividly described the lengths to which he went in order to pursue his anatomical studies, and to emphasize his commitment and dedication to the task, even when little support was forthcoming. He demonstrated his expertise in the use of surgical instruments and his willingness to learn from manual workers – something that Galen himself was prepared to do.

All these efforts bore fruit: shortly after publication of the *Fabrica*, Vesalius was appointed physician to Charles V.

3.7 Vesalius' legacy

You have seen so far how Vesalius' published works were initially inspired by the humanist controversy over bloodletting, and how they formed part of a quintessential Renaissance project concerned with the 'revival' of the practice of Galenic anatomy. In the process, Vesalius advanced new and often controversial theories surrounding the inner workings of the human body, which threatened to undermine some of the most cherished beliefs of the educated medical profession. But what impact, if any, did his Renaissance programme have on his contemporaries?

Through Vesalius' efforts, anatomy became an academically respectable subject, able to cast off its earlier, inferior status, which resulted from the manual character of the anatomist's work. Anatomy indeed became central to the study of medicine. The *Fabrica* itself had an immediate impact on the learned medical world. Pirated copies of its spectacular illustrations spread rapidly throughout Europe – much to the annoyance of Vesalius, who was helpless to alter the fact that many were copied erroneously and were used alongside misplaced and incorrect text that differed from Vesalius' original. But the popularity of his work did not secure the approbation of all his fellow anatomists. Those that followed in his footsteps were just as critical of Vesalius' errors and oversights as he had once been of his ancient mentor, Galen. Bartolomeo Eustachio (*c*.1500–74), for example, corrected Vesalius' work on the kidneys, while Gabriele Fallopia (1523–63), Vesalius' successor at Padua, pointed out that his predecessor had erred in stating that the **sacrum** consisted of six parts, rather than five. Both men also described parts of the human anatomy that Vesalius had overlooked, ignored or misunderstood. Eustachio described the tube that links the throat to the middle ear; Fallopia discovered the third ossicle of the ear and the uterine tubes.

Among more conservative-minded physicians, Vesalius' claim that Galen had erred because he had never dissected human bodies caused a storm of protest. His former teacher, the humanist Sylvius, argued that if what was seen in a dissected body did not correspond with Galen's description, then this was due to changes in the nature of the human body over time. This theory helped to explain why ancient heroes were capable of much greater feats of strength and endurance than were sixteenth-century men, as well as accounting for the vast ages of biblical figures like Methuselah. Others, such as the English humanist physician John Caius (1510–73), who was instrumental in reviving the practice of anatomy in England, sought to defend Galen's reputation by pointing out passages in his work where it is suggested that he must have dissected human cadavers. On this issue, the medical world split into two camps, for and against Vesalius. Several respectable humanist physicians disagreed with Vesalius, a fact that provides important evidence for the multifaceted nature of medical humanism. It was never a fixed ideology, pointing in one direction, but rather a set of values and attitudes, inspired by the example of the ancients, that might lead to many different, and sometimes mutually exclusive, positions.

Let us now return to the issue with which I began: what impact did Vesalius' work have on the practice and the theory of bloodletting? Evidence for the former is hard to come by. Although surgical manuals in this period, including those written in the vernacular, began to include reference to Galen and Hippocrates, with the occasional sprinkling of Greek terms and phrases, Vesalius was rarely cited as an authority on the subject. There is little evidence to suggest that the practice of bloodletting changed dramatically as a result of his observations, or that surgeons uniformly followed his advice on treating pain in the side.

More significant was Vesalius' impact on the theory of bloodletting – in particular, on the learned controversy over venesection. He reorientated the debate in such a way that those after him, although they continued to quote from Galen and Hippocrates, would now have to shore up their argument on anatomical grounds. An example is Eustachio's response to Vesalius' description of the azygos vein: he challenges the description point by point, showing that it was contrary not only to the Galenic text, but also to the evidence of human anatomy. It is important to remember that, at this time, bloodletting was an extremely serious business – a matter of life and death. Not surprisingly, then, Vesalius' work prompted ever closer scrutiny of the inner workings of the human body, and in this case, a renewed interest in the structure and function of the all-important azygos vein, as witnessed by the deposition of the Portuguese physician Johannes Amatus Lusitanus (d.1568), writing in 1551:

> Vesalius of Brussels, the distinguished anatomist and physician to the Emperor Charles V, published some years ago a discussion on this subject in which he argued that pleurisy [i.e. pain in the side], whether the inflammation be on the right or left side, the internal vein of the right side must always be opened ... The reason given by him is as follows: since the vein called azygos, that is 'without a fellow', arises near the heart from the right side of the vena cava and in its passage downward along the spine, nourishes the eight lower ribs of either side and is distributed to the diaphragm and separating membrane, hence (so he said) the matter causing [pain in the side] would be eradicated and evacuated far better if the blood is withdrawn by venesection from the right arm rather than the left, because the basilic vein of the right arm is furthermore more directly in accord with the azygos than the basilic of the left ...

> Forsooth, this teaching should be excluded as an error and eliminated from practical procedure as a menacing danger. In this connection it is easy to see that the argument of Vesalius is utterly erroneous because the azygos vein does not once again return the blood which it receives from the vena cava. On the contrary, it is so constructed at its orifice where it is

joined to the vena cava as to possess certain **ostiola** which are opened to permit their inhibition of blood and which are later so closed that they no longer allow the blood which has been received, to return. Thus the azygos vein operates in this regard like the orifices of the urinary bladder or of the vessels of the heart. That this is a characteristic feature of the azygos, that is to say, that it no longer returns along the same channel the blood which it has received, we have determined from the dissection of bodies.

(quoted in Vesalius, [1539] 1948, pp.22–4)

Lusitanus' discovery was subsequently discredited, but the passage neatly illustrates the increasing emphasis that was placed on the anatomical structure of the veins and the heart as a result of Vesalius' contribution to the bloodletting controversy.

Ten years after Vesalius' death, the lecturer in surgery and professor of anatomy at Padua (the position once held by Vesalius) was Hieronymous Fabricius of Aquapendente (*c*.1533–1619). Fabricius carried on the tradition of original research begun by his illustrious predecessor and discovered the *ostiola* ('little doors') in some of the veins, which he believed had the function of delaying blood flow (Figure 3.11). Fabricius' discovery, however, was in many respects antipathetic to, and different from, that research programme initiated by Vesalius. Though he shared Vesalius' passion for humanism and the learning of the ancients, Fabricius' research was inspired not by Galen but by Aristotle. This in turn meant that Fabricius – despite his academic position at Padua – was not solely interested in exploring human anatomy. His aims were more universal, embracing the earlier vision of Aristotle, who wished to provide a general account of all animal life in which man was one example among many.

Exercise

Now read 'Fabricius and the "Aristotle Project"' (Source Book I, Reading 3.6). How did Fabricius' account of the 'little doors' in the veins represent a different approach to anatomy from that conducted by Vesalius?

Discussion

On the surface, Fabricius appeared to be following closely in Vesalius' footsteps. His discovery of the 'little doors' in the veins resulted from his dissection of human bodies. However, unlike Vesalius, Fabricius placed far more stress on understanding the function or causation of the structures he described, whereas Vesalius was more interested in simple observation and description. As a student of Aristotle, Fabricius actively sought to explain, in general terms, the physiological attributes common to all animal life. He adopted a philosophical approach to his subject, constantly seeking to explain causation in nature, and in the process elevated the work of the anatomist to a higher plane in the academic pantheon.

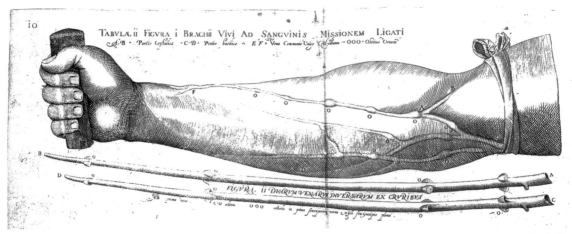

Figure 3.11   Fabricius' drawing of the 'little doors' in the veins, from H. Fabricius, *De Venarum Ostiolis*, 1603, as reproduced in his *Tractatus Quatuor*, 1625. The drawing is of an arm, its upper part tied up with a ligature, as was usually done in bloodletting. This ligature allows the 'little doors' (labelled *O*) to become visible on the surface of the skin. This finding was crucial for the work of Fabricius' student, William Harvey (1578–1657), who later reproduced this illustration in his *On the Motion of the Heart and Blood in Animals* (1628) to prove a different point. Wellcome Library, London

In his work on the 'little doors', as in his earlier work on the eye, larynx and ear, Fabricius was preoccupied with establishing 'universally true explanatory accounts of the causes of phenomena' – that is, in Renaissance parlance, principles that have the status of *scientia* (Cunningham, 1985, pp. 203–4). Fabricius' project was different from that of Vesalius. It sought to explain, rather than describe, the structure and function of all animal life, not just human beings, and as such was deeply indebted to the revival of Aristotelian natural philosophy that was widely taught in the universities of early modern Europe. This approach has traditionally been seen by historians of science and medicine as representing something of a dead end in terms of scientific and medical progress. And yet, as we shall see when we look more closely at the work of Fabricius' student, William Harvey, in Chapter 7, the desire to complete the projects of the ancients continued to provide a crucial impetus to innovatory medical research well into the seventeenth century. The legacy of Vesalius and those who followed him was substantial, though the routes to medical enlightenment were rarely unilinear.

References

Cunningham, A. (1985) 'Fabricius and the "Aristotle Project" at Padua' in A. Wear, R.K. French and I.M. Lonie (eds) *The Medical Renaissance of the Sixteenth Century*, Cambridge: Cambridge University Press, pp.195–222.

Porter, R. (1999) *The Greatest Benefit to Mankind: A Medical History of Humanity from Antiquity to the Present*, London: Fontana.

Talbot, C.H. (1967) *Medicine in Medieval England*, London: Oldbourne.

Vesalius, A. [1539] (1948) *Andreas Vesalius Bruxellensis, the Bloodletting Letter of 1539: An Annotated Translation and Study of the Evolution of Vesalius's Scientific Development*, ed. and translated by J.B. de C.M. Saunders and C.D. O'Malley, London: Heinemann.

Vesalius, A. [1543] (1999) *On the Fabric of the Human Body*, translated by W.F. Richardson with J.B. Carman, 2 vols, San Francisco: Norman Publishing.

Source Book readings

V. Nutton, 'The rise of medical humanism: Ferrara, 1464–1555,' *Renaissance Studies*, 1997, vol.11, pp.1–8 (Reading 3.1).

N.G. Siraisi, *Medieval and Early Renaissance Medicine: An Introduction to Knowledge and Practice*, Chicago and London: University of Chicago Press, 1990, pp.136–41 (Reading 3.2).

Andreas Vesalius' First Public Anatomy at Bologna 1540, an Eyewitness Report by Baldasar Heseler Medicinae Scolaris, ed. and translated by R. Eriksson, Uppsala and Stockholm: Almquist & Wiksells, 1959, p.237 (Reading 3.3).

A. Cunningham, *The Anatomical Renaissance: The Resurrection of the Anatomical Projects of the Ancients*, Aldershot: Scolar Press, 1997, pp.102–16 (Reading 3.4).

A. Vesalius, *On the Fabric of the Human Body*, translated by W.F. Richardson with J.B. Carman, 2 vols, San Francisco: Norman Publishing, 1999, vol.1, pp.87, 378, 382–3; vol.2, pp.147, 150 (Reading 3.5).

A. Cunningham, 'Fabricius and the "Aristotle Project" at Padua' in A. Wear, R.K. French and I.M. Lonie (eds) *The Medical Renaissance of the Sixteenth Century*, Cambridge: Cambridge University Press, 1985, pp.206–9 (Reading 3.6).

4
Medicine and Religion in Sixteenth-Century Europe

Ole Peter Grell

Objectives

When you have completed this chapter you should be able to:

- understand the relationship between religion and medicine in the early modern period;

- appreciate the impact of the Reformation and the Counter-Reformation on various aspects of medical theory and practice;

- understand how a new type of medicine, Paracelsianism, emerged as a consequence of the Reformation.

4.1   Introduction

In standard textbooks on the history of medicine, the **Reformation** is considered of minor significance, coinciding as it does with the revival of anatomy and the preceding innovations of the so-called '**scientific revolution**'. This in part reflects the approach of earlier generations of medical historians, who have accorded little importance to the role of religion generally in the development of western medical knowledge. Traditionally, science and medicine have been viewed as proceeding in isolation from, and in some cases in opposition to, the religious preoccupations of the early modern period. Recently, however, historians have begun to reassess the relationship between medicine and religion and to demonstrate that the fate of the former was radically affected and shaped by the latter. In this chapter, I wish to explore this relationship in more detail, particularly with reference to the changes that came about as a result of the religious upheavals of the sixteenth century initiated by the Protestant Reformation.

Broadly speaking, the Reformation saw a major confessional divide in Europe, which split the continent into two warring religious factions: Protestantism, which became most firmly established in northern Europe, and Catholicism, which remained dominant in the south. These changes – as I shall show in this chapter – were to impact on attitudes to both medical practice and medical knowledge. In the Protestant north, for example, they promoted a new approach to the provision of health care as well as providing fertile conditions for the emergence of a new, specifically Christian, form of medicine: Paracelsianism. Meanwhile, in southern Europe, the **Counter-Reformation**, too, initiated a revival of interest in various aspects of health care in Catholic communities.

4.2   Medicine and religion in the later Middle Ages

Before the Reformation, the only Christian church in the medieval west was the Catholic church. Although the Catholic church was, first and foremost, concerned with the saving of souls, it also took a considerable interest in the body and in those who cared for it. There was considerable suspicion of non-Christian medical practitioners, with particular emphasis placed on midwives being Christian – Jews and heretics were explicitly excluded. This, of course, had more to do with the Christian midwife's ability to perform an emergency baptism, thereby ensuring the newborn child's entry into heaven, rather than a belief in her superior medical expertise. More importantly, however, the medieval church held a virtual monopoly on learned medicine. Before the rise of the universities in the thirteenth century, religious institutions such as monasteries and abbeys served as repositories of medical knowledge, and were home to some renowned medical scholars. Until the fifteenth century, the involvement of monastic establishments with medicine remained greater than that of any other institution. Thus, it was in the monastery of Monte Cassino in Italy that the definitive version of the so-called *Articella* [Little Art of Medicine], the standard collection of authoritative medical texts, was finally put together.

The interest of the church in learned medicine meant that it also played a leading role in providing medical services. Monasteries had established hospitals to provide medical care for members of their order who had fallen ill, and these rapidly began to serve lay people too. These hospitals were staffed by monks trained as healers, with the occasional support of physicians from outside the monasteries. However, despite the medical services they offered, these early hospitals were very different from the modern equivalent. They were primarily religious institutions, dedicated to saving souls – both those of the patients and those of the individuals who cared for the sick or who financed such care. Accordingly, most of the income of these hospitals was spent on the machinery and fabric of religion, such as masses or decorative altar screens; only a fraction was spent on medicine.

The majority of medieval hospitals were small, and were situated in and around centres of pilgrimage, such as shrines and holy sites associated with healing properties. Such sites were a rapidly expanding phenomenon in the later Middle Ages, and there was intense competition between them. There was no conflict in people's minds between religious healing and the dispensing of medicine. God was the ultimate source of all healing, and, if He so chose, could provide a cure by either route. A host of saints could be called on to cure a variety of diseases, and saintly relics or pictures of saints were believed to have curative powers. Some, such as St Michael or St Luke, might cure a range of complaints; others were more specialized: St Radegund and St Roch, for example, were invoked against ulcers and the plague, respectively.

During the fifteenth century, a number of new and much larger hospitals came into existence. These were often independent foundations, established by individual merchants or by trade organizations such as guilds. However, even hospitals that did not come under the direct influence of the church still continued to operate in a religious context. Despite their size and quality, these new, larger hospitals, like their smaller predecessors, were still first and foremost intended as religious institutions. The medical services they offered developed only gradually, and as an adjunct to the provision of religious care.

The fifty universities that were founded in Europe between 1200 and 1500 gradually came to supplement many of the monastic institutions as repositories of medical knowledge. However, throughout the Middle Ages – and beyond – the church exerted a powerful influence on the universities too. Furthermore, university faculties of medicine were slow to establish themselves. They came into being only when physicians realized the extent to which the prestige and professional standing of legal practitioners and theologians had been raised by the roles they played in these new institutions.

As you read in Chapter 1, in the fifteenth and sixteenth centuries, university-educated physicians were not only taught about the physical human body, but also instructed in the basic principles of natural philosophy. This complex set of doctrines was sustained by the rules of logic, which were ultimately subordinate to theology. A fundamental principle of natural philosophy was the idea that nature was God's creation, with the human body seen as part of the wider natural world. In a medical consultation, therefore, a physician not only took account of an individual's constitution, diet and environment, but also sought to understand the hidden influence of nature, especially the workings of the heavens – in other words, he practised astrology. Medical astrology already had a long history by the Middle Ages, and continued to play an important role in medical practice after the Reformation. Throughout the Middle Ages and the sixteenth century, astrology was considered a highly useful tool for physicians, who often attended their patients armed with tables to help them calculate the position of the planets, and their relationship to the body and its ailments.

4.3   Medicine and the Reformation

The Reformation and the study of anatomy

In 1517, the German monk Martin Luther posted his **ninety-five theses** on the door of the university church at Wittenberg, condemning the Roman Catholic church's system of **indulgences**. This was the first in a series of challenges to the papacy that eventually resulted in the Reformation and the emergence of Protestantism. Luther saw his mission as reviving the true church. He rejected many of the beliefs, practices and institutions of the Catholic church as additions made by humans to the true Christian faith. Luther argued that salvation did not depend on good works or on the intercession of the church, but solely on faith and grace.

What effect did this rejection of papal authority have on medicine? Naturally, many areas remained unaffected. Diseases, of course, struck both Catholics and Protestants alike, and in their medical treatment and practice they differed little, if at all. Likewise, students in both Catholic and Protestant universities used the same medical textbooks. However, one area of medical knowledge where it may be possible to detect the influence of reformist ideas is the study of anatomy. You have seen in the previous chapter how Vesalius' ambition to revive the anatomical project of Galen was partly driven by his deep-seated attachment to the humanist values of the Renaissance. Humanism was equally important in helping to shape and drive the religious changes that culminated in the religious reformations of the sixteenth century. Many of the earliest critics of the Catholic church, such as Desiderius Erasmus and Thomas More (1478–1535), were inspired by their deep-seated attachment to humanist methods of scholarship and their reading of the classics. Though both Erasmus and More remained within the Catholic church, other humanist-inspired critics opted to reject papal authority and promote root-and-branch reform in the church.

Part of Luther's ambition to take the church back to its apostolic roots was the undertaking to retrieve the unadulterated word of God – that is, a Bible based on the best Hebrew and Greek sources. This return to pristine sources was an endeavour Luther shared with many Renaissance scholars, especially Christian humanists. Luther also advocated the study of the natural world, and of the human body. A renewed interest in human beings as the pinnacle of God's creation was a feature of the Renaissance, and the dissection of the human body was frequently justified in religious terms.

Until the first decades of the sixteenth century, the public dissection of human bodies had taken place only occasionally, and within a university medical faculty. In the middle of the sixteenth century, however, a revolution took place in the way anatomy was studied. The publication in 1543 of Andreas Vesalius' great illustrated volume *De Humani Corporis Fabrica* [On the Structure of the Human Body], in which realistic drawings of the dissected human body were printed for the first time, firmly established the importance of anatomy in the teaching of medicine. Because anatomical dissection was believed to reveal God's work, it can be seen as a religious endeavour that was important for both Catholics and Protestants. But did Vesalian anatomy have a specific link with **Lutheran Protestantism**? In his book *The Anatomical Renaissance*, Andrew Cunningham (1997) claims that it did, arguing that Vesalius was primarily motivated by religious concerns generated by Lutheran Protestantism. Although Cunningham admits that his evidence is inconclusive, he makes a strong case. From its beginnings in Wittenberg, Protestantism spread rapidly throughout northern Europe. Vesalius grew up in the Netherlands during the turmoil of Luther's confrontation with Rome, and he received his medical education at the University of Paris, at a time when Luther's ideas were making a serious impact in the French capital. Cunningham thinks it impossible that Vesalius could have remained untouched by Lutheranism.

Cunningham also suggests that there is a close connection between Luther and Vesalius, both in their intellectual preoccupations and in their methods. Just as Luther rejected the Catholic church's interpretation of God's words, exhorting people instead to read for themselves the literal word of God in the Bible, so Vesalius argued against accepting unquestioningly the interpretation of God's work (the human body) given in traditional medical texts, exhorting students instead to 'read' the text itself – that is, the dissected human body. An indication of the close links between the work of Vesalius and that of Luther is the fact that, around the time of the publication of the *Fabrica*, Vesalian anatomy was quickly taken up in the new Lutheran universities. This was largely through the efforts of Luther's assistant, Philip Melanchthon (1497–1560), who was influential in creating and propagating a reformed curriculum. In these new universities, anatomy was studied not only by medical students, but by all students, as part of the philosophy course undertaken at the beginning of their university career.

Historians are divided on the extent to which Luther and the Protestant faith influenced Vesalius and the study of anatomy. The circumstantial evidence is strong: it does seem unlikely that Vesalius was unaffected by the social and religious turmoil around him at the time he was developing his radical new ideas, and the similarity in approach between Luther and Vesalius is remarkable. Perhaps, as Cunningham says, whether or not Vesalius actually converted to Protestantism matters little. Instead, what is important is the fact that Vesalius, consciously or unconsciously, acted like a Lutheran.

Luther and medicine

It is evident from the statements Luther made about medicine that he saw medicine and religion as closely connected. Like most people in the sixteenth century, he saw God as the ultimate source of all healing, with the physician acting on God's behalf to effect a cure. The physician healed the body just as the minister healed the spirit. Luther believed that God would reveal medical knowledge to those who searched for it, but that this required the diligent study of the natural world. Like Vesalius, he held the view that such knowledge could not be acquired from the study of books alone.

Exercise

Now read 'Luther and medicine' (Source Book 1, Reading 4.1) and then answer the following questions:

1   Who or what, according to Luther, was the cause of all serious illnesses?

2   How did Luther believe diseases were cured by physicians?

Discussion

1   Luther believed that the devil was at the root of all serious illnesses, stating that 'all dangerous diseases are blows of the devil'. Further, he said that, to serve his purposes, Satan is prepared to use all the 'instruments of nature' – in other words, he makes use of whatever he can find in the natural world.

2   Luther regarded physicians as acting on God's behalf. To effect a cure, the physician, too, might make use of whatever God has provided in the natural world. Luther was clear, therefore, that it was allowable for humans to use medicine when they fell ill, because drugs were created by God for this purpose. However, since Luther considered medicine an inexact science, and was convinced that only physicians who sought God's assistance in their tasks could

hope for success, he emphasized that if a physician 'acts of his own righteousness, he is of the devil'.

Luther's personal experience of serious illness had done little to give him great faith in professional medicine. During a stay in Schmalcalden in Thuringia (Thüringen in modern-day Germany) in 1537, for example, he nearly died from a bad case of bladder or kidney stones. His physicians had forced him to drink large quantities of water, which caused him considerable discomfort, and the treatment had rendered his body battered and lifeless. He had obeyed his doctors from necessity, adding: 'Wretched is the man who relies on the help of physicians. I don't deny that medicine is a gift of God and I don't reject this knowledge, but where are the physicians who are perfect?' (Luther, [1538] 1967, p.266).

Medical reform in Denmark

The Reformation that had begun in Germany quickly spread until it extended throughout most of northern Europe. Wherever the reforming zeal arrived, the existing Catholic religious institutions and systems were replaced by those of the new Protestant order. Monks and nuns were expelled from their convents and the buildings themselves were put to different use; new schools were set up to replace those run by the church; church funds were seized and used to set up new systems of poor relief and health care, to be administered by secular bodies. In each locality, the reforms took a slightly different form. To see how medicine was viewed in the context of religious reform, and to assess the effect of reform on medical provision, let us look at what happened in Denmark.

The Reformation reached the kingdom of Denmark in 1536, and, not surprisingly, the first institution to be reformed was the church. The reform of the study and practice of medicine was soon to follow. The University of Copenhagen had nominally incorporated a medical faculty since its original foundation in 1479, but, on the university's refoundation, in 1537, it acquired a medical faculty in more than name. The first Protestant vice-chancellor of the university, Christian Torkelsen Morsing (c.1485–1560), was also the first professor of medicine, and his Lutheran credentials were impeccable.

Morsing considered the reform of the study and practice of medicine to be part of the wider Reformation of church and state. He viewed medicine as a religious vocation, which should be practised in order to serve one's fellow beings and not to further the physician's political or social ambitions. In an introduction Morsing wrote for a herbal written by his friend Henrik Smith (1495–1563), he stated that:

> among those chosen for the holy office of preacher, only a few are powerful and noble. Similarly, not many wealthy and mighty but only poor and simple people are chosen to become physicians, thereby serving Man's bodily needs, as his soul is served through the preaching of the Gospel.
>
> (Smith, 1556, fol.Aij; reprinted in Brade, 1976; my translation)

Clearly, Morsing was rooted in the values of Protestantism, with its emphasis on a return to what was perceived to be the original apostolic tradition. In this tradition, people were called by God to become preachers and physicians, not encouraged to take up such positions by political and social ambitions. He later emphasizes the duties of the pious physician:

> To know the herbs and other healing plants which God allows to grow on Earth for the use and benefit of man, and to see several human bodies dissected, part by part, in order better to understand how the inner parts of man are created, in order to know what remedies are needed for that part of man's body which is found to suffer from want and damage.
>
> (ibid.)

Like Morsing, Henrik Smith had been an early convert to Protestantism. His first medical publication, in 1536, was a pamphlet about the plague, its causes and treatment. This was followed by his *Home Medical Adviser* (1540), a medical manual for domestic use. It is clear that Smith and his Protestant friends had high hopes that the new, Protestant government would carry out a general reform of medicine and health care. Smith dedicated his herbal to the royal chancellor. He wrote his dedication at a time when the government was issuing the first medical regulations for the country, and seeking to employ physicians for each of its regions. The sentiments expressed in it are clear:

> Dear Lord Chancellor, We find written that every city which has been endowed with a Christian and godly magistracy, with good ministers and preachers, who teach and preach the Word of God purely to the people; likewise, also with pious and learned schoolmasters who correctly chastise the young children in piety, teaching them to read and write and good manners; similarly, with good, learned and faithful physicians and midwives, who can assist the people when they are sick, distressed and destitute – that city is blessed and well provided. These first three, which are Christian government, good ministers and preachers, pious and learned schoolmasters, are now, God be praised, provided in most of the Kingdom's towns, but learned and faithful physicians and midwives are missing in many places.
>
> (Smith, 1556, preface; reprinted in Brade, 1976; my translation)

According to Smith and other Protestants, a proper reformation of the Christian community was a hierarchical affair. It should start from the top, with the reform of the government, continue with the reform of the church and of the education system, and conclude with the reform of medicine. The provision of a reformed system of health care was seen as essential, but this entailed making sure that there were enough physicians and midwives to serve the reformed territory. In Denmark, by 1540, the reformation of the first three – government, church and education – had succeeded reasonably well. The fourth – the provision of doctors and midwives in most of the kingdom's towns – was still to be achieved. Catholic clerics could be re-educated to serve in the new Protestant church and in the schools; medical practitioners, however, were simply not yet available in significant numbers to help bring about the envisaged changes in medical provision.

The case of Denmark demonstrates that the introduction of the Lutheran Reformation was accompanied by widespread support in political and religious circles for a broader educational and social reform, including the provision of health care. In practical terms, however, the aspirations of the reformers more often than not failed to materialize. Lack of resources, both human and material, often made major changes impossible. This, however, was not purely a Danish problem. Many of the recently reformed communities within the Holy Roman Empire also found it difficult to implement their ideals.

4.4   The Reformation, the Counter-Reformation and attitudes to popular and sacred healing

An essential task for the Protestant reformers was to cleanse Christianity of everything that in their opinion had served to corrupt the true faith. This meant ridding it of such practices as the adoration of saints, the veneration of relics and pilgrimages to holy sites, many of which were closely associated with healing. The Protestant church tried to discourage belief in sacred and miraculous healing as a dangerous superstition, but this was easier said than done, and the popular demand for holy sites and relics did not disappear overnight. Many of the new Lutheran churches struggled, for at least a generation after the Reformation had been introduced, to convince their parishioners that pilgrimages to popular shrines were the inventions of the devil, and that images and altars no longer held healing power.

Denmark represents a good example of how the Protestant church responded to this demand for sacred healing. The popularity of healing sites continued unabated after the Reformation, in the form of holy springs, of which there were a considerable number in Denmark by the seventeenth century. In most cases, these springs seem to have become important only after the Reformation. Significantly, though, most of them were located at sites that had been important places of Catholic worship, pilgrimage and miraculous healing. In 1570, King Frederik II issued the first royal decree prohibiting superstitious belief in the healing power of holy springs. It was specifically directed to the royal administrator in Aalborg, who was ordered to stop the idolatry practised in a nearby rural parish by a number of worshippers around a spring and chapel dedicated to the Holy Trinity. This was to be done by cutting off the spring and tearing down the chapel. The edict, however, had little or no effect. By the beginning of the seventeenth century, although some Protestant bishops persisted in trying to discourage visits to holy springs, most had given up the attempt. Instead, they emphasized that it should be explained to those who sought a cure from the holy spring that its healing power was due solely to the grace of God and not to some mystical healing power inherent in the spring itself. Likewise, they recommended that regular sermons should be offered at these springs, explaining how the healing grace of God could work indirectly, through nature. Thus, the vicar of Elsinore thought it probable that water from a local spring – the Helene Spring – could cure eye problems, as was popularly believed. However, he emphasized that 'no monkish superstition' should be allowed to explain the cures. Those who benefited were told to praise Jesus Christ for the healing power God had granted the water (Johansen, 1997, p.63).

Another strategy was to harness natural explanations for a spring's healing properties, and thus give them a medical rationale. In 1639, for example, King Christian IV himself visited the Helene Spring to drink the water. Shortly afterwards, he commissioned seven of the kingdom's leading medical experts to check the water for its medicinal qualities. Only the professor of medicine at the University of Copenhagen, Ole Worm, had doubts about the beneficial effects of the water. His medical colleagues appear to have been confident about its healing potential, and the spring was given royal approval. As a consequence, its popularity appears to have increased, indicating that the vote of confidence in the medicinal benefits of water from a holy spring had made this popular form of sacred healing even more acceptable. Thus, having initially sought to ban holy springs, the Danish church recognized the difficulties inherent in such an enterprise, and reconsidered its position. The decision was made instead to regulate their use along acceptable religious and medical lines (Johansen, 1997, pp.59–69).

Now let us turn to the reaction of the Catholic church to popular and sacred healing. The healing power of saints, either directly, through their miraculous intercession with Christ, or indirectly, through the inherent quality of their relics, had long been part of the medical pluralism of the Catholic world. The church's response to the threat posed by the spread of Protestantism included an increased anxiety about possible breaches of Catholic orthodoxy. The **post-Tridentine** Catholic church thus continued to encourage this form of healing while simultaneously trying to regulate and control it. Counter-Reformation Catholicism was often deeply hostile to, if not directly opposed to, local attempts to make use of sacred healing, especially if these were not channelled through the proper religious avenues. Particularly troublesome were so-called 'living saints' – that is, individuals who were recognized locally for their miraculous healing powers, but who rarely achieved sainthood in their lifetime. Within the church, there was a deep-seated suspicion that such individuals, rather than being holy, might instead be the tools of the devil. The church, therefore, had to keep up its vigilance: consequently, large numbers of living saints were examined by that major guardian of post-Tridentine orthodoxy, the Congregation of the Holy Office of the Inquisition, founded in 1542. As pointed out by David Gentilcore (1998, pp.156–7), the devotion to saints and relics continued to thrive after the **Council of Trent**. Despite the much more rigorous procedures for saint-making laid down by the Counter-Reformation church, it continued to sanction a constant stream of new canonizations. One of the new institutions set up to police the making of new saints was the Congregation of Sacred Rites and Ceremonies, established in 1588. Records of the Congregation reveal the part played by miraculous healing in this process. In 1621, for example, a certain Giulia Pagano described to the Congregation the terrible pain and loss of vision she had recently suffered in her left eye. Her doctors were convinced her symptoms were caused by a cataract, which if not quickly cured would result in her permanent blindness. Pagano used the various remedies prescribed by her doctors, but she also obtained a relic of Camillo de Lellis, the founding father of the Ministers of the Sick (a Catholic nursing order that I shall discuss in more detail below), who was widely considered to be a saint. She put her faith in the intercession of de Lellis, rather than in the skills of her doctors, and thus attributed her successful cure to the influence of the saintly man.

Now read 'The church, the devil and living saints: the example of Maria Manca' (Source Book I, Reading 4.2). According to Maria's **hagiographer** Paticchio, why were the surgeons she consulted unable to help her?

The surgeons tried all their remedies, including 'the knife and the flame', but all in vain. Meanwhile, Manca's wounds grew worse. She also developed ulcers, which emitted a dreadful stench, and drove her visitors away. Shunned by the local community and her friends, Manca 'held up her wounds to the Celestial Doctor' and placed all her faith in God. Instead of consulting medical practitioners, she began to attend a dilapidated chapel where she prayed to an image of the Virgin and Child. Shortly afterwards, the Virgin Mary appeared to her and she was miraculously healed. The root of Manca's disease was diabolical, and as such, according to her hagiographer, all medical knowledge and intervention was useless, the cures of the physicians and the surgeons consequently proving ineffective. Contemporary learning distinguished between illnesses due to natural causes, where medical intervention could work, and illnesses due to supernatural causes, where it could not, because it was caused by the devil. In such cases, the only cure was religious intervention, in the form of prayers and exorcisms.

Clearly, therefore, throughout sixteenth-century Europe, popular demand for sacred or miraculous healing remained strong in Protestant, as well as in Catholic, areas. However, in the minds of church leaders of both faiths, such popular beliefs could easily develop into dangerous superstition and even witchcraft. For the Counter-Reformation Catholic church and for the new, Protestant churches, the need to control and channel this demand remained a major preoccupation.

4.5 Paracelsus and Paracelsianism

Given the dramatic social, political, and religious changes that took place in Europe in the first decades of the sixteenth century, it is hardly surprising to learn that a challenge was also issued to orthodox, western medicine. To some extent, as you have seen, the type of medicine practised remained unaffected by the turmoil of the Reformation. In the mid-sixteenth century, the centuries-long Galenic tradition was still the mainstay of a university medical curriculum, with its emphasis on qualities, elements and humours. However, the sixteenth century witnessed the birth of a new type of natural philosophy and medicine, which came to be known as Paracelsianism, after its leading advocate, the Swiss medical reformer Paracelsus (Figure 4.1). Paracelsus rejected traditional Galenic medicine because of its heathen roots, claiming that his was a medicine based on Christian

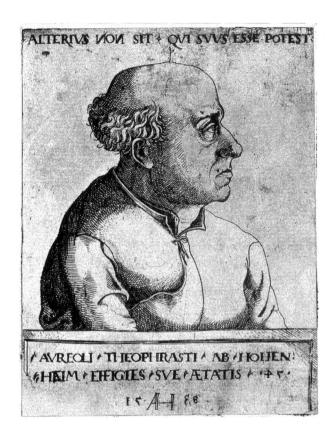

Figure 4.1   Paracelsus, aged 45, etching by
Augustin Hirschvogal, 1538. Wellcome
Library, London

principles. Just as Luther and his followers wanted to create a truly Christian
church, so Paracelsus and his followers wanted to do the same for medicine. Not
surprisingly, Paracelsus was nicknamed 'the Luther of medicine' by his opponents.
Paracelsian medicine was praised by historians in the nineteenth and early
twentieth centuries, who saw in it the beginnings of a new type of medicine based
on chemical properties. Paracelsus was hailed for his innovative views of the
chemical workings of the human body, and for his new and effective drugs, both of
which were seen as contributing to modern medicine. At the same time, the deeply
spiritual basis of his work was dismissed as irrational. However, Paracelsus' ideas
about medicine spring directly from his religious beliefs – these cannot simply be
ignored.

By rejecting Galenic medicine, Paracelsus was also discarding traditional
Aristotelian natural philosophy. He replaced its four elements (earth, air, fire
and water) with his own primary substances of salt, sulphur and mercury. (He
chose these particular substances because they had been important in earlier
Arabic alchemical studies.) These primary substances were chemical in origin, but
Paracelsus saw them not as material substances but as spiritual principles, which
represented solidity (salt), metallicity (sulphur) and liquidity (mercury). He also
introduced new spiritual forces, and used these to explain bodily processes. Thus,
he talked about *archei*, which were alchemical principles that controlled internal
processes such as digestion.

You know from previous chapters that in the Galenic tradition, disease was seen as caused by an imbalance in the bodily humours. Paracelsus, however, believed that disease was not the result of an internal imbalance, but that it was a condition caused by external factors. Thus, diseases might be caused by poisonous emanations from the stars or from minerals in the earth. In comparison with humoral theory, the view that every disease has a specific cause and is an entity in its own right may seem modern; however, it is important to remember that for Paracelsus the essence of a disease was of a spiritual nature. He built on the existing belief that there was a close correspondence between the macrocosm (the universe) and the microcosm (the human body), arguing that humans did not merely resemble the heavens and the earth, but were composed from them, as a result of what he saw as God's great alchemical act – the creation of the world. Humans therefore consisted of both mineral and astral components – the so-called *semina* (seeds) – which had both mortal and immortal elements. He called these elements *essentia*, or spirits, and each had a particular **signature**, by which it could be identified. In direct opposition to Galenic theory, Paracelsus stated that like cured like. A disease entity could be fought by knowing what was appropriate to the affected part, rather than by giving something contrary. This also led him to develop chemical remedies as cures for specific ailments, in place of the traditional herbal remedies of Galenic medicine.

Paracelsus' ideas are often difficult to pinpoint, not least because they are deeply rooted in Neoplatonic mysticism and the ideas of the mythical sage Hermes Trismegistus. Also, information relating to his life is hazy; very little is known about his upbringing, education and career. According to Paracelsus, he was educated by his physician father, who taught him botany, medicine, mineralogy and mining. He also claims to have been educated by the famous abbot of Sponheim, Johannes Trithemius (1462–1516), who may well have inspired him to take an interest in magic and mysticism. However, he received no formal secondary schooling and, while he may briefly have attended a couple of Italian universities, he at most received only a minor medical degree from the University of Ferrara. He seems to have travelled widely, chiefly as a military surgeon. He went to the Mediterranean and the Middle East in the service of the Venetian Republic, and later visited Scandinavia, possibly in the service of the Danish king, Christian II (1513–23). Lacking social connections, not to mention proper academic credentials, Paracelsus developed a deeply anti-authoritarian and iconoclastic outlook that served to make him a highly volatile individual. His eccentric behaviour made it difficult for him to settle in one place for long: he was constantly falling foul of his friends and running into trouble with the local authorities, who more often than not wanted to be rid of him as quickly as possible.

Undoubtedly, Paracelsus' peregrinations also had their roots in a thirst for new knowledge and experience, which meant that his views were constantly developing and changing. However, his opposition to established knowledge meant that he repeatedly clashed with both lay and ecclesiastical authorities wherever he went.

Now read 'Paracelsus on the medical benefits of travel' (Source Book 1, Reading 4.3) and then answer the following questions:

1　How did Paracelsus justify the virtues of travelling for a physician?

2　Why did he feel such a strong need to justify it in this way?

1　Paracelsus put forward two reasons why he regarded travelling as essential for a good physician. First, he saw it as religiously justified, comparing it to a Christian's journey to seek God. According to Paracelsus, travel offered the opportunity not only to see places, cities and people, but also to learn about 'the nature of heaven and the elements' – that is, about the created world. Second, he saw it as educationally enriching. Extensive travel afforded a physician the opportunity to learn about different diseases that might appear in different places, and at different times. Just as those who wanted to understand the Bible had to read it for themselves, so those who wanted to understand the 'book of nature' (*Codex Naturae*) had to study and experience it for themselves, by visiting different places.

2　Paracelsus' justification of his itinerant life was a veiled criticism of the established medical profession. By declaring that travelling was imperative for a good physician, Paracelsus was therefore implicitly accusing most physicians of being sedentary and idle, relying on their 'learned' status.

Why did Theophrastus Bombastus von Hohenheim self-consciously adopt the nickname Paracelsus around 1527/8? Clearly, he wanted to imply that he surpassed (from the Greek *para*, meaning 'beyond') the famous Aulus Cornelius Celsus (25 BCE–50 CE), who, early in the first century CE, had written a comprehensive encyclopedia covering the whole of medicine. Apart from referring to Paracelsus' own encyclopedic interests, which ranged across the whole of natural philosophy, medicine and much more, it also refers to the fact that Celsus had been a layman writing for other lay people. Paracelsus emulated him by writing in vernacular German, rather than in the Latin of the learned medical establishment. His aim was thus to communicate with a broader and less educated audience than the small group of university-trained physicians he so despised. This was, of course, an aim he shared with Luther, and it was around this time that Paracelsus' enemies began calling him 'the Luther of physicians'. The implication of heresy in this epithet did not worry him. In fact, he argued that Luther's enemies were also 'the very rabble that hates me', and that this 'rabble' hoped to see both of them burned at the stake. Furthermore, Paracelsus claimed that God alone had made him a physician, and he rejoiced 'that rogues are my enemies for the truth has no enemies except liars' (Paracelsus, 1990, pp.72–4).

There is no doubt that Paracelsus promoted a new and deeply religious type of natural philosophy and medicine, which presented a Christian alternative to traditional Galenic medicine. What is less clear is whether he was a Protestant or a Catholic. Historians have found it difficult to agree on where to place him in relation to the Reformation. For example, while acknowledging that Paracelsus had sympathies for the radical reformers in particular, Gerhild Scholz Williams maintains that he never left the Catholic faith (1996, pp.211–13). Given Paracelsus' close links with several of the leading reformers of the day and his fierce critique of the Catholic church and the pope, it is somewhat perplexing that so many scholars continue to emphasize his Catholicism, based on the fact that he never left the Catholic church. But why should Paracelsus have chosen to leave the church? After all, he had enough difficulties already with both lay and ecclesiastical authorities. Publishing his theological works, which contained his most pronounced criticisms of Catholicism (he described the Catholic clergy, indulgences, sacraments and fasts as the works of Antichrist, a name he repeatedly used for the pope), would have added to his problems, and so he may well have avoided publication for this reason. Such considerations were important for most reformers of the period, whether radical or moderate. Indeed, Catholicism's most fervent critic during the Reformation – Martin Luther – never left the Catholic church. It left Luther, excommunicating him in January 1521. It is true that, hostile as he was to any formal ecclesiastical structure, Paracelsus was critical of most of the leading reformers and their theology. However, despite his disagreement with many of the Protestant leaders, Paracelsus not only respected but was close to several of them. His fiercest attacks were reserved for the Catholic church and the pope.

Exercise

Now read 'The religion of Paracelsus' (Source Book 1, Reading 4.4) and answer the following questions:

1   What was Paracelsus' debt to the Reformation?

2   Is it possible, or desirable, to place Paracelsus in either the Protestant or the Catholic camp?

Discussion

1   The links between the Reformation and Paracelsus were clearly many and significant from the outset. According to Charles Webster, there is a close link between Paracelsus' writings and the protest literature of the Reformation. Paracelsus' fierce attack on the Catholic church and its practices demonstrates how close his thinking was to that of the Protestant reformers. At the same time, despite his remaining aloof from all organized religion, his social concerns and emphasis on the significance of the Holy Spirit, not to mention his strong apocalyptic and millenarian beliefs, place him close to the more radical and spiritual wing of the Reformation. Webster sees Paracelsus' medical ideas as being firmly rooted in the upheavals of the Reformation.

2   It is difficult, if not impossible, to place Paracelsus firmly in any religious camp. Like so many of the early Protestant reformers, he clearly straddles religious

boundaries, which were themselves fluid and open to negotiation in this period. Sometimes, Paracelsus appears as a dissenting Catholic; at other times, he seems indebted to aspects of evangelical Protestantism. Unorthodox and deeply individualistic, he defies simple categorization, but his anti-authoritarian stance and critique of the established church and the pope would point to him having been close to the more radical elements of evangelical Protestantism.

The links between Paracelsianism and Protestantism remained strong throughout the sixteenth century and appear to have intensified around 1570, when a number of hitherto unpublished works by Paracelsus appeared in print. This tendency was enhanced by the fact that the post-Tridentine Catholic church rejected Paracelsianism as a part of what it perceived to be a dangerous Neoplatonic, hermetic philosophy. In 1599, Paracelsus' books were included in the **Index** of forbidden books.

Another difficulty in assessing Paracelsus' position is that only a few of his works were published during his lifetime. By the time he died in 1541, Paracelsus had published only his surgical work, *Grosse Wundartzney* [Big Book of Surgery] (1536), two pamphlets on the pox and two booklets containing astrological predictions of a prophetic and an apocalyptic nature. The vast majority of the works that incorporate the ideas of Paracelsus were not edited and published until a generation after his death. An additional complication is that the provenance of the texts published under Paracelsus' name is often far from clear. Many scholars consider a fair number of them to be pseudo-Paracelsian – that is, texts written by the followers of Paracelsus in imitation of their master. It is quite possible that, when preparing his work for publication, later editors made significant changes to texts they saw as being incomplete and contradictory.

From this, it is clear that the set of ideas labelled Paracelsianism is, in fact, full of contradictions. Paracelsus was an anti-authoritarian radical, challenging the establishment with his startling new ideas about natural philosophy and medicine. However, when Paracelsian ideas finally won through, at the end of the sixteenth century, it was within the princely courts, among the rich and powerful to whom Paracelsus had been so deeply opposed. By that time, Paracelsianism had become part of the establishment. However, Paracelsus' ideas had been largely deradicalized. Let us take as an example one of the most influential Paracelsian texts of the late sixteenth century, Peter Severinus' *Idea Medicinae Philosophicae* [Medical and Philosophical Ideas]. Published in Basel in 1571, this work promoted an urbane and eclectic variety of Paracelsianism. Unlike the vernacular texts written by Paracelsus, *Idea Medicinae Philosophicae* was written in Latin, and so was aimed at the learned. The work integrated the ideas of Hippocrates into Paracelsianism, and it proved acceptable to both lay and ecclesiastical powers in many Protestant states.

The legacy of Paracelsus is discussed in Chapter 5.

4.6   Religion and epidemics

The sixteenth century was a period of demographic growth. This was a new experience for Europeans, who had become used to stagnation since the disaster of the **Black Death** (1348) had decimated the population. Accompanying this population expansion the century witnessed an increased urbanization, which did much to generate and spread many of the epidemic diseases that came to characterize the age. To contemporaries, what these epidemics had in common apart from dramatically raised mortality rates, be they pox, 'sweating disease' or plague, was that they were all seen to have a divine cause: they were God's arrows sent to punish sin. This view, of course, raised the question of what people should or could do in such circumstances: should they passively await their fate, or should they take action and use medical remedies? These were questions that deeply concerned theologians as well as physicians of the age.

Chapter 6 explores responses to these epidemic diseases in more detail.

In 1527, Luther wrote his highly influential pamphlet 'Whether you are allowed to flee the plague'. This tract not only went through numerous editions, but also continued to be quoted by subsequent writers on the plague, in various translations as well as in the original German, well into the seventeenth century. Luther's words were made more powerful by the fact that he himself had experienced a serious outbreak of the plague shortly before he published his work. The disease had broken out in Wittenberg in the summer of 1527 and Luther had been ordered by the Duke of Saxony to leave the town for the safety of Jena. He decided to disregard the order and remain in Wittenberg with his assistant, Johannes Bugenhagen (1485–1558), where he ministered to the sick and frightened population. Luther believed he had acted as a good Christian should, and in his pamphlet he commended those who refused to flee the plague: 'They uphold a good cause, namely a strong faith in God, and deserve commendation because they desire every Christian to hold to a strong, firm faith' (Luther, [1527] 1968, p.20). He recognized that not everyone had sufficient strength to bear such a burden, but he firmly believed that ministers of the church and others who held public office were obliged to remain 'steadfast before the peril of death'. Only when they could be relieved by others might such people be allowed to seek their own safety. The same applied to all individuals who were bound by service or duty to people who had been infected by the plague. In this connection, Luther specifically mentioned the duty of 'paid public servants such as city physicians' not to flee. His message was simple. A doctor was obliged to stay and care for his patients, unless a colleague was prepared to cover for him. Christian charity obliged the physician to fulfil such minimal requirements, which were a natural consequence of Luther's theology of faith and grace (Luther, 1968, pp.115–38, especially pp.120–2).

Did Luther's views on the duties of the physician influence a later generation of Protestants? In the next extract, you will read what the Protestant physician Johan Ewich wrote on the same subject. Like Luther, Ewich had personally experienced a severe outbreak of the plague in the German city of Bremen before he ventured to present his views in print in 1582.

Now read 'The Christian physician in time of plague: Johan Ewich' (Source Book 1, Reading 4.5). Did Ewich's views correspond with those of Luther?

Ewich agreed with Luther that the Christian physician's obligation was to remain with his patients during an epidemic. He called for town officials to employ physicians and surgeons in times of crisis, and recommended that these individuals should be upright Christians of good repute. When the outbreak ended, he stated that they should be well rewarded for their services. Like Luther, Ewich also strongly emphasized the obligation of the Christian physician to show care and commitment to his community. In particular, he emphasized the physician's obligation to be charitable and provide assistance to the poor. Similarly, Ewich emphasized the duty of the officials to police their medical personnel during an epidemic, to make sure that they met the necessary Christian standards. Ewich, too, was fully aware of the difficulties involved in such challenging demands, and realized the dangers and fears that physicians had to overcome in the course of carrying out their obligations to God and to the Christian community.

The impetus to provide practical care for less fortunate individuals was born out of the deep commitment of the first generation of Protestant reformers to teach their followers that charity and neighbourly love were civic duties, which had to be offered to the whole Christian community or commonwealth. In this they differed from their Catholic counterparts, who saw charitable acts as a route to salvation. Not until the middle of the sixteenth century was there a similar imperative within the Catholic church, and even then the driving force remained the salvation of souls. In the following section, I shall look at what effects the Reformation and the Counter-Reformation had on the provision of practical health care.

4.7   Health care

Another significant aspect of sixteenth-century medicine that was affected by the Reformation, as well as by the Catholic Counter-Reformation, was health care. It is important to understand that early modern health care was closely connected with the wider provision of material assistance for poor people. In the context of this system of poor relief, health care was offered either internally, by admitting poor patients into hospitals, or externally, in the recipients' homes, by the free provision of medicine and medical care. For nearly a century, historians have debated the role and importance of the Reformation in the restructuring of charity, charitable organizations and hospitals that took place in the sixteenth century. Since the late 1960s, the conventional or predominant view has been that these changes were mainly necessitated and brought about by the considerable social and economic changes that affected most of western Europe in this period, and that had begun before the Reformation. This interpretation has probably found its most articulate expression in the work of Natalie Zemon Davis, who concluded: 'The context for

Health care and poor relief are discussed further in Chapter 6.

welfare reform, it seems to me, was urban crisis, brought about by a conjuncture of older problems of poverty with population growth and economic expansion.' She is convinced that 'reform of poor relief cut across religious boundaries' and was primarily shaped by the 'vocational experience of businessmen and lawyers and certain humanist concerns' (Davis, 1991, pp.59–60).

However, I would argue that the role of the Reformation and of Protestantism was seminal in providing a rationale for the changes that took place. As I state elsewhere: 'Even if Protestantism and the Reformation cannot lay sole claim to having caused the reforms of poor relief and health care which occurred in the sixteenth and seventeenth centuries in Protestant, Western Europe, the speed and thoroughness with which they were undertaken would not have been imaginable without the theological rationale which the Protestant Reformers gave to these reforms' (Grell, 1997, pp.43–65). I have emphasized throughout this chapter that the sixteenth century was a period profoundly dominated and shaped by faith, and find it difficult to believe that religion played little part in the way societies treated their sick and their poor. The fact that some reforms to poor relief and health care pre-date the Reformation does not necessarily mean that the Reformation did not decidedly shape and accelerate these changes.

To get a clearer picture of how Protestant reforms to the provision of health care and poor relief worked in practice, let us look at those undertaken by Luther's friend and collaborator, Johannes Bugenhagen (Figure 4.2). Born in Pomerania in 1485, Bugenhagen became the leading Protestant reformer in northern Europe. His influence can be seen in the fact that he helped to institute reforms in no less than six locations: Braunschweig (1528); Hamburg (1529); Lübeck (1531); Pomerania (1535); Denmark (1537–9); and Schleswig-Holstein (1542). Luther had called for reform of the system of poor relief, to make it part of an integrated system of general welfare provision. Bugenhagen took these reforms further, and added many innovations in the field of health care provision.

Exercise

Now read 'Protestantism, poor relief and health care in sixteenth-century Europe' (Source Book I, Reading 4.6). What were the main areas of concern for health care in Bugenhagen's church orders?

Discussion

For the modern reader, perhaps the most surprising area of concern is baptism. In his church orders, Bugenhagen was primarily concerned with preserving the health of the child that was to be baptised; the sacramental rite came second. Apart from simplifying and shortening the rite of baptism, emphasizing that it should be done only by scooping water over the head of the child, he pointed out that children being baptised in cold weather should remain swaddled in order to protect them. The other three areas of concern were more directly connected with what we would understand to be health care, namely midwifery, nursing and hospitals. In all three areas, Bugenhagen emphasized the Protestant community's obligation to provide for their poor and unfortunate members. For women who

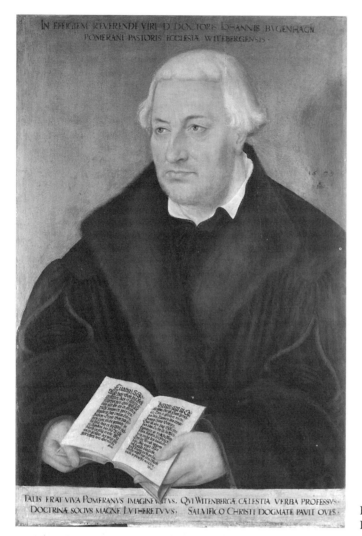

Figure 4.2   Johannes Bugenhagen.
Leipzig Museum. Photo: AKG-Images

could not afford the services of a midwife, free assistance was to be provided. Likewise, free nursing care was to be provided for the sick poor. The aim was for this nursing to be done by poor women in return for assistance they themselves had received from the common chest. They thus were obliged to put something back into the community that supported them. Likewise, Bugenhagen's suggestions for hospital reforms were primarily aimed at the poor. He paid particular attention to sufferers of syphilis, specifying that money from the common chest was to be used to pay for everything they needed – beds, food and medicine. It is also noteworthy that Bugenhagen emphasized the obligation of the Christian community to constantly supervise these new arrangements.

Changes to health care and poor relief, however, were not restricted to northern, Protestant Europe. Southern, Catholic Europe, too, experienced moves to reform the practices and standards of health care. These were specifically related to the general desire to revitalize traditional Catholic practices and beliefs in the wake of the Counter-Reformation. Renewed emphasis was placed on the redemption of sinners and the salvation of souls, and more effort was invested in caring for and nursing the sick poor. Hospitals in particular provided a convenient location for the merging of these two functions. Here, the physical and the medical requirements of the poor were easily ministered to, together with their spiritual needs. Moreover, hospital beds provided priests with important opportunities to ensure that patients were received into the Catholic communion before death. The Counter-Reformation hospital therefore constituted a convenient site of 'missionary' activity as well as tending to the physical needs of the sick poor and dying.

Perceptions of and responses to the plague and the pox are discussed in Chapter 6.

In the 1490s, a terrifying new sexually transmitted disease had broken out – a form of syphilis, otherwise known as the great pox, or the French disease. The new hospitals for the incurables that had come into existence as a response to the horrors of this disease proved particularly fertile ground for the work of the new Counter-Reformation orders and brotherhoods that were increasingly being founded to provide nursing care for the sick. Their preoccupation with sin and its consequences meant that they were particularly concerned with rescuing those who were considered to be in moral danger because of their way of life, such as prostitutes. The Counter-Reformation Catholic church, like the Protestant church, considered both the plague and the pox to be general scourges sent by God as a punishment for sin. Where the two faiths differed was in the emphasis placed by Catholicism on confession. The Catholic church insisted on patients confessing their sins before and during medical treatment, and great importance was placed on the patient taking the sacrament of penance. This was not only an essential preparation for the afterlife, but also ensured the efficacy of the treatment. Without this act of contrition, the church considered medical intervention to be of little or no consequence. An indication of how seriously the church regarded this aspect of medical care is the fact that medical practitioners who failed to comply with it were threatened with excommunication.

Among the most important of the new nursing orders that came into existence during the Counter-Reformation was that of San Giovanni di Dio. The order began life in Spain and rapidly spread throughout Europe in the late sixteenth century, founding no less than seventy-nine hospitals and running another twenty-nine. Another important order was that of the Capuchins. This was an existing order that had become more militant as a result of the Counter-Reformation. In Italy, in particular, the Capuchins played a major role in the care and nursing of plague victims, and won fame for their work in Milan with the influential Counter-Reformation bishop, Carlo Borromeo, during the plague epidemic of 1576–7.

Let us now look in more detail at one of these Catholic nursing orders. The Ministers of the Sick was founded in 1586 by Camillo de Lellis (1550–1614) (Figure 4.3). Members of the order were also known as the Camillans, or the fathers of the little cross, owing to the small red cross they wore on their habits. De Lellis was a soldier in the Venetian army until his religious conversion drew him to become a novice in the Capuchins in 1575. Ill health quickly forced him to leave the Capuchins, but later that same year, he joined San Giacomo, a hospital for incurables in Rome, where he remained until 1584. Here de Lellis came under the influence of the priest Phillipo Neri, who became his spiritual adviser. After a second failed attempt to join the Capuchins, he was ordained as a priest and, with the assistance of Neri, he founded the order of the Ministers of the Sick, a male nursing order. The members of the order were expected to combine pastoral duties with the more menial tasks of nursing. Perhaps because of his military background, de Lellis portrays them in military terms, as crusaders against the devil. In the following extract, de Lellis explains the significance of the small red cross they wore:

> All other religious, lords, and knights who wear the cross on the left side, bear it as a defensive weapon like a shield to defend themselves from the blows and temptations of enemies from hell. But our congregation has the special task of helping souls in their final battle at the time of death, and so we wear the cross on the right side, as if it were the blade of a sword and an offensive weapon to subdue the devils who are the most deadly enemies of so powerful a symbol.
>
> (quoted in Pullan, 1999, p.31)

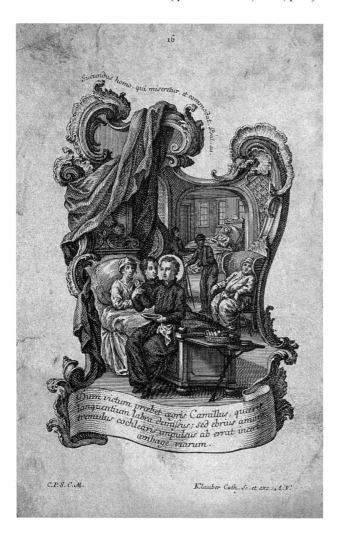

Figure 4.3   An eighteenth-century engraving, by C. Klauber, of St Camillo de Lellis (he was canonized in 1746) comforting patients in a hospital. Wellcome Library, London

The Ministers of the Sick did not restrict their activities to hospitals, but also visited the sick in their homes. His charitable activities soon earned de Lellis a reputation as a saint, and, after his death, sick people began to ask members of his order to bring a relic with them on their house visits. Thus, nursing care was combined with miraculous healing.

De Lellis's biographer paints a grim picture of hospital life before the arrival of the Camillans. With no one to assist them, patients were said to have suffered from hunger and thirst, and to have been confined to their beds 'amidst vermin and filth'. Whether the situation was really as bad as this is difficult to say. However, the rules for Milan's Maggiore Hospital, where the Ministers of the Sick had made their cautious beginnings in 1594, confirm that the order focused on these areas.

Exercise

Now read 'Rules for ministering to the sick in the Maggiore Hospital, Milan (1616)' (Source Book 1, Reading 4.7). What were the most important tasks of the Camillans?

Discussion

The statutes from Milan stated that members of the order should attend the sick according to the physicians' instructions, informing them of any changes in the patients' circumstances. They also stated that they should help feed and wash the sick, make their beds and help them die 'a good death'. The statutes differentiated between two groups of brothers, each group subdivided into hospital nurses and nursing assistants. One group was to deal with the physical needs of the patients, clearly concentrating on nursing care; the other group was to attend to their spiritual needs, taking confessions and offering the sacrament.

The statutes, however, leave no doubt that the paramount duty of the Ministers of the Sick was to make sure that patients made a good confession and were well prepared for communion. It was particularly important to make sure that they actually swallowed the communion wafer, as it was only by swallowing the wafer that the patient received the benefits of the sacrament. This was necessary not only for salvation but also for the efficacy of any subsequent medical treatment (Gentilcore, 1998, pp.134–8).

4.8 Conclusion

In the sixteenth century, medicine and Christianity were closely connected, as they had been since Christianity's birth. In many respects, the events that resulted in the break-up of western Christianity – the Reformation – did little to disrupt this relationship. Thus, the texts used in teaching medicine remained the same in Protestant and Catholic universities, while medical treatment and practice differed little, if at all. Likewise, despite the attempts of the Protestant reformers to root out all superstitious practices that they saw as connected to Catholic malpractice, popular demand for sacred and miraculous healing remained strong in Protestant areas. While both the Counter-Reformation Catholic church and the new Protestant churches sought to control this demand, it is noteworthy that in Protestant countries in particular it was often channelled into new avenues, where natural explanations might serve to make such practices more palatable.

However, as you have seen, a particular Protestant interest in and approach to human anatomy and dissections may have emerged with the Reformation. This interest in man – the pinnacle of God's creation – was largely driven by the ambition to retrieve a true and unadulterated Christianity. This was done by studying both God's word, the Bible, and the book of nature, the created world – especially human beings, who alone were created in the image of God.

The importance of the study of nature was emphasized by many of the reformers, including Luther, even if some of his statements were often little more than commonplaces. In this context it is important to bear in mind that many of the reformers considered a reform of medicine and medical provisions to be an important part of a full Reformation, as we have seen in the case of Denmark. Likewise, the emphasis on practical charity and neighbourly love engendered by the Reformation and later taken up by the Counter-Reformation Catholic church resulted in changes and improvements in poor relief and health care in Protestant, as well as in Catholic, countries.

Finally, the emergence in the sixteenth century of a new, specifically Christian medicine, known as Paracelsianism, would hardly have been imaginable without the religious and social turmoil of the Reformation.

References

Brade, A.E. (ed.) (1976) *Henrik Smiths Laegebog*, vols I–IV, facsimile reprint of 1577 edition together with the introduction to the 1556 edition, Copenhagen: Rosenkilde og Bagger.

Cunningham, A. (1997) *The Anatomical Renaissance: The Resurrection of the Anatomical Projects of the Ancients*, Aldershot: Scolar Press.

Davis, N.Z. (1991) *Society and Culture in Early Modern France*, Stanford: Stanford University Press.

Gentilcore, D. (1998) *Healers and Healing in Early Modern Italy*, Manchester: Manchester University Press.

Grell, O.P. (1997) 'The Protestant imperative of Christian care and neighbourly love' in O.P. Grell and A. Cunningham (eds) *Health Care and Poor Relief in Protestant Europe 1500–1700*, London: Routledge, pp.43–53.

Johansen, J.C. (1997) 'Holy springs and Protestantism in early modern Denmark: a medical rationale for a religious practice', *Medical History*, vol.41, pp.59–69.

Luther, M. [1527] (1968) 'Whether you are allowed to flee the plague' in *Luther's Works*, 55 vols (1957–72), vol.43, ed. by J.Pelikan and H.T. Lehmann, Philadelphia: Fortress Press, pp.115–38.

Luther, M. [1538] (1967) 'Smalcald' in *Luther's Works*, 55 vols (1957–72), vol.54 *Table Talk*, ed. and translated by T.G. Tappert, Philadelphia: Fortress Press, p.266.

Paracelsus (1990) *Paracelsus: Essential Readings*, ed. and translated by N. Goodrick-Clarke, Wellingborough: Crucible Press.

Pullan, B. (1999) 'The Counter-Reformation, medical care and poor relief' in O.P. Grell, A. Cunningham and J. Arrizabalaga (eds) *Health Care and Poor Relief in Counter-Reformation Europe*, London: Routledge, pp.18–39.

Williams, G.S. (1996) 'Paracelsus' in *The Oxford Encyclopaedia of the Reformation*, vol.3, Oxford: Oxford University Press, pp. 211–13

Source Book readings

M. Luther, *Table Talk*, ed. and translated by T.G. Tappert, in *Luther's Works*, 55 vols, Philadelphia: Fortress Press, 1957–72, vol.54, 1967, pp.53–4, 102–3, 237 (Reading 4.1).

D. Gentilcore, *Healers and Healing in Early Modern Italy*, Manchester: Manchester University Press, 1998, pp.159–60 (Reading 4.2).

Paracelsus, 'Seven defensiones, the reply to certain calumniations of his enemies. the fourth defence: concerning my journeyings' in *Paracelsus: Four Treatises*, ed. by H.E. Sigerist, Baltimore and London: Johns Hopkins University Press, 1941, pp.24–9 (Reading 4.3).

C. Webster, 'Paracelsus: medicine as popular protest' in O.P. Grell and A. Cunningham (eds) *Medicine and the Reformation*, London: Routledge, 1993, pp.64–74 (Reading 4.4).

J. Ewich, *Of the Duetie of a Faithfull and Wise Magistrate, in Preserving and Delivering of the Common Wealth from Infection, in the Time of the Plague or Pestilence ... newlie turned into English by John Stockwood Schoolemaister of Tunbridge*, London: Thomas Dawson, 1583, fols13v–15r (Reading 4.5).

O.P. Grell, 'The Protestant imperative of Christian care and neighbourly love' in O.P. Grell and A. Cunningham (eds) *Health Care and Poor Relief in Protestant Europe 1500–1700*, London: Routledge, 1997, pp.50–60 (Reading 4.6).

P. Mario Vanti, *S. Giacomo Degl'Incurabili di Roma nel Cinquecento: Dalle Compagnie del Divino Amore a S. Camillo de Lellis*, Rome: Tipolitografia Rotarori, 1991, pp.139–41; translated by S. De Renzi (Reading 4.7).

5

Chemical Medicine and the Challenge to Galenism

The legacy of Paracelsus, 1560–1700

Peter Elmer

Objectives

When you have completed this chapter you should be able to:

- understand the nature of the challenge posed to Galenic medicine and the medical establishment by the proponents of chemical medicine in early modern Europe;

- assess the contribution of the chemical physicians to the emergence of new forms of medical practice in early modern Europe;

- appreciate the significance of non-medical criteria in the debates surrounding the reception of new medical ideas and modes of practice in this period.

5.1 Introduction

In the previous chapter, you encountered the first major challenge to the early modern medical establishment in the form of the Swiss medical reformer Paracelsus. Despite the fact that he published little during his own lifetime, the medical works of Paracelsus were rapidly disseminated in print after about 1560 by his enthusiastic supporters, who sought both to elaborate and to build on the foundations laid down by their master. In the process, a new approach to medical practice and theory came into existence in the second half of the sixteenth century that threatened to overthrow the old medical order. The Paracelsian revolution, however, never quite materialized in the way that Paracelsus, and some of his more radical followers, had envisaged. In the century after 1560, aspects of the Paracelsian programme were slowly integrated into orthodox medical practice, while others, especially Paracelsus' critique of Galenic humoralism, were studiously avoided by those physicians who sought to effect a compromise between the old and the new. Even in the most conservative of medical schools, such as that at Paris, the efficacy of chemical remedies was finally accepted.

From about the middle of the seventeenth century, however, a new threat to orthodox medicine emerged in northern Europe, which some historians believe constituted a more radical challenge than Paracelsianism. Joan Baptista van Helmont (1579–1644), like Paracelsus, published little in his own lifetime. With the posthumous publication of his collected works in 1648, however, a new phase was initiated in the chemical physicians' conflict with the Galenic medical establishment. Helmontianism was rapidly adopted throughout much of northern Europe and once again provoked a furious rearguard action by the defenders of medical orthodoxy, whose theoretical conservatism was further undermined by the

Mechanistic explanations of natural phenomena are discussed in Chapter 7.

emergence of the new mechanical philosophy and the demise of Aristotelianism in academic circles. In the event, the Helmontian revolution, like its Paracelsian predecessor, failed to conquer the medical faculties of Europe and, by 1700, its influence on medical debate was largely peripheral. Nonetheless, its long-term legacy was far from negligible, particularly in the case of medical practice and attitudes to the medical profession, both of which were the subject of heated discussion throughout this period.

In this chapter, I explore in more detail the nature of Paracelsianism and Helmontianism, or the **iatrochemical revolution** as it is often termed, and its impact on the medical world of the late sixteenth and seventeenth centuries. In particular, I look in some detail at the nature and depth of the challenge to the status quo posed by these new medical philosophies, as well as the response of medical traditionalists to the reformers' programme. In Section 5.2, I investigate how Paracelsianism was able to shake off the subversive legacy bequeathed to it by its founder, Paracelsus, and achieve a modicum of respectability in the medical world. In Section 5.3, I look more closely at the impact of van Helmont's thought on the medical reform movement that arose in England after 1650, and investigate why, despite widespread support, the English Helmontians failed to achieve their goal of wholesale reform of the organization, practice and theory of medicine. An essential and consistent theme of both sections is the seemingly endless capacity of Galenic traditionalists to adapt to the challenges posed by the chemical physicians, and to preserve traditional methods of healing, which in most instances survived into the eighteenth century.

5.2   The Paracelsian revolution, 1560–1640

The legacy of Paracelsus

When Paracelsus died in 1541, he left behind a rich legacy of unpublished manuscripts. Mostly written in German, these covered a range of topics, from astrology, medicine and mineralogy to works of a religious or mystical nature – highly critical of both Catholic and Protestant orthodoxy – that defy easy categorization. For nearly twenty years, the bulk of these works remained undisclosed to the wider public, despite clear evidence of a growing interest in his thought among scholars and intellectuals in the German-speaking lands. If they had remained unpublished, it is quite possible that Paracelsus' reputation as a healer and medical iconoclast might have sunk without trace. In 1560, however, the printing presses of central Europe began to produce countless editions of Paracelsus' hitherto unpublished writings, in particular his medical works, which, in typical fashion, were highly critical of Galenic medicine and its practitioners. Between 1560 and 1570, eighty editions of **Paracelsiana**, many in Latin, were printed at Basel, Frankfurt and Strasburg. These were then sold and disseminated to the rest of Europe through the highly developed and efficient network of booksellers that was characteristic of the period. Within a decade, the Paracelsian challenge to medical orthodoxy had been resurrected, and once again Paracelsus' ideas posed a renewed threat to the continuing supremacy of the Galenic system.

The response of the medical community to this new phenomenon was mixed. Most physicians reacted with hostility to Paracelsus and his latter-day followers. The most hostile were those who had been trained in the humanist atmosphere of the medical schools and who had gone on to become pillars of the medical establishment in their various faculties and incorporated colleges. A significant minority, however, were sufficiently intrigued by the furore created by the first generation of Paracelsians to purchase the new publications and to react positively to various aspects of the emerging reform programme. In the process, a significant debate arose in medical circles, which soon spread beyond the university faculties into society at large, as supporters and opponents eagerly sought to enlist powerful patrons in church and state in defence of their respective positions.

I shall look at the outcome of this debate shortly. Before I address this issue, however, it might be helpful to remind yourself of some of the basic tenets of Paracelsus' medical philosophy, and how and why these were so eagerly adopted by a range of enthusiasts after 1560. In Chapter 4, Ole Grell emphasized the extent to which Paracelsus' world-view, including his specifically medical beliefs, emerged out of the maelstrom that was the Reformation. Putting to one side the thorny subject of Paracelsus' own religious position, and his attitude to Protestantism, it is nonetheless clear that his hostility to traditional medicine was founded on his profound distaste for the paganism of Galen and Galenic medical philosophy. In its place, Paracelsus argued for a Christian medicine, based on the two books of divine revelation, the Bible and nature. The implications of such thinking were eagerly taken up by Paracelsus' followers after 1560, as Galen and his 'tribe' were frequently stigmatized as 'heathen' and 'antichristian'. The message comes across loud and clear in one of the first defences of the Paracelsian system to be published in England; it was written by Richard Bostocke (d.1606) in 1585.

Exercise

Now read 'Paracelsianism in England: Richard Bostocke (1585)' (Source Book 1, Reading 5.1) and then answer the following questions:

1   On what grounds did Bostocke reject Galenic medicine?

2   What rhetorical strategies did he adopt in order to persuade his audience of the greater virtue of the medicine of Paracelsus over that of Galen?

Discussion

1   The chief source of Bostocke's opposition to traditional medicine was its absence of a spiritual or Christian core. According to Bostocke, it was impossible to trust the therapeutic regime of the Galenist since it was not sanctioned by God. As a good Christian, Bostocke was forced to question the whole basis of Galenic medicine, both in theory and in practice, because it was founded on the false principles of those arch pagans, Aristotle and Galen. In particular, their obsession with secondary or natural causes to the detriment of the first cause, God, and their rejection of some of the most basic tenets of Christianity, including the story of the creation, made them highly suspect as reliable guides to

curing the afflictions that beset the 'little Worlde' of man. Under the circumstances, he saw it as hardly surprising that they were unable to cure even the most simple and common of ailments.

2   First and foremost, Bostocke adopted a deeply pious and evangelical tone, addressing his concerns not to men, but to God. In addition, in order to allay fears surrounding the novelty of Paracelsus' ideas, he stressed the latter's role as a restorer or reformer in the mould of a Luther or a Calvin – a strategy that was bound to hit the right note in a country that had recently undergone Protestant reform. In opposition to traditional medical thinking, particularly that taught in the humanist-inspired medical faculties of Europe, Galen was dethroned as the ancient fount of wisdom, and an older, and more pure, source for medicine was proposed in his place. Though Bostocke's title did not allude to individuals, it is clear that what he had in mind related to an earlier, biblical tradition of healing, which predated the Greeks by many centuries. Turning traditional thinking upside down, Bostocke implied that it was the heathen, Galen, who was the newcomer, with whom lay the responsibility for perverting the original purity of medicine – a point that was made explicit in the title of the tract.

In focusing on the Christian roots of a reformed medicine, some of Paracelsus' followers proceeded to argue that the creation itself was a chemical act, described in some detail in the book of Genesis (for example, Joseph Duchesne in Reading 5.3). If this was the case, it logically followed that the whole superstructure of Renaissance natural philosophy, in particular its debt to Aristotle, was erroneous. Paracelsus himself had rejected the four elements (earth, air, fire and water) as the basic building blocks of creation and argued in their stead for a new dispensation, the **tria prima**, composed of salt, sulphur and mercury. In the process, he also jettisoned the humoral system and rejected the Galenic view that opposite or contrary qualities cured. According to Paracelsus, disease was not the result of an imbalance of humours, but rather a specific condition caused by external factors (described by Bostocke as 'impure seeds') that required specific remedies. These, characteristically, were to be produced by chemical distillation, so that all impurities were removed, and were prescribed on the principle of *similia similibus curantur* ('like cures like'). Typically, these included chemically prepared minerals and vegetables, especially drugs compounded from mercury, antimony and gold, which were administered as purges (Figure 5.1).

Paracelsianism appealed to a broad audience, then, for a number of reasons, not all of which were simply related to medicine. In religious terms, it seemed to offer an alternative, more Christian, approach to nature and natural philosophy – one that was consonant with the teachings of the Bible. Such thinking was reinforced by the emphasis that Paracelsus and his followers placed on the divine nature of the physician's calling. Here, the apocryphal text from Ecclesiasticus 38:1 – 'Honor the physician for the need thou hast of him: for the most high hath created him' – was frequently cited by the Paracelsians as evidence of the sacred vocation of the physician and as a justification for their own incursion into the medical marketplace. In addition, the procedures of the chemists, and the language they

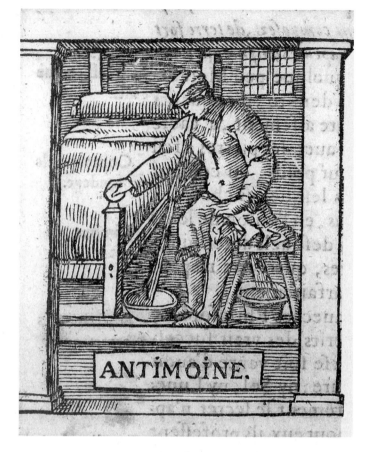

Figure 5.1 *Antimoine* [Antimony], from Hannibal Barlet, *Le vray et methodique cours de la physique resolutive, vulgairement dite chymie,* 1657. The powerful effect of antimony on the body is graphically illustrated in this simple woodcut. Debate over the efficacy of this metallic medicine as a purge was at the centre of the controversy between French Galenists and Paracelsians for almost a century. It was finally resolved in favour of the latter in the late 1650s, when the young King Louis XIV was successfully prescribed the drug in a concoction known as *vin émétique*. Wellcome Library, London

used to describe their operations, were saturated with religious imagery. For example, the separation of pure, spiritual seeds from impure bodies – a central feature of Paracelsian chemistry – possessed obvious parallels in Christian teaching concerning the relationship between soul and body, and the separation of the good and the evil at Judgement Day.

Moreover, Paracelsianism possessed great appeal for a growing band of natural philosophers who were no longer satisfied that the Aristotelian world-view, based as it was on excessive respect for book-learning and the wisdom of the ancients, provided an answer to the mysteries of the natural world. As you saw in Chapter 3, in the case of Vesalius, there was a new emphasis in some circles on the need to pursue a more experimental and observational approach to the study of man and nature. During the second half of the sixteenth century, the move towards such an approach was gathering pace and was frequently lauded by the followers of Paracelsus, who saw advantages beyond the medical in the pursuit of such goals. In particular, many natural philosophers were attracted to Paracelsianism as part of a wider revival of interest in Renaissance Europe in alchemy and the **occult sciences** (Figure 5.2). The traditional goal of the alchemist – the search for the philosopher's stone that might turn base metals into gold and provide a panacea for all humanity's ills – remained a key objective for many who were attracted to Paracelsus' innovative writings.

In many parts of Europe, the mystical and alchemical associations of Paracelsianism fused with other currents of thought – in particular the **eirenicist** aspirations of some rulers and intellectuals – in such a way as to promote yet further interest in the new medicine among a broad and often powerful audience. In particular, Paracelsianism became hugely popular at the courts of many central European princes, including that of the Holy Roman Emperor, Rudolf II (1576–1612), at Prague. For such rulers, the Paracelsian vision of a harmonious creation, in which man, nature and God were intimately connected by a universal spirit, or *spiritus mundi*, represented an ideal image of unity that they wished to see replicated in their war-torn and religiously divided principalities. As a result, the devotees of the

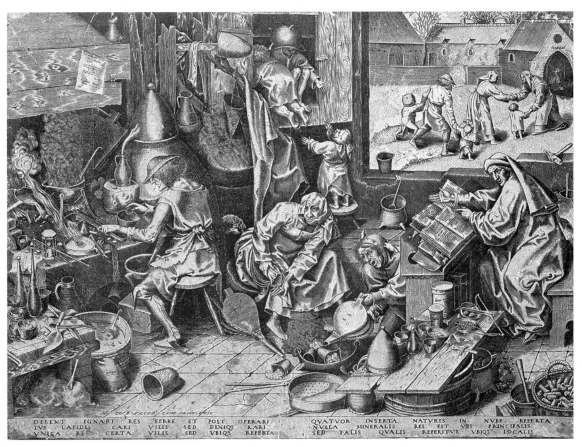

Figure 5.2 *L'Alchimiste*, after Pieter Brueghel. In this popular allegorical print, the alchemist (shown seated on the right at his desk, pointing to an alchemical book) is satirized not only for his vain pursuit of the philosopher's stone, but also for reducing a poor couple to poverty by inducing them to sacrifice their goods and children (seen running amok) in the elusive search for gold. The unhappy outcome – the pair are forced to receive charitable support from a hospital (top right) – stands as an indictment of the alchemist's art. Through their association with such commonplace images, the Paracelsian physician was frequently stigmatized as a charlatan and a cheat, as much the butt of popular criticism as that levelled against him by the defenders of medical orthodoxy. Wellcome Library, London

new chemical medicine were increasingly attracted to the courts of men such as Rudolf and Maurice, **landgrave** of Hesse-Kassel (1572–1632), where they were provided with both financial and moral support, as well as with important outlets for the promotion of the Paracelsian programme of medical reform (Moran, 1991).

Exercise

Now read 'Sanitising Paracelsus: the Paracelsian revival in Europe, 1560–1640' (Source Book 1, Reading 5.2). How, according to Hugh Trevor-Roper, did the Paracelsians achieve a degree of respectability for their radical beliefs in the period after 1560?

Discussion

Trevor-Roper emphasizes in particular the importance of princely patronage as the key to the survival and spread of Paracelsian ideas and practices. Princes offered the ultimate form of protection to medical innovators in an age in which incorporated bodies – whose ultimate source of authority also lay in princely patronage – jealously sought to defend their privileges from interlopers and outsiders. In addition to providing protection from harassment, princes sponsored research and publications, as well as providing the vital resources and equipment, including laboratory facilities, that were the lifeblood of the Paracelsian practitioner.

In order to accommodate itself to the needs of its new, wealthy patrons, Paracelsianism also began to shed its radical religious and social trappings. Trevor-Roper stresses the fact that it was largely Paracelsus' medical writings that were published after 1560 and not his more radical works of social and religious criticism. By the early 1570s, Paracelsianism 'became respectable', an outcome that Trevor-Roper accords not only to princely patronage but also to the fact that Paracelsus' works were now appearing in polished Latin, the language of the learned.

The obstacles faced by the Paracelsians in their search for acceptance and respectability were nonetheless considerable. Objections to the new medicine ranged from disapproval of its founder, and his semi-mystical religious leanings, to a concerted attempt by the medical establishment to stigmatize his supporters as social subversives whose real aim was to overthrow the corporate power exercised by the various schools, faculties and colleges of medicine in Europe. Paracelsus himself was the object of intense scrutiny. By the early 1570s, a popular stereotype had emerged in conservative circles that characterized him as a moral debauchee and drunkard, who consorted with demons and devils and dabbled in black magic in his search for medical wisdom. He never quite managed to escape this caricature.

Worse still, his disciples too fell under a similar spell. From 1560 onward, they were consistently accused of holding a variety of heretical opinions by both

Catholic and Protestant theologians, and were accused in particular of responsibility for spreading the new heresy of **Arianism** in central and eastern Europe (Webster, 1990, pp.18–20). In Catholic Europe, the plight of Paracelsus' followers grew yet more difficult when in 1599 his works were placed on the papal Index.

Though doubts surrounding the religious orthodoxy of Paracelsus and his followers were expressed by members of the medical establishment, the primary concern of this group was to demonstrate that the ultimate goal of the Paracelsians was the destruction of the medical hierarchy. The Paracelsians were accordingly depicted as quacks and charlatans, who were eager to undermine the orderly medical marketplace and to create in its stead a state of anarchy. To the extent that many Paracelsians wished to see an end to the monopolistic powers exercised by the Galenists in the field of medical education and licensing, this was a fair assessment. However, it is doubtful that the majority, who had themselves enjoyed a university education, were in favour of a complete medical free-for-all. Indeed, by the end of the sixteenth century, many Paracelsians, or those sympathetic to certain aspects of the Paracelsian reform programme, were beginning to infiltrate the very bodies that they had formerly criticized. In the process, the scene was set for a major showdown between the forces of medical conservatism and those of medical reform, which led in most cases to a gradual reconciliation between the two sides.

Confrontation or compromise? The case of France

The speed with which Paracelsus' medical teachings spread throughout Europe was uneven. In the German-speaking territories of the Holy Roman Empire, acceptance of key elements of the new approach to medicine began at an early date, thanks largely to the promotion and protection of Paracelsians by many of the ruling princes of this region. Following the lead of the emperor, Rudolf II, figures like Maurice, landgrave of Hesse-Kassel, invested both time and money in promoting the cause of the iatrochemists. A highly learned man, with a profound interest in alchemy and the occult sciences, Maurice was the first European prince to promote the academic study of chemistry when he established the inaugural chair in the subject at the University of Marburg in 1612. Maurice himself even engaged in the manufacture of new drugs. Heinrich Petraeus (1589–1620), who held the chair of anatomy and surgery at Marburg, paid a glowing testimony to his prince in 1617 when he described Maurice's endeavours in this respect:

> But one thing I must mention, namely that Your Grace … has diligently practised and questioned in the [medical] arts, has prepared medicines with his own hands, especially the ingenious chemical sort, which his servants have used for the good of their health. He has thereby improved his understanding of medicine to such an extent that he himself is able to converse with the most experienced Masters and occasionally compre-hends a matter better than they … In addition he has followed the example of his father, Wilhelm IV, and has had the most learned and most experienced physicians at his court in Kassel. For these he has provided the opportunity to increase their art and experience in his well known princely laboratory … Your Grace has also propagated this wonderful and

necessary art for posterity, supporting, loving, and protecting the medical faculty of Your university ... and especially You have raised and extended the true chemical art, which until now had remained hidden, and have caused it to be taught publicly and to be practised in a laboratory built for this purpose.

(quoted in Moran, 1990, p.100)

In adopting such a hands-on approach, Maurice of Hesse-Kassel was clearly an exceptional prince. He was by no means alone, however, in princely circles in promoting the cause of the Paracelsians (Trevor-Roper, 1990). One of the first courts in sixteenth-century Europe to adopt the new medicine was that of the Valois kings of France. Here, however, courtly patronage of Paracelsianism met with considerable opposition in the shape of the medical faculty of Paris, a corporation with a royal charter, which jealously guarded its right to police medical practice in the capital. The outcome of this conflict provides an excellent case study in the difficulties involved in promoting new medical theories and practices in early modern Europe.

Paracelsian ideas first entered France in the 1560s via two main routes. First, they were imported into the country by army doctors and surgeons returning from the various wars that had torn Europe apart in the previous two decades. And second, they were encouraged and disseminated by returning **Huguenot** exiles, many of whom had sought refuge in the Protestant territories bordering France during the same period of conflict. Significantly, both received encouragement and support at the royal court, particularly under the patronage of the queen mother, Catherine de' Medici (1519–89). At first, the response to Paracelsus was muted. Few royal physicians openly promoted his ideas, preferring instead to debate their potential usefulness in a liberal and tolerant atmosphere. Slowly, however, Paracelsianism gained ground within court circles, and many medical men who attended on the royal entourage became partially converted to the new medical philosophy. At the same time, the same individuals were suspected, sometimes unfairly, of promoting or tolerating religious heresy. Consequently, the defenders of Paracelsus came under fire from various quarters in French society, including the premier bodies representing the legal, theological and medical authorities: the ***parlement* of Paris**, the Sorbonne and the faculty of medicine. Matters came to a head in 1578, when these three bodies colluded to bring a test case against one of the foremost French Paracelsians of the day – Roch le Baillif, a Huguenot, who held the impressive title of *médecin ordinaire du roy*.

The outcome was inconclusive. However, with the accession to the throne of Henry of Navarre as Henri IV (1553–1610) in 1589, the prospect for further reform on Paracelsian lines looked decidedly favourable. Unlike the last Valois kings, Henri, the first of the Bourbon line, was a Huguenot sympathizer – his conversion to Catholicism in 1589 was politically inspired in order to secure the throne – whose power base lay in the Protestant stronghold of Navarre, in southern France. At his small court at Nérac, he employed numerous physicians, all Huguenots, most of whom were dedicated supporters of the new medical heresies of Paracelsus. Indeed, many had trained in Germany or Switzerland, the home of Paracelsianism, while others were educated at the local university of Montpellier, whose important medical faculty was soon to be dominated by supporters of the new medicine. The defenders of medical traditionalism in France now faced their sternest challenge.

Now read 'Challenging the medical status quo: the fate of Paracelsianism in France' (Source Book 1, Reading 5.3) and then answer the following questions:

1 Briefly summarize the nature of the opposition to Paracelsianism in France in the period from about 1590 to 1650.

2 How was a compromise between the proponents of the old and the new medicine finally achieved?

1 The chief source of opposition to the Paracelsians clearly came from the Paris medical faculty. Not only did members of the faculty oppose the introduction of what they saw as harmful drugs, but they were also clearly concerned with the threat that Paracelsianism posed to the whole philosophical basis of contemporary medicine and natural philosophy. Moreover, Duchesne's conception of the creation as a chemical process, and his attempt to inaugurate, on Paracelsian lines, a new Christian natural philosophy based on chemical precepts, was anathema to the medical faculty. Furthermore, it was also likely to face stern opposition from the conservative theologians within the University of Paris. The Protestant background of so many of the Paracelsians, fostered by their training in Montpellier, added to such doubts. Most important of all, however, the medical faculty objected to Paracelsianism because of the threat it posed to the preservation of hierarchy in the medical marketplace. As was evident in the case brought against Duchesne, Renaudot and others, many defenders of the status quo felt that Paracelsianism encouraged quackery and charlatanism, which in time threatened to subvert the whole structure of organized medicine and to topple the Paris-trained physicians from their position of professional and social eminence. For the defenders of legal, social, religious and political tradition, these were powerful arguments that the Paracelsians struggled to overcome, despite the protection that they received from influential patrons at court.

2 A compromise was ultimately achieved because of the willingness of medical men on both sides of the debate to concede ground. In the case of the iatrochemists, this is most evident in their subtle manipulation of the language they used to describe the pedigree of their ideas. Duchesne, for example, claimed that he was not a Paracelsian, and he denied that Paracelsus was the founder of chemical medicine. Instead, he acknowledged Hippocrates and Galen as the true originators of this art, thus establishing an ancient and respectable ancestry for the 'new' medicine. At the same time, his condemnation was reserved for the modern-day disciples of these two ancient authorities in medicine, whom he lampooned as stick-in-the-mud 'dogmatists'. Equally important, however, was the fact that the Paracelsians' opponents were increasingly willing to admit a limited role for chemically prepared medicines in the official list of drugs, or

pharmacopoeia. The position of the Paris medical faculty in this respect was symptomatic of a broader recognition that was taking place in medical faculties all across Europe at this time. Though many 'orthodox' Galenists fought strenuously to demolish the philosophical claims of men such as Duchesne, the same individuals frequently acknowledged the usefulness of chemical medicines, which they incorporated into their everyday practice. The case of Palmarius highlights the way in which members of the conservative faculty were slowly but surely integrating the new therapies into their otherwise conventional modes of practice.

The fate of Paracelsianism in France, where the opposition to medical change was deep-rooted, is symptomatic of the general rapprochement that took place in Europe between the proponents of the old and the new medicine during the course of the sixteenth and seventeenth centuries. In England, a similar process was at work, in which it is evident that the advocates of chemical medicine were more than happy to jettison the radical trappings of Paracelsian dogma in return for official recognition of the efficacy of chemically prepared remedies. As in France, this was partly facilitated by the appointment of moderate Paracelsians to influential positions. The French émigré Theodore Turquet de Mayerne (1573–1655), for example, became physician to the court of James I (1603–25). Mayerne's election to a fellowship of the College of Physicians in 1616 may have further assisted the gradual acceptance of chemical medicines among the collegiate physicians, all of whom had been trained in the Galenic tradition. A testament to this new spirit of compromise was the inclusion of Paracelsian mineral-based receipts in the first published edition of the official pharmacopoeia of the college in 1618 (Figure 5.3). In the same year, James I agreed to the creation of a separate incorporated body for the apothecaries, whose professional conduct in preparing drugs was henceforth to be regulated by the college. In both cases, Mayerne played an important role as go-between and adviser to the Crown and the college, thus ensuring official support within the latter for Paracelsian iatrochemistry (Cook, 1986, pp.95–7).

The fate of Mayerne lies in stark contrast to the treatment received by the college's earliest and most prominent convert to Paracelsianism, Thomas Mouffet (1553–1604). Mouffet, who played only a peripheral role in the college's activities, was largely ostracized by its leadership. Within a generation, however, his most important publication, the *Theatrum Insectorum* (1634), appeared in print with the imprimatur of a former president of the college. The contrasting fates of Mouffet and Mayerne is perhaps indicative, once again, of the crucial importance of patronage in the promotion of new medical thinking, but it is equally apparent that by about 1620 attitudes to Paracelsian medicine in English medical circles were changing. Lower down the medical hierarchy, many influential surgeons, such as William Clowes (1544–1603) and John Woodall (d.1643), also began to popularize Paracelsian remedies in vernacular handbooks that were designed for a wide audience (Figure 5.4). Despite the fact that few original works by Paracelsus or his followers were published in England before 1650, they circulated widely in private and university libraries prior to this date. Virtually unknown in England

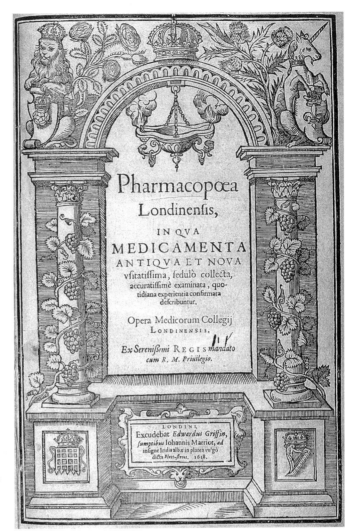

Figure 5.3   Title page of *Pharmacopoea Londinensis*. The publication of the official pharmacopoeia of the London College of Physicians in 1618 marked an important stage in the recognition of the value of chemical drugs by the Galenic physicians of the college. Published in Latin, it was not translated into English until 1653, when the medical publisher Nicholas Culpeper issued it as a vehicle to undermine the monopolistic powers exercised by the college. Wellcome Library, London

before 1560, Paracelsus' ideas, according to Charles Webster, 'had been largely assimilated by 1600' (Webster, 1979, p.323).

It is easy to see, with hindsight, why the advocates of Paracelsianism were tempted to soften their criticisms of Galenic methods and theories of treatment in order to secure professional recognition and status. It is less easy to determine why their opponents gradually mellowed in their opposition to Paracelsus. Clearly, there is evidence of moderation on both sides, a fact which might lead us to conclude that the two contesting systems of medical thought, Paracelsianism and Galenism, were perhaps more readily reconcilable than we might have been previously led to believe. The ease with which Paracelsians were able to claim, in all sincerity, that if Galen or Hippocrates were alive today they would subscribe to chemical medicine, or Galenists to argue that chemistry was perfectly compatible with traditional humoral therapeutics, is highly suggestive. After all, Paracelsian therapeutics was based on essentially the same methodology as that of the Paracelsians' Galenic

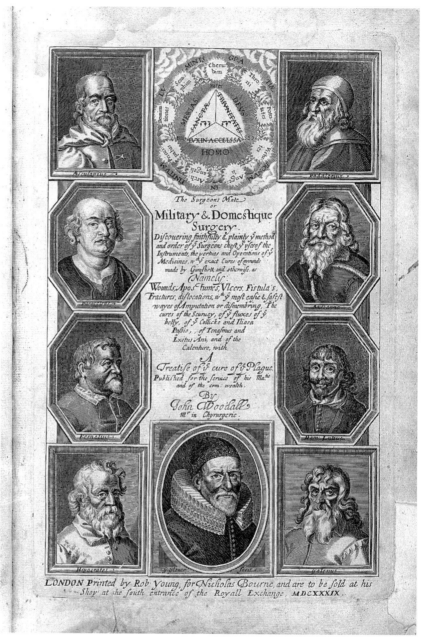

Figure 5.4   Title page of John Woodall, *The Surgeon's Mate*, 1639 edition. This edition of Woodall's popular treatise on common surgical operations, first published in 1617, depicts Paracelsus (second from the top on the left) alongside such other medical giants as Hippocrates (bottom left) and Galen (bottom right) – a powerful visual and emblematic statement of the position Paracelsus now occupied in medical circles. Woodall (in the larger portrait, seated between Hippocrates and Galen) himself was surgeon-general of the East India Company and recommended numerous oils and unguents that owed much to Paracelsian remedies. Wellcome Library, London

opponents, namely the need to purify the body by evacuative procedures. In the last resort, it is tempting to concur with Laurence Brockliss and Colin Jones, who, in their assessment of French Paracelsianism, have argued that it was 'sometimes far closer to orthodox medical teaching than might be thought at first sight' and that Galenism was 'a much more plastic and eclectic doctrine than it appeared to be on the surface' (1997, pp.126, 129). Regardless of how such a compromise was managed, it was undoubtedly the case that Galenism remained the dominant medical philosophy in Europe in the first half of the seventeenth century.

5.3   The new challenge of Helmontianism, 1650–1700

Joan Baptista van Helmont

During the second half of the seventeenth century, the world of medical ideas and practice was once again thrown into turmoil by the emergence of a new medical philosophy. This time, it was based on the ideas of the Flemish iatrochemist and natural philosopher Joan Baptista van Helmont (Figure 5.5).

Van Helmont was born in Brussels in 1579, the son of an eminent nobleman and state counsellor in Brabant. He studied at Louvain University and was awarded a medical degree in 1599, though he subsequently repudiated the quality of education he had received at university, condemning it as empty, vain and fruitless. Thereafter, his career followed a similar trajectory to that of the physician he most admired, Paracelsus. He turned his back on academia and travelled widely in Europe, visiting among other places Switzerland, Italy, France and England. On his return to what is today Belgium, he refused to accept any public office, either at court or at university, and opted instead to dedicate his life to private study and research in the laboratory he established in his own home. Armed only with the two books of God and nature, he set out to unravel the mysteries of man and the creation through the twin processes of chemical distillation and analysis, seeking, in the words of his most eminent modern biographer, 'to make visible the invisible, which to him meant the real' (Pagel, 1982, p.6).

Although van Helmont was clearly preoccupied for much of the time with elucidating theoretical chemistry, as it was then known, there was also a very practical side to his research. In particular, he wished to see a complete reform of medical practice and theory, and he dedicated his life to providing cheap and pure medicines for the poor and sick, to whom he dispensed these medicines free of charge. Like Paracelsus, van Helmont published little during his lifetime and, again like his mentor, when he did venture into print it frequently got him into trouble with the medical and religious authorities. He made powerful enemies with the Jesuits (van Helmont himself was a Roman Catholic, who lived in the Counter-Reformation stronghold of the Spanish Netherlands), who accused him of dabbling in black magic and other superstitious and ungodly practices. This brought him to the attention of the **Spanish Inquisition**, which placed him under virtual house arrest for the best part of two decades. He continued, nonetheless, to write and research in private, as well as to communicate with some of the most important medical and scientific figures of his age. He died in 1644, a nominal Roman Catholic, having been released from the supervision of the church. However, he

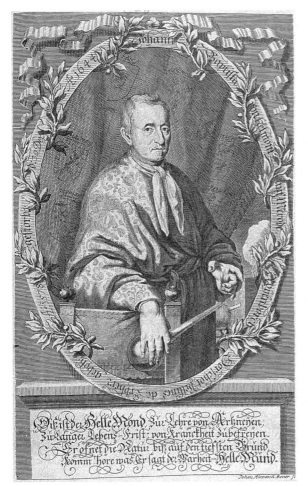

Figure 5.5   This engraving of Joan Baptista van Helmont, by Johann Alexander Baener, is the only extant portrait of the medical reformer and is taken from the German translation of his *Ortus Medicinae* [Origin or Garden of Medicine], *Aufgang der Artzneykunst*, published in 1683. The inscription on the plaque begins and ends with a play on van Helmont's name – 'Helle Mond' (bright moon) and 'Helle Mund' (bright speech). The verse itself reads: 'For the knowledge of medicines, for long life, the eradication of disease he opens Nature to her deepest vault, come hear what speaks truth'. Wellcome Library, London

appears never to have recanted from some of his more mystical and unorthodox opinions, which subsequently found their way into his published writings.

Little known outside academic circles in his own lifetime, van Helmont's radical approach to medicine only acquired a wider audience with the posthumous publication of his collected works in 1648 by his only son, Franciscus Mercurius van Helmont (1614–99). The *Ortus Medicinae* [Origin or Garden of Medicine] was highly critical not only of Galenic medicine, but also of many of the most cherished beliefs of the Paracelsians. In many respects, Helmontianism represented a more purified form of Paracelsianism, which studiously avoided some of the more abstruse elements associated with the great Swiss reformer (Figure 5.6). Not only did van Helmont reject the belief in the interaction of the macrocosm and the microcosm, but he was also critical of astrological medicine and denied the **doctrine of signatures**. Van Helmont's originality as a natural philosopher is evident in the emphasis he placed upon revising the theoretical framework of early modern chemistry. Critical of much of the terminology of medieval and Renaissance alchemy, he attempted to create a new language with which to describe the operations of nature and their impact upon the human body. In the

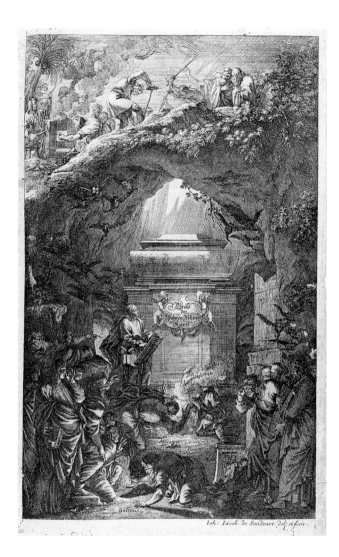

Figure 5.6 *Van Helmont's vision of the Sepulchre of Truth*, from the frontispiece to his *Aufgang der Artzneykunst*, 1683. This print was the work of Johann Jacob Sandrart and appeared as the frontispiece to the German edition of van Helmont's works. It depicts a vision discussed in the work itself (p.530), and shows van Helmont inside a bat-infested cave, where poisonous vapours have reduced his illustrious medical forebears, Galen, Avicenna and Paracelsus, to crawling on all fours in the dark. Van Helmont alone stands in the light, adjacent to the Sepulchre of Truth. The powerful imagery of the light as a form of spiritual and intellectual awakening was particularly apt given the emphasis that van Helmont's medical teaching placed on knowledge gained through ecstatic 'enlightenment'. Wellcome Library, London

process, he invented new terms, such as ***blas*** and ***gas***, as well as revising older ones, such as the Paracelsian concept of the ***archeus***. In the process, he rejected both the Aristotelian elements and the Paracelsian *tria prima* as the prime matter in the universe, arguing instead that water and *semina* (seeds or seminal spirits) were the essential constituents of all natural phenomena.

Van Helmont's originality as a theoretical chemist is now widely acknowledged by historians of early modern science, who have traced the impact of his ideas upon some of the leading scientific and medical writers of the age, among them Robert Boyle (1627–91), Thomas Willis (1621–75) and the influential Dutch natural philosopher Franciscus Sylvius (Franz de le Boë) (1614–72). It was in the field of medicine, however, that Helmontianism was to have its most profound and immediate effect. On the basis of his new chemical theories and investigations, van Helmont proposed a new model of the body and of disease that radically challenged medical orthodoxy, particularly that of the diehard Galenists. Van Helmont and his followers claimed that the 'dogmatic' Galenists were obsessed with the symptoms of disease, which they sought to treat by recourse to a range of interventionist and, in van Helmont's eyes, very dangerous practices, including purges and blood-letting. In place of the humours and qualities, van Helmont argued for an ontological approach to disease – that is, one that acknowledged the existence of disease as an entity (*ens*) in its own right. Elaborating on Paracelsus, he maintained that most diseases were the work of invisible spirits or gases. These spirits entered the body from outside and attached themselves to the *archei*, or governing forces, which oversaw the efficient running of the various organs and parts of the body. In most cases these spirits were benign, but under the influence of the **imagination**, they transmuted into specific diseases, which in turn required specific remedies. Alternatively, illness was the product of acid–alkali ferments in the body, processes that under normal circumstances were considered essential for the proper functioning of the digestive system and the production of the vital spirits, including blood. Helmontian treatment thus focused on the need to restore harmony to the chemical processes of the body, and to assuage the influence of the imagination, an outcome that was most readily achieved by the use of simple, chemically prepared, drugs. Nature, according to van Helmont, thus provided humans with a vast storehouse of remedies, which it was the work of the iatrochemist to locate, refine and prescribe.

The Helmontian revolution in England, 1650–80

Following the publication of the collected works of van Helmont at Amsterdam in 1648, his ideas were rapidly adopted and promoted by large numbers of practising physicians throughout northern Europe. Nowhere, however, were they more enthusiastically received than in England, where in the 1650s the religious and political upheavals of the previous decade had created a highly congenial atmosphere for medical innovation and reform. As a result of the civil wars (1642–6; 1648) and the execution of Charles I (1625–49), the new republic ushered in an age of change and great uncertainty in the social, religious and political life of the nation. With the demise of an effective system of licensing and censorship, the presses rang with the call for root and branch reform of just about every aspect of early modern life. Not surprisingly, medicine was high on the agenda of the reformers.

Enthusiasm for Helmontian medicine was soon all the rage. In 1651, for example, the otherwise unknown author Noah Biggs produced a searing critique of the contemporary medical establishment. In it, he called for sweeping reforms in university education, particularly in relation to the training of physicians and the promotion of chemistry, which he termed the *terra incognita* ('unknown land') of traditional medicine. Medical knowledge, like other forms of learning, should be both useful and widely available, he advised; likewise the secrets of chemistry. To this end, like so many other would-be reformers of the day, he published in the vernacular. His most severe criticisms, however, were reserved for the College of Physicians in London. Biggs lambasted the collegiate physicians as ignorant 'dogmatists', whose perfunctory approval of chemical remedies in their recently published pharmacopoeia was dismissed as too little, too late.

Now read 'Helmontianism and medical reform in Cromwellian England: Noah Biggs (1651)' (Source Book 1, Reading 5.4) and then answer the following questions:

1   How radical a challenge did Biggs's Helmontianism pose to both Galenism and Paracelsianism?

2   What evidence can you find here for the debt of van Helmont and his followers to religious and scriptural arguments?

1   Biggs's full-blown adoption of van Helmont's medical philosophy is manifest in his complete rejection of both the theory and the practice of Galenism. The humours are cast as figments of the imagination that had no foundation in reality. Consequently, all forms of Galenic intervention in the regular or natural operation of the body are rejected, including phlebotomy, or bloodletting, purges and other evacuative methods. More surprising, perhaps, is the inclusion of traditional Galenic notions of diet in Biggs's broad-ranging critique. These are stigmatized as expensive, worthless and contrary to nature – in short, they are used by practitioners as an excuse for their own failure to heal in the first instance.

It is equally evident, however, that Biggs's subscription to Helmontianism leads him to reject many facets of the Paracelsian medical system. He not only rejects the Paracelsian *tria prima* of salt, sulphur and mercury as the essential building blocks of life, but also extends his criticism of the Galenic reliance on cure by contraries to Paracelsus' faith in cure by similarities. In doing so, Biggs reflects van Helmont's profound adherence to the idea that the qualitative approach to medicine and natural philosophy is flawed. The natural world is not made up of warring properties which require the intervention of the physician. On the contrary, the most excellent cures are the simplest and most natural. The task of the gifted physician, then, is only to improve on those remedies that already exist, and for this, pyrotechny, or 'the art of the fire', is needed so that impurities can be removed.

2   Van Helmont's debt to religion and the Bible is manifest in numerous ways. At the heart of his thinking lies the belief that God has endowed his creation with everything necessary for the cure of humankind. Nature, unlike humans, was unaffected by the fall of Adam and Eve. Everywhere, it contains beneficial seeds and seminal powers, which it is the job of the skilful chemist to unlock through the chemist's art. Alternatively, most remedies are abundantly available in the form of simples – that is, drugs produced from readily available herbs and plants. On the basis of such thinking, van Helmont, as we have seen, rejected some of the main elements of Galenic therapeutics, including the recourse to purgative medicines. The debt of van Helmont's medical philosophy to Scripture, albeit the **Apocrypha**, is also evident in his rejection of bloodletting on the grounds that the blood is the chief receptacle of the 'life' (Biggs's shorthand for the soul). But perhaps most damaging of all is his critique of Galenic dietetics, which runs

directly counter to van Helmont's belief in a benign and uncorrupted natural world. Unlike the Galeno-Aristotelian view of nature, and that of Paracelsus, van Helmont banishes warring principles and notions of 'contrariety', and proposes in their stead a beatific vision of a peaceable and untainted creation that has been placed at the disposal of humankind by the goodness of its Creator.

Van Helmont is equally indebted to scriptural authority on the question of the making of the physician. Like Paracelsus, he maintains, citing Ecclesiasticus 38:1, that the true physician is made in heaven, not by the academies. Van Helmont goes one stage further, however, in arguing that a physician's knowledge is the fruit of spiritual illumination, and that the greatest enemy of the medical scholar is the corrupt faculty of human reason. It is little wonder that his ideas were taken up with so much enthusiasm in England in the 1650s, since they very much parallel those put forward by religious radicals at this time in their struggle against the authority of a state church staffed by university-trained clergy.

The appearance of Biggs's manifesto for medical reform constituted part of a wider appeal for intellectual, social, religious and political change that characterized so many books and pamphlets published in England at this time. It is no coincidence, for example, that Biggs's work was addressed to the new ruling body of England, Parliament, which had recently authorized the abolition of the monarchy, the bishops and the House of Lords. His work was studded with allusions to the recent conflicts between Crown and Parliament, and between Anglicans and Puritans, the supporters of the old regime being consistently associated with the forces of medical conservatism. Biggs's views were echoed by the radical exponent of university and educational reform, John Webster (1611–82), who in 1654 castigated the universities for promoting forms of learning that produced no new knowledge and encouraged intellectual inertia. The training of physicians, in particular, came under Webster's scrutiny, the art of medicine having been

> turned into a way of meer formality, flattery, cunning, craft and covetousness, nothing being so much sought after by its professors as popular applause, repute, and esteem with rich and mighty men, that thereby the larger fees may be drawn from them, while in the mean time, the poor are neglected and despised ... and must these things have the countenance of Law, and confirmation by Charters?
>
> (Webster, 1654, p.72)

Meanwhile, the art of healing had fallen into decay. New diseases went unchecked, and old ones were inadequately treated by traditional therapies that were generally ineffective and in some cases positively harmful. Webster advocated a new approach to medicine, one informed by the **Baconian** principle of utility, which he believed had reached its maturity in the form of Helmontian chemistry. He therefore demanded that the Galenic system, 'a path that hath been long enough trodden to yield so little fruit', should no longer 'be the prison that all men must be inchained in', and that it was now time to entertain a 'more sure, cleer and exquisit way of finding the true causes, and certain cures of diseases, brought to light by those two most eminent and laborious persons, Paracelsus, and Helmont' (Webster, 1654, pp.106–7).

In the 1640s and 1650s, various individuals and groups actively campaigned for the reform of all aspects of the art of healing. Peter Chamberlen, for example, a radical Fellow of the College of Physicians, had encountered stiff opposition before the civil war when he proposed the creation of a new body to supervise and license the practice of midwives (their activities were traditionally overseen by the church). In 1648, he was finally expelled from the college after his attempt to introduce a scheme of public bathing was opposed, partly on the grounds that the evil influence of Paracelsus was once again detected at work. Others, such as the lawyer John Cook, campaigned for free medical assistance for the poor and an end to the college's monopolistic powers in London. In addition, he suggested that doctors should make their own medicines (this, of course, was the work of socially inferior apothecaries) and write their prescriptions in clear and legible English (Webster, 1975, pp.289–90, 298). Characteristically, those campaigning for reform emphasized the futility of traditional modes of practice and sought to undermine the monopolistic powers exercised by bodies such as the College of Physicians in London in the regulation of the profession. The latter, for example, came under consistent fire from Nicholas Culpeper (1616–54), the celebrated herbalist, who published dozens of medical works and translations that were predicated on the simple premise that each man and woman might be their own physician. At the same time, chemical clubs sprang up in Oxford and London, dedicated to the pursuit of new knowledge in natural philosophy and medicine. In true Baconian fashion, such individuals and groups were united in the belief that the crucial test of such knowledge was its potential use for humanity. They argued for a new theoretical approach to medicine – one that was based on utility, experimentation and observation – and in the process won converts from all quarters of society.

Whereas the earlier challenge to the medical establishment of Paracelsianism was either thwarted, diluted or absorbed by the dominance of the Galenic physicians, who were able to point to the philosophical and religious unorthodoxy of their opponents, the threat posed by the Helmontians was less easily contained. In England in the 1650s, the religious mood of the nation was clearly more receptive to the radical theological and intellectual implications of van Helmont's thought. Cromwellian England was perhaps, with the exception of the **United Provinces**, one of the most tolerant regimes in Europe. In the wake of the civil wars, and the consequent breakdown of religious authority and censorship, religious experimentation flourished. Radical groups such as the Baptists and the Quakers rejected the notion of a university-educated and salaried clerical elite. Other more moderate puritans, Cromwell included, argued that the essence of organized religion lay in a voluntary association of like-minded men and women, whose faith was founded upon an intense and often semi-mystical relationship with God. Such developments were in stark contrast to traditional forms of worship and organization, and as such they alarmed many in authority, who feared the social and political consequences of religious sectarianism. As the debate raged in Cromwellian England as to the extent to which religious dissent should be accommodated, there is little doubt that the general climate of the times was conducive to the spread of the message of the Helmontian reformers.

Van Helmont's rejection of reason in the acquisition of medical knowledge, coupled with his, and his followers', denunciation of the authority of university-educated physicians, was clearly complementary to the radical sectarian rejection of a university-educated and state-salaried church. It is hardly surprising, then, that when van Helmont's medical writings were translated into English in 1662, the work was performed by a Quaker, John Chandler. There were other points of contact, too, between the religious radicals and the proponents of medical reform and innovation. The 1650s witnessed a revival of interest in the imminent return of Christ to earth – either in body or in spirit – which many believed would be accompanied by wholesale social, religious and political upheaval. Many of the would-be medical reformers shared in this sense of millennial excitement and optimism. It was widely believed in alchemical and iatrochemical circles, for example, that the long-awaited millennium would be accompanied by medical regeneration. These aspirations were picked up by a number of the medical reformers, including the Helmontians, who loudly proclaimed that, come the millennium, new medicines would be discovered and people would live longer as the old system and practices of Galenic medicine were swept away. These ideas had a long pedigree in iatrochemical circles. Paracelsus, himself, had imbibed the vision of a new millennial awakening, and millennial notions were given renewed vigour in the second decade of the seventeenth century with the emergence of the **Rosicrucian movement** in Europe. Expectations associating moral and spiritual revival with medical regeneration were always likely to arise in early modern Europe during periods of religious and political upheaval. The immediate aftermath of the English civil war witnessed one such episode. In the event, though, little of any lasting value was achieved, as the new rulers of England found themselves unwilling or unable to meet the demands of the radicals.

In addition to the encouragement that Helmontianism received from the religious and political atmosphere of the 1650s, it also undoubtedly benefited from the support it obtained from a large group of influential physicians and natural philosophers in England, who shared the Baconian vision of a general programme of intellectual reform. At the heart of this network of enthusiasts was a Polish émigré, Samuel Hartlib (c.1600–62), who perhaps did more than anyone else to popularize and disseminate the cause of medical reform in seventeenth-century Europe. Though Hartlib wrote little and was, until fairly recently, a largely forgotten figure in the history of medicine and science, his vast collection of papers and correspondence provides invaluable evidence for the huge enthusiasm that greeted the reception of Helmontianism in northern Europe during the middle decades of the seventeenth century. It was Hartlib who was chiefly responsible for popularizing the work of van Helmont's influential European followers in England, in particular the practical writings of the German chemist Johann Rudolph Glauber (1604–70) (Young, 1998, especially pp.183–216). He was also partially responsible for introducing the young Robert Boyle to the chemistry of van Helmont, which ultimately proved a seminal influence on the fledgling career of the celebrated natural philosopher (Clericuzio, 1993, pp.314–16). Hartlib's chief claim to historical significance, however, lies in the fact that he played a crucial role in fostering contact and communication among numerous individuals from a wide range of social, religious and political backgrounds who shared his vision of a world transformed by scientific and medical progress. Throughout the 1640s and 1650s, he relentlessly pursued the goal of what he termed 'universal reform', petitioning and cajoling those in authority, with the aim of securing governmental support and money for his ambitious programme. In the end, however, all his efforts came to nothing and at the time of his death in 1662, little in practical terms had been achieved (Webster, 1975, especially pp.246–323).

The Society of Chemical Physicians, 1665

In May 1660, King Charles II (1660–85) was restored to the throne of England, thus bringing to an end nearly two decades of religious and political experimentation. With the return of the Crown and the resumption of the Church of England, bishops and all, it was widely expected that any further discussion of broad-ranging plans for social, educational and intellectual reform would vanish, and that the old medical hierarchy and order would likewise be restored. The Restoration, however, proved to be a mixed blessing for the medical establishment. Buoyed by the creation of the Royal Society in 1660 (officially chartered in 1662), a group of English iatrochemists with powerful contacts at the court of Charles II now sought to revise plans for the wholesale reform of the medical profession in the form of a new body calling itself the Society of Chemical Physicians, which was intended to replace the authority of the College of Physicians in London.

The composition of this group, and the impressive cross-section of support that it managed to attract in the summer of 1665, is indicative of the continuing vitality and appeal of the new chemical medicine in the post-revolutionary era. Some commentators, not surprisingly, have sought to locate the roots of the nascent society in the 1650s. Just as the origins of the Royal Society have been traced to this period, likewise it is possible to see the Society of Chemical Physicians as an outgrowth of earlier schemes, for example that of William Rand, an ally of Hartlib and Boyle, to create an alternative College of Graduate Physicians in 1656 (Webster, 1967). Among the various signatories to the petition requesting the king to create a new Society of Chemical Physicians, there were many with connections to the Hartlib circle, who were potentially tainted by their loyalty to the old regime. The prospective membership of the new society was certainly drawn from a wide spectrum of the social and medical world and included empirics and graduates, both of whom were intent on undermining and ultimately destroying the privileged position of the collegiate physicians in London.

Harold Cook (1987), however, has argued that the proposal to create a new college of chemical physicians owed more to the enthusiasm with which Helmontian medicine was received in court circles than it did to the earlier connections of many of those physicians who signed the petition. The ringleader and central figure here, who acted as an intermediary between the Helmontians and the court, was Thomas O'Dowde, who in addition to practising medicine was groom of the royal bedchamber. As a former royalist, who had suffered for his beliefs prior to the Restoration, he occupied a powerful position from which to lobby for medical change. In March 1665, he produced a 100-page pamphlet, dedicated to Gilbert

Sheldon, archbishop of Canterbury, in which he attacked the Galenists of the college. Appended to the pamphlet were two petitions: the first requested the king to give official recognition to the Society of Chemical Physicians, and was signed by thirty-five of the Helmontians; the second supported their aims, and was signed by thirty-eight of the most prominent noblemen and gentlemen at Charles's court. Shortly thereafter, the leaders of the fledgling society were given an audience with the king. In the event, though, the chemists failed to achieve official recognition and incorporation. The following exercise contains readings relating to the contemporary debate surrounding the merits of chemical medicine and the campaign to create a new Society of Chemical Physicians.

Exercise

Now read 'A new threat to medical orthodoxy: the Society of Chemical Physicians (1665)' and 'Defending the status quo: William Johnson and the London College of Physicians (1665)' (Source Book 1, Readings 5.5 and 5.6) and then answer the following questions:

1   Comment on the tone of this debate, in particular the language used by the two adversaries to get their views across.

2   To what extent do these two readings suggest that the outcome of this controversy would depend exclusively on purely medical or scientific criteria?

Discussion

1   One of the most obvious differences in tone between the two men is the markedly more restrained and conciliatory approach adopted by Johnson. Though he is not averse to the use of innuendo, he nonetheless comes across as the voice of reason. As chemist to the College of Physicians, he speaks with a degree of authority that his adversary clearly lacks. Thomson, on the other hand, is acutely conscious of his inferior status and seeks to make up for this by peppering his discourse with jargon and Latinate terms such as 'Entellechie', 'Polyarchical government', 'Philomatheis' and 'Amathie'. To some extent, this is foisted on Thomson because of his need to rebut the charge, laid by Johnson and others, that the chemists are obscurantists, opposed to all formal learning and the social decorum that goes with the attainment of such knowledge.

2   Thomson's aggressive condemnation of the college and the failure of its Galenic members to effect true cures is grounded upon an uncompromising adherence to the insights of van Helmont. Phlebotomy is rejected as positively harmful to the body, and those traditionalists who claim to have adopted some of the practices of Paracelsus and van Helmont – the 'Galeno-Chymists' – are dismissed as hopeless hybrids, as 'monstrous and Anomalous as a Centaure or Syren'. There was clearly little room in Thomson's medical world-view for accommodation or compromise. Unlike his opponent, Thomson would much prefer to focus the debate on scientific and medical criteria. This was not possible, however, as he was constantly forced to return to the charge laid against the society that it contained men of dubious social, religious and political

backgrounds. In particular, the charge of illiteracy and quackery levelled against some of his colleagues clearly touched a tender spot, and perhaps helps to explain much of the high-flown language used by Thomson in his, and the society's, defence. Thomson's own loyalty to church and Crown, however, is never in doubt. Indeed, he makes a point of emphasizing that one of the advantages of adopting learned Helmontian medicine is that it might effect a cure not just of bodies but also of society at large, and of 'those rebellious and enormous Vices of the Minde, too grassant at this day among us'.

Typically, Johnson's reply to Thomson adopts a two-pronged approach, combining medical and scientific objections to the Helmontian cause with polemical arguments designed to undermine the social, religious and political respectability of Thomson and his colleagues. Thus, he stresses the great advances that have been made in medicine in the last twenty years, and the role of the college's own members in that process. In ways that are highly reminiscent of the earlier accommodation between Galenic and Paracelsian medicine, he also underlines the extent to which modern Galenists have incorporated the best elements of chemistry into their regular practice (Johnson's own career as chemist to the college is eloquent testimony to this process). At the same time, however, he consistently casts doubt on the religious and political orthodoxy of his opponents, as well as stressing the social inferiority of so many of those who have signed the chemists' petition.

5.4   Conclusion

The year 1665 marked the high point in the campaign of the iatrochemists to overthrow Galenic medicine, and along with it the monopolistic corporate structures that enabled medical traditionalists to impose their will on the medical marketplace. Despite the heroic actions of many of those chemical physicians who stayed in London during the last great epidemic of the plague in 1665–6 (Figure 5.7; most of the college's physicians took their own advice to their wealthy patients and fled to the sanctuary of the countryside), the chemists failed to gain official approval. Within thirty years, the Helmontian cause was extinct in England, as well as throughout much of the rest of Europe. The Galenic system of therapeutics had survived yet another challenge to its supremacy, demonstrating remarkable vitality and flexibility in the process.

Is it fair, however, to describe the demise of the iatrochemists' cause as a failure, fit to be consigned to the dustbin of history? Many, in the past, have tended to see it in these terms. Historians more recently have tended to adopt a more positive evaluation. Despite, for example, the ultimate failure of the chemists to dislodge the Galenists from their privileged position at the top of the medical hierarchy, the pressure they brought to bear on the medical establishment was not without effect. Not only were chemical medicines widely adopted and integrated into traditional Galenic therapeutics, but by the end of the seventeenth century it was not uncommon for physicians to prepare their own medicines, thus conflating the role of apothecary and physician. In addition, the medical optimism of the Paracelsians

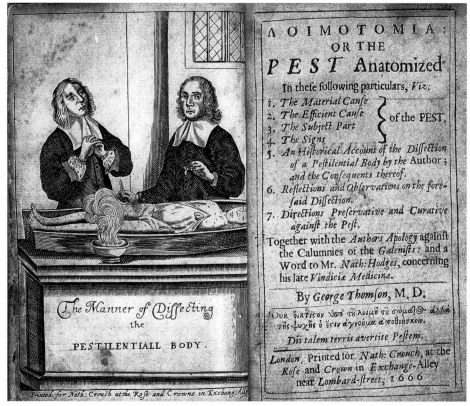

Figure 5.7 Title page of George Thomson, *Loimotomia: or the Pest Anatomized*, 1666. Unlike most of their Galenic opponents, many of the Helmontian advocates of a new college for chemical physicians in London stayed in the capital during the last great outbreak of the plague in 1665–6, ministering to the sick and the poor. Among them was George Thomson, who is portrayed here in the act of dissecting a plague victim. Like many of his colleagues, Thomson contracted the plague, but he survived to tell the tale. The actual dissection is described in some detail in the text of *Loimotomia*, Chapter 5. Wellcome Library, London

and Helmontians – their belief in the curability of all ills, as epitomized by their refusal to flee the plague – and their willingness to practise without payment among the poor helped improve the image of the profession in the public eye. Finally, the example of van Helmont showed that it was possible to conceive of a system of medicine that was largely non-interventionist, eschewing all traditional forms of therapy based on purgatives and bloodletting.

Despite all this, however, in the last resort the Helmontians and their Paracelsian predecessors failed to break the Galenic stranglehold on medicine, which survived into the eighteenth century. Various factors account for the failure of the iatrochemists, not all of which were medical in nature. On a non-medical level, their cause was always prone to attack because of the esoteric and semi-mystical language favoured by Paracelsus and van Helmont. Despite the fact that their medical ideas appealed to a wide religious constituency, their opponents frequently and successfully stigmatized them as subversive and heretical. In the case of English Helmontianism, such fears were further exacerbated by the social diversity of its supporters. Despite the fact that some Helmontian practitioners were able to call upon the support of powerful and well-connected men at court, as a group they lacked the social cohesion and learning which, as in the case of the Royal Society, won official respect and acceptance. The subsequent failure to establish an institutional base or centre for further research was a major blow to the chemists' aspirations.

The failure of the followers of both Paracelsus and van Helmont to effect a medical revolution was, then, partly the product of the iatrochemists' inability to secure professional and institutional recognition and partly the result of factors that lay outside the medical sphere. But in focusing on its failure we may be in danger of underestimating the success of the Galenic system, and its practitioners, in facing down the challenge of the chemical physicians. Another way of looking at this phenomenon, and perhaps a more accurate one, would be to ask how it was that Galenism survived as long as it did. Andrew Wear, for example, has located the failure of the Helmontian challenge in the resistance of patients to novelty and their support for tried and trusted therapeutic regimes based on the age-old principles of evacuation and dietetic intervention. In dismissing the value of such methods, especially those involving diet and close attention to the six non-naturals, the Helmontians were bucking the trends of a medical market in which the clout of the consumer was all-powerful (Wear, 2000, pp.399–433).

Finally, the Helmontians, like their professed enemies, the Galenists, were themselves forced to confront broader developments that were taking place at this time in the field of medicine and natural philosophy. During the second half of the seventeenth century, chemistry itself was undergoing evolution, as men such as Thomas Willis in England and Franciscus Sylvius in Holland sought to refine and apply chemical methodology to the new mechanistic conception of the human body. Both Willis and Sylvius likened the body to a distillation unit in which 'all physiological processes could be explained chemically – primarily through fermentation, effervescence and putrefaction' (Debus, 1991, p.138). The debt of such advocates of the 'new philosophy' to van Helmont is beyond question. Equally, however, it is apparent that these advocates, many of whom did acquire official recognition and status, were taking chemistry in a new direction – one that was shorn of the occult and semi-mystical overtones of the older alchemical and iatrochemical traditions. By 1700, chemistry was fully integrated into the newly emerging and dominant model of the body proposed by such iatromechanists as Hermann Boerhaave (1668–1738). In the process, the seminal work of Paracelsus and van Helmont was largely forgotten, only to be rediscovered in the twentieth century by historians eager to reconsider the dynamic role played by the earliest proponents of chemotherapy in reshaping the world of early modern medicine.

References

Brockliss, L. and Jones, C. (1997) *The Medical World of Early Modern France*, Oxford: Clarendon Press.

Clericuzio, A. (1993) 'From van Helmont to Boyle: a study of the transmission of Helmontian chemical and medical theories in seventeenth-century England', *British Journal for the History of Science*, vol.16, pp.303–34.

Cook, H.J. (1986) *The Decline of the Old Medical Regime in Stuart London*, Ithaca and London: Cornell University Press.

Cook, H.J. (1987) 'The Society of Chemical Physicians, the New Philosophy, and the Restoration court', *Bulletin of the History of Medicine*, vol.61, pp.61–77.

Debus, A.G. (1991) *The French Paracelsians: The Chemical Challenge to Medical and Scientific Tradition in Early Modern France*, Cambridge: Cambridge University Press.

Moran, B.T. (1990) 'Prince-practitioning and the direction of medical roles at the German court: Maurice of Hesse-Kassel and his physicians' in V.Nutton (ed.) *Medicine at the Courts of Europe, 1500–1837*, London and New York: Routledge, pp.95–116.

Moran, B.T. (1991) *The Alchemical World of the German Court: Occult Philosophy and Chemical Medicine in the Circle of Moritz of Hessen (1572–1632)*, Stuttgart: Franz Steiner.

Pagel, W. (1982) *Joan Baptista van Helmont: Reformer of Science and Medicine*, Cambridge: Cambridge University Press.

Trevor-Roper, H.R. (1990) 'The court physician and Paracelsianism' in V. Nutton (ed.) *Medicine at the Courts of Europe, 1500–1837*, London and New York: Routledge, pp.79–94.

Wear, A. (2000) *Knowledge and Practice in English Medicine, 1550–1680*, Cambridge: Cambridge University Press.

Webster, C. (1967) 'English medical reformers of the puritan revolution: a background to the "Society of Chymical Physitians"', *Ambix*, vol.14, pp.16–41.

Webster, C. (1975) *The Great Instauration: Science, Medicine and Reform 1626–1660*, Duckworth: London.

Webster, C. (1979) 'Alchemical and Paracelsian medicine' in C. Webster (ed.) *Health, Medicine and Mortality in the Sixteenth Century*, Cambridge: Cambridge University Press, pp.301–34.

Webster, C. (1990) 'Conrad Gessner and the infidelity of Paracelsus' in J. Henry and S. Hutton (eds) *New Perspectives on Renaissance Thought: Essays in the History of Science, Education and Philosophy in Memory of Charles B. Schmitt*, London: Duckworth, pp.13–23.

Webster, J. (1654) *Academiarum Examen, or the Examination of Academies*, London: Giles Calvert.

Young, J.T. (1998) *Faith, Medical Alchemy and Natural Philosophy: Johann Moriaen, Reformed Intelligencer, and the Hartlib Circle*, Aldershot: Ashgate.

Source Book readings

R. B[ostocke], *The Difference Betwene the Auncient Phisicke ... and the Latter Phisicke*, London: Robert Walley, 1585, sigs. A5v–A7r, H6v–H7v (Reading 5.1).

H. Trevor-Roper, 'The court physician and Paracelsianism' in V. Nutton (ed.) *Medicine at the Courts of Europe, 1500–1837*, London and New York: Routledge, 1990, pp.79–84, 87 (Reading 5.2).

A.G. Debus, *The French Paracelsians: The Chemical Challenge to Medical and Scientific Tradition in Early Modern France*, Cambridge: Cambridge University Press, 1991, pp.48–51, 53–5, 56–9, 65, 84–5, 88–91, 93, 94–5, 100–1 (Reading 5.3).

N. Biggs, *Mataeotechnia Medicinae Praxews: The Vanity of the Craft of Physick*, London: Giles Calvert, 1651, pp. 77–8, 136, 161–2, 193–4, 200–1, 213–14, 216–17, 219, 221 (Reading 5.4).

G. Thomson, *Galeno-pale: or, a Chymical Trial of the Galenists*, London: R. Wood, 1665, sigs A2r–A4r; pp.19–20, 48–9, 55, 103–6 (Reading 5.5).

W. Johnson, Ἀ'γυρτο-Μα'ζιξ. *Or, Some Brief Animadversions upon Two Late Treatises ... Galeno-pale ... [and] ... The Poor Mans Physitian*, London: T. Mabb, 1665, pp.6–8, 67–9 (Reading 5.6).

6

Policies of Health

Diseases, poverty and hospitals

Silvia De Renzi

Objectives

When you have completed this chapter you should be able to:

- describe how past societies responded to contagious diseases;

- assess the specific problems concerning the health of a community;

- outline major health policies, and their medical, social and political implications;

- distinguish the various functions of hospitals in early modern societies and outline some recent approaches to their history.

6.1 Introduction

The 'welfare state' and its future is frequently a topic of passionate debate. Its philosophy, best embodied in the expression 'from the cradle to the grave', is based on the principle that one of the duties of the state is to care for the well-being of its citizens at each stage of their lives. Health is now recognized, at least in most European countries, as a universal right and many agree that its costs should be met by society as a whole and not just by those who are sick. Furthermore, one of the criteria by which we judge a society is its ability to maintain an environment that is clean and safe. All this, however, is very recent, and is the fruit of struggles and controversies in the nineteenth and twentieth centuries. But what happened in earlier times? What did 'disease' and 'health' mean to communities regularly decimated by epidemics? What measures, if any, were taken? What happened to poor people, dependent on their ability to work, who could not afford the costs involved in falling ill? In this chapter, I provide some answers to these and related questions.

I begin, in Section 6.2, by looking at how historians seek to understand past diseases. In particular, I focus on two major contagious diseases that devastated early modern societies, the plague and the great pox (now called syphilis), exploring how they were understood at the time and the different responses they triggered. Epidemics of contagious diseases had social and political, as well as medical, implications, as they inevitably damaged the economic resources of a community. I examine the measures taken by authorities to deal with such periodic scourges, looking in particular at how these measures affected the poor, and explore the links between health care provision and poor relief schemes. In Section

6.3, I discuss the role of hospitals in early modern Europe. Originally intended as shelters for the destitute and needy, hospitals performed an increasingly complex role as they became one of the main institutions in which communities confronted the broader implications of diseases – that is, their social, economic and political consequences. The preservation of the health of a community became an area of growing public intervention towards the end of the seventeenth century, and was later bound up with processes of political centralization and with a booming economy. In Section 6.4, I look at the development of state-promoted health policies in the age of **Enlightenment**.

6.2 Diseases and society

In early modern Europe, epidemics which devastated whole communities were an all too familiar experience. For those living in modern western societies, it is difficult to recapture this collective experience of disease. Occasionally, epidemics of contagious diseases, such as influenza, reach newsworthy status, but in general, illnesses tend to be regarded as individual occurrences. Perhaps the nearest the modern world has come to the experience of the early modern epidemics was in the 1980s, when a new disease called acquired immune deficiency syndrome (Aids) appeared. Like the earlier epidemics, Aids provoked fear in society at large because of its sudden appearance and apparently unstoppable spread. It, too, caused devastation in the communities that were most affected by it and gave rise to political controversies over how best to tackle it.

The history of diseases

Until recently, historians dealing with past epidemics tended to focus on specific issues relating to the scale of the crisis, patterns of contagion and cycles of outbreak. In the process, they combed official documents and quantified the effects of epidemics, transforming them into graphs and numerical tables of mortality. Numerical tables based on contemporary data can certainly help us to apprehend the impact of an epidemic, but such tables are notoriously deceptive and rarely tell the whole story. For example, while an outbreak of plague was raging through a community, the disease was frequently blamed for any sudden death that might have occurred. Moreover, in the early modern period, records of the incidence of other illnesses are simply much less abundant and there is little that historians can do to correct this distortion. These problems are exacerbated by the fact that scholars have tended to focus on the plague to the exclusion of most other diseases. Consequently, we know much less, for example, about mortality from childhood diseases in the period, despite its very high incidence. (It has been argued that in early modern France there were more deaths from childhood diseases than from the plague; Jones, 1996a, p.100.) In other words, while producing numerical data appears to be the most objective and direct way of dealing with the past, it often provides only a very limited and often distorted perspective.

Traditionally, historians of medicine have also put much effort into deciphering descriptions of symptoms in historical sources in order to give the condition in question a label consistent with modern medical knowledge: in this way they have been at pains to distinguish pulmonary from bubonic plague, and typhus from influenza. The implication of this approach is that by transferring *our* categories and *our* understanding to the past, we can decide what really happened – a possibility denied to contemporary observers. More recently, historians have questioned the value of this form of 'retrospective diagnosis', arguing that concepts and perceptions of disease change enormously over the centuries according to both broad cultural assumptions and specific medical knowledge. The concept of disease with which we are familiar today – that is, as a clearly identifiable and classifiable entity linked to a material cause – is completely different from the notion of humoral imbalance specific to an individual, which was the working definition of disease until the nineteenth century. In relation to the plague, awareness of this fundamental difference has led scholars such as Andrew Cunningham to claim that

Retrospective diagnoses are discussed further, in relation to mental illness, in Chapter 9.

> the laboratory construction of plague [that is, the isolation of the bacillus *Yersinia pestis* in a microbiological laboratory in 1894] means that there is an unbridgeable gap between past 'plague' and our plague. The identities of pre-1894 plague and post-1894 plague have become incommensurable. We are simply unable to say whether they were the same.
>
> (1992, p.242)

What it now means to talk about the modern disease that we call 'the plague' is of little or no use in making sense of what past people experienced when they were struck by what they called 'the plague'.

To recapture what past people meant and experienced, we need to look beyond tables of mortality and retrospective diagnosis and investigate how the meanings that they attached to disease were shaped by the social and the cultural, as well as the medical, expectations of their age. For the early modern period, therefore, we have to engage with religion as well as medicine. In the remainder of this section, I shall examine contemporary perceptions of, and responses to, two major epidemic diseases of this period: the plague and the great pox.

The plague

When the plague struck in Venice in 1630, the municipal authorities responded in the following way. They ordered that the mortal remains of the first patriarch (that is, bishop) of Venice, who was renowned as a successful healer, were first to be displayed in three of the city's churches, and then taken in procession at intervals through the neighbouring streets. At the same time, magistrates were ordered to clamp down on inappropriate behaviour in the city, including gambling, blasphemy and excessive expenditure on clothing. Measures were also taken against begging, and poor people were removed from the places where they habitually gathered. Shortly afterwards, regulations were introduced to control the food trade and the provision of fresh water, and decrees were issued to order the segregation of the sick from the healthy (Pullan, 1992). Thus, religious, moral and medical concerns combined in the measures taken by the Venetian authorities to contain the disease. At one and the same time, the plague was perceived as a divine punishment for sin and immorality, and as a phenomenon that could be controlled by a series of carefully designed medical, religious and political interventions, among which policing the poor was one of the first. Rotten food and dirty water were seen as the secondary causes through which God (the first cause) was believed to act. While accepting His will, it remained incumbent on humans to try any measures that might reduce the impact of such diseases.

The public display of the patriarch's remains is a good illustration of how different healing elements, both spiritual and material, coexisted in Catholic Venice. Expressing religious devotion by viewing the sacred relics was believed to offer spiritual benefits, while the **effluvia** emanating from the relics were believed to have a material effect by counteracting the poisonous air that was so often blamed for the disease (Figure 6.1). In the early modern period, a disease was understood as a warning or a punishment sent by God. Epidemics of contagious diseases such as the plague afflicted whole communities, and so the belief was that God was admonishing the whole community for its sinful behaviour. This is why laws regarding urban morality were usually tightened up and, in Catholic countries, communal rituals were organized, including penitential processions and public prayers. When the epidemic was over, towns often promised to build a new church, as a form of collective votive offering, to give thanks for the ending of the scourge (Plate 7).

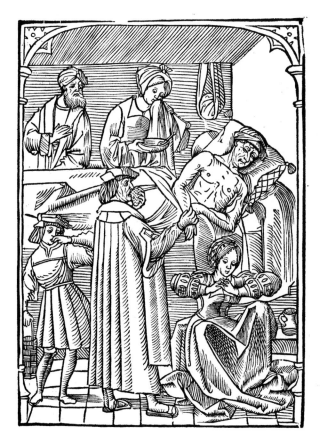

Figure 6.1 This woodcut graphically depicts the stench emitted by those suffering from the plague. While taking the sick man's pulse, the physician holds to his nose a sponge that is probably soaked in vinegar. This was believed to purify the air. The nurse and the young boy are also affected by the smell, which was thought to be not only unpleasant but also dangerous. From *Fasciculo Medicinae te Antwerpen*, 1512; reproduced from Cunningham and Grell (2000), p.282

In the mid-fourteenth century, the Black Death had reduced the population of Europe by between one-fifth and one-third. Frequent, if less devastating, outbreaks of plague epidemics followed and communities across the continent were on constant alert for signs of the disease (looking out, in particular, for sudden deaths and the appearance of **buboes**). But it was in the states and cities of the Italian peninsula that sophisticated policies to fight such epidemics were implemented most effectively. This remarkable interest in preserving the health of the community was doubtless the result of the civic pride and robust political life that had characterized the numerous *comuni* of late medieval Italy and was still vigorous in the regional states of the seventeenth century. Pistoia, a middle-sized town under the rule of the Grand Duchy of Tuscany, is a good case in point. Note that in the following exercise, the terms 'pesthouse' and 'lazaretto' are used interchangeably to mean a hospital for people suffering from a pestilential and contagious disease – in this case, the plague.

Exercise

Now read 'Fighting the plague in seventeenth-century Italy' (Source Book I, Reading 6.1) and then answer the following questions:

1 What was the nature of the work of the health deputies, and what actions did they take to combat the disease?

2 What role did medical experts play in fighting the epidemic, and how would you describe their relationship with the local magistracy?

Discussion

1 The health deputies were not doctors but administrators. Among their first actions was the establishment of a cordon sanitaire around the city: they restricted the movement of people and goods, and banned foreigners, beggars and sick people from entering the city's boundaries. Their actions were designed to strike a balance between health concerns and the needs of the local economy (in this case the grape harvest). The deputies were diligent in the financial aspects of the task: they were active in raising funds, engaged a bank to manage the money and appointed an official called a *provveditore* (general manager) to oversee the whole business. They were keen to avoid unnecessary expenditure and undertook to revise their plan as soon as conditions improved. The deputies also took a series of very specific measures. These included: the appointment of a physician; the establishment of pesthouses and makeshift hospitals; and the implementation of general programmes of social welfare and public hygiene (for example, providing the poor with clean clothes and food, and ensuring the streets were cleaned).

2 At the first signs of the outbreak, the deputies asked local physicians for their advice, and, when the plague reached the countryside around Pistoia, they hired a physician (Stefano Arrighi) and a surgeon (Francesco Magni) to establish and run a pesthouse outside the gates of the city. It is revealing that Arrighi, who had already served as a community physician, was the youngest of the local physicians.

He probably accepted this risky job in the hope that the dedication he showed would boost his future career prospects. Arrighi corresponded regularly with the deputies about the running of the pesthouse, mostly with requests for more money and supplies. His reports show that he knew what he was doing, and yet he was not asked to sit on the health board, and so had no say in the financial decision-making.

Apart from the emphasis on financial matters – hardly surprising in a region renowned for its long-established and highly sophisticated tradition of banking – the measures taken by the health deputies in Pistoia were not particularly original or innovative. The rationale for their course of action rested on contemporary understanding of what caused the plague and how it was spread. The most popular theory was that the disease originated from a malign quality in the air. This putrid air, termed 'miasma', might be caused by earthquakes, by unfavourable conjunctions of the stars or planets or by a range of other environmental factors, for example the putrefaction of organic matter. A miasma rising from, say, a particularly swampy, smelly or dirty place, was thought to enter the body and disturb the balance of the humours. The theory that the disease could be spread by contagion from person to person gained force, though it was combined with, and in the early modern period never displaced, the theory of miasma (Nutton, 1990). Bear in mind that all these theories about the cause of the plague, and of other contagious diseases, coexisted with the fundamental notion that ultimately, whatever its origin, a disease led to an imbalance of humours in the individuals who contracted it. However, when hundreds of people were struck by a disease at the same time, there had to be some sort of intervention at the level of its less immediate causes. Even those who supported a miasmatic origin of the plague believed that once a person was sick, he or she could spread the disease in various ways. Thus, it made perfect sense to control the disease by fencing off the most affected areas and quarantining the sick in special places, so as to limit their contact with healthy citizens. The successful implementation of measures such as these, though, required a tight political control over the whole community – or at least the administrative ability to mobilize and coordinate a range of resources. This was the case in Pistoia, which meant that the procedures set up by the authorities operated relatively smoothly and were effective. It was often not the case elsewhere in Europe.

Let us now look at how the authorities in London handled the problem. Since the mid-sixteenth century, efforts had been made to tackle outbreaks of the plague. However, conflicts frequently arose between the City – that is, the self-governing body of the largest and oldest part of London – and the crown. In essence, while the **Privy Council**, following the example of foreign political authorities, argued for a comprehensive and coordinated policy of containment to be implemented, including segregation of the sick and the establishment of a pesthouse, the City's aldermen, who were expected to implement such policies, were reluctant to levy the necessary taxes to finance such measures. In their eyes, the costs should have been met by private charity, usually channelled through the numerous and financially independent parishes of London. The City was no doubt also aware of the difficulties in imposing a central policy onto the collection of autonomous institutions that formed the administrative backbone of London. As a result, poor neighbourhoods, which were often more seriously hit by such epidemics, were forced to rely on much smaller budgets than richer areas, where private philanthropy guaranteed a constant flow of cash into the parish's coffers. In 1630, Charles I decided to push the issue further and asked the College of Physicians to intervene in the controversy by providing directions for the prevention and cure of the plague.

The College of Physicians, which had been established by royal decree in 1518, was a loyal ally of the crown and could provide much needed weight to its political measures. At the same time, the special relationship between the college and the monarchy endowed the former with greater authority in its attempt to control and police medical practice in and around the capital. In the 1630s, the king's French physician, Theodore Turquet de Mayerne, also entered the arena and urged that a board of public health with unlimited powers should be established. While he obviously had in mind something very similar to what we have seen in action in Pistoia, he went further, and demanded a strong presence of physicians on the board. The proposed board was to consist of twelve members appointed by the king, four of whom were physicians, and was to take over responsibilities previously delegated to the City. In the event, this public health board never materialized, though the College of Physicians was called upon to provide further advice about measures to fight the plague. Some historians have seen the king's intervention and call for medical advice as evidence that he was using health policy as a blueprint for his larger project of subjecting the independent bodies that ran London (parishes, guilds, the City) to centralized, royal authority (Cook, 1989, p.31). In the eyes of many of his subjects, Charles's motives in this and many related schemes in the 1630s were highly controversial and potentially divisive. While public health policies remained patchy in London, control over the plague offered an important model for schemes of political centralization.

A similar process was evident in seventeenth-century France. Here, coordination of health policies was in the hands of *intendants*, administrative officials who represented the growing **absolutist** power of the king in the provinces: as Laurence Brockliss and Colin Jones have argued, by the mid-seventeenth century 'plague had become a matter of state' (1997, p.352). The political implications of health policies, however, went well beyond these important questions of administrative organization or negotiations between centre and periphery.

Medical care, social control

In discussing the policies implemented in Pistoia by the health deputies, Carlo Cipolla contrasts the treatment of the poor with that of the rich. Whereas poor people were forced into pesthouses, rich people were allowed to live in their own homes, but urged not to go out.

> If the health deputies managed to break down the resistance of the poor, they encountered insurmountable difficulties when it came to people of consequence ... Rationalising on this common practice, the deputies argued that the poor lived in crowded quarters, and thus it was imperative

in their case to remove the infected. The well-to-do, it was argued, had abundance of space and rooms, and even if locked up together in the same house, the infected and the healthy could keep at a safe distance from one another.

(Cipolla, 1981, p.76)

The social tensions generated by the plague have been the focus of much research (Slack, 1985). Contemporaries had a contradictory attitude towards possible links between social conditions and the disease. On the one hand, the plague was often portrayed as an indiscriminate calamity, from the horrors of which no one was immune. On the other hand, links between poverty and sickness were routinely discussed in the abundant literature on the plague, and provided the basis of most health policies during outbreaks of the disease.

Exercise

Now read 'Plague and the poor in early modern England' (Source Book 1, Reading 6.2) and then answer the following questions:

1   What were the reactions of the common people to the regulations that were enforced in times of plague?

2   What links does Paul Slack see between health policies and policies designed to enforce social control?

Discussion

1   By examining episodes of social unrest in cities struck by the plague, Slack shows the deep resentment of various sectors of the population toward the strict measures taken by the local authorities. The shutting up of houses and the restrictions on customs surrounding death were especially unpopular, as they undermined strong communal bonds and practices of mutual support. Women in particular were active in resisting these measures.

2   Slack shows how the wealthy and those in authority came to the conclusion that the plague was a disease spread by the poor, and that health policies should thus form part of a broader drive to deal with problems of poverty and disorder. Plague epidemics acquired a political significance in that they were used to justify and reinforce the harsh treatment of the poor and to impose what was perceived as social and moral order. The authorities thus used health policies to implement broader policies of social exclusion, which became increasingly popular in both Protestant and Catholic states in seventeenth-century Europe.

There is a general consensus among historians that the plague played an important role in shaping seventeenth-century attitudes towards poverty. Instead of being seen in a religious light, as a vehicle of salvation, the poor gradually came to be seen as the source of moral and physical corruption. This change of perception in turn led to the design and implementation of new forms of poor relief. As a result of the restrictions that applied during outbreaks of the plague, the recipients of charity were increasingly subjected to bureaucratic oversight, discipline and moral reproach. Moreover, the new purpose-built institutions, in which the poor were increasingly confined as the seventeenth century drew on, were based on the earlier experience of warehousing the plague-infected poor in pesthouses.

So far, I have discussed the plague largely from a social perspective, focusing on the perceptions and responses of the governing authorities. But how did the medical establishment respond to the disease? Since the time of the Black Death, a vast body of literature on the plague had been produced throughout Europe, both in Latin and in the vernacular. These works ranged from highly specialized medical books to publications that addressed a more general audience. To take just one example from among many, Stephen Bradwell's *Physick for the Sicknesse, Commonly Called the Plague* appeared in 1636. It contained a short but clear explanation of the nature and causes of the plague, followed by practical advice on how to avoid the contagion.

Exercise

Now read 'Medical advice in time of plague: Stephen Bradwell (1636)' (Source Book 1, Reading 6.3) and then answer the following questions:

1   Who was Bradwell writing for?

2   How did he characterize the plague as a disease?

Discussion

1   Bradwell wrote his book in English rather than in Latin, and so was probably writing for a general rather than a specialized readership. However, he cited numerous other medical authorities, both ancient and modern, and quoted sources in the original Latin and Greek. He clearly assumed, therefore, that his readers had at least a basic knowledge of medicine and of the learned languages.

2   Bradwell explained that, unlike other contagious diseases, which were transmitted in a singular way (either by touching or by breathing), the plague could be caught in many different ways. He maintained, though, that air was the main medium of infection. Bradwell discussed the 'seminarie tincture' of the plague – a very thin mix of particles that mingled with air and penetrated the pores of the body, where it interacted with the humours and spirits. He vividly described the power of odourless and invisible particles to stick to garments and bedding, thereby making them vehicles of contagion. The notion that the plague was spread by poisonous particles was very popular, although in some respects it ran against the common view about the origin of diseases. According to Galenic medicine, a disease was the outcome of an alteration in the patient's distinctive balance of humours, and therefore was unique to each individual. That an external cause could have the same effects on everyone clearly challenged this assumption. Bradwell himself engaged with this debate when he argued that there were as many types of plague as there were types of constitution; the existence of different temperaments and lifestyles explained why some people got ill and some

did not. This was reassuring to physicians. Despite the intervention of an external agent, they could still apply their traditional expertise, take into account temperaments and constitutions, and prescribe individually tailored treatments. Bradwell also drew a fine distinction between categories of people, including the poor. In fact, he seems to have regarded being poor almost as part of an individual's physical make-up, like being choleric or phlegmatic.

In discussing how to avoid the contagion, Bradwell emphasized the importance of the six non-naturals, the regulation of which formed a major part of the Galenic armoury against disease. He also urged his readers to exercise a strict control over space – both the space immediately surrounding their bodies, and the broader environment in which they lived. He recommended the following precautions in particular: carefully monitoring the air that was breathed, checking its origin and qualities (its temperature and degree of humidity); keeping garments and bedding clean; keeping lozenges in the mouth; avoiding stinking odours; keeping the house clean and well ventilated; making sure that any possible source of putrefaction was removed from one's neighbourhood or burnt. But Bradwell's main piece of advice was to 'keep oneself as private as he may', by which he meant that it was best to shun crowds and potentially infected places. Like most contemporary literature on the plague, Bradwell's book was about the precautions that individuals should take. However, it was on arguments like his that health boards would base their policies, not only those that concerned the general cleanliness of the urban environment, but also those that involved keeping a tight control over the movements of the sick, and segregating those believed to be particularly prone to the disease. Bradwell himself claimed that, because of their bad and insufficient diet, the poor had their bodies 'much corrupted ... and become (of all others) most subject to this Sicknesse' (quoted in Wear, 2000, p.284).

How far can the measures adopted to fight plague epidemics in early modern Europe be regarded as part of broader policies concerning public health? Bear in mind that health boards were not active all the time. They convened only during times of crisis, and the health policies they introduced were usually temporary measures, designed to fight the immediate threat of plague. Nevertheless, apprehension about the condition of the environment did lead to the regulation of a range of urban activities that were widely regarded as hazards to health. These included the closer supervision of foul-smelling crafts such as tanning, stricter controls over the movement of food and animals, and orders enforcing the clearance of rubbish and excrement from cellars and streets. Although partly stirred by aesthetic concerns, these rules and regulations also had a medical rationale: they were meant to reduce the formation of dangerously putrefied and polluted air, which, as you have seen, was regarded as the main vehicle of contagious diseases.

By the middle of the eighteenth century, the plague had disappeared from Europe: the last epidemic occurred in Marseille in 1720–2. Historians disagree as to why this should have been so. Some have argued for the efficiency of the cordon sanitaire that was established during the eighteenth century by the Austrian government along the borders of the Ottoman Empire, from where the plague usually originated. Others have highlighted the general economic improvement in most European countries and the growing resistance of a better-nourished population to the disease. You may notice that the role accorded to health policies is decisively different in these interpretations: in the former, it is central; in the latter, it is marginal.

The great pox

The plague was by no means the only contagious disease in the early modern period: smallpox, for example, was a great killer too, though many more people survived it than survived the plague (Brockliss and Jones, 1997, p.44). At the beginning of the sixteenth century, a new disease started to spread uncontrollably. It was painful and unpleasant – it made the flesh gradually rot away – and it killed many people, though it was much less rampant than the plague and sufferers seemed able to live with the condition for a long time. Wherever it struck, it was characteristically blamed on foreigners – foreign armies helped to spread it – and it was therefore frequently given different names in different countries. It generally came to be known, however, as the 'French disease' (*morbus gallicus*), or the great pox. A vast literature, both of a medical and of a moral nature, soon started to appear, which discussed its origins, causes and apparently incurable nature.

Medical approaches to the French disease are discussed in Chapter 1.

Descriptions of the disease focused on its most obvious symptoms – pustules, rapidly turning into ulcers, which first showed in the genital area and then spread to the whole body. The skin of the affected person quickly became pock-marked and started to emit a terrible stench. Nothing like this had been seen before, and there were great debates about whether it would go as quickly as it had come, or whether it would stay to torment communities forever. There were various theories on its origin. Some claimed that the disease had originated in sexual intercourse between people with skin diseases, with the offspring of such liaisons being the first to be affected. The Italian practitioner Leonardo Fioravanti, whom you met in Chapter 2, argued that the disease was rooted in cannibalism, episodes of which had allegedly occurred among some armies during the recent European wars (quoted in Eamon, 1998, pp.10–11). Both theories encapsulate the contemporary feeling that it was the transgression of boundaries of decent behaviour that had generated such a devastating disease. A more naturalistic interpretation, which claimed that a particular conjunction of planets and stars had brought about a dramatic corruption of the air and ignited the disease, was also very popular. This theory coexisted with the belief that the pox was a punishment for sinful behaviour – the evident link of the disease with sex made God's message very clear this time – with the stars' conjunction seen as the medium via which God had acted. The theory that the disease ultimately came from the newly discovered land of America acquired a broad consensus. The pox was highly contagious; it was known to be transmitted by sexual intercourse, but the stinking and suppurating bodies of syphilitics were also seen as vehicles of contamination. A great moral stigma was thus attached to the new disease, and sufferers tried hard to hide their condition. All these aspects – medical, religious and moral – combined to give the pox its particular character (Figure 6.2).

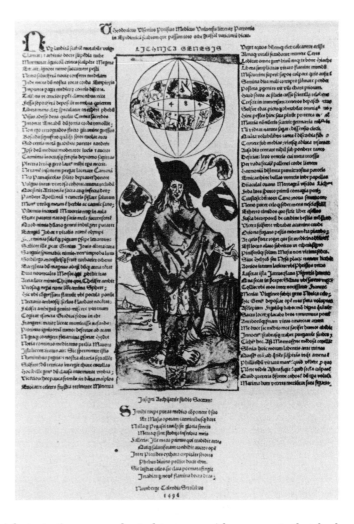

Figure 6.2   This broadside, produced by the municipal authorities of the German city of Nuremberg in 1496, is the first visual representation of a sufferer of the pox. It consists of a poem written by the physician Theodoricus Ulsenius, which surrounds a woodcut by Albrecht Dürer. The ulcers on the syphilitic's legs are clearly visible, as are his enormous, plumed hat, voluminous cloak, fashionably slashed shoes and flowing hair. He is thus portrayed as a man of extravagant tastes and, by implication, intemperate habits. Alongside this condemnatory portrayal of the origins of the sufferer's plight, however, is another suggested cause: the astrological diagram at the top refers to a specific conjunction of planets that occurred in 1484, which was widely believed to have caused the outbreak. Reproduced from Gilman (1988), p.249

What medical and social strategies were adopted to cope with a scourge that had such an impact on the life of communities? Since the Middle Ages, skin conditions had been treated with applications of mercury, and, because this new disease had a visible effect on the skin, it was to mercury that people first turned. Mercury-based ointments and inhalations of the metal's hot vapours were generously prescribed: they were thought to help the body get rid of the corrupted matter that caused the disease, and the abundant salivation they induced was considered evidence of their efficacy. What we now call the side effects of a treatment were, in this case, horrific. Painful ulcers, loss of teeth, and uncontrollable trembling were common and dreaded consequences. It was, then, with a sense of relief and wonder that news of an alternative, painless treatment was received in Europe by the 1520s. The remedy was concocted from the bark of a particular tree, *Guaiacum officinalis*, known colloquially as 'holy wood'. It could be taken as a liquid draught or applied to ulcers and sores. The only disadvantage was its cost. A monopoly over its importation from America was soon established by a family of German bankers, the Fuggers, who made a fortune by selling the drug at a huge profit. Initially, this meant of course that only the very wealthy could afford the treatment. However,

This remedy is discussed further in Chapter 12.

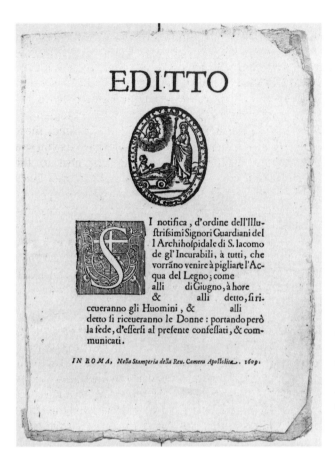

Figure 6.3   Bill advertising the distribution of holy wood to those affected by the pox at the hospital of San Giacomo, in Rome, 1609. Bills such as this were posted across the city to advertise this event, which occurred once every two years. Gaps were left in the printed text, so that the exact date and time when the holy wood would be distributed could be inserted at the last moment. Archivio di Stato di Roma

making the drug available to the poor became the focus of many large-scale charitable operations, especially in Italy and Germany (Figure 6.3).

People sick with the pox could not work. If they were poor, therefore, they quickly joined the large throngs of beggars who were omnipresent in sixteenth-century Europe, and who were increasingly presented as a source of infection, disorder and immorality. Even if in the case of the pox it was not possible to establish a clear link with poverty, the disease was soon represented as a social as much as a medical problem and, once again, the sick poor were the target of the measures taken by many authorities to deal with its spread. Among the first of these measures were the prohibition of prostitution and the isolation of sufferers in purpose-built hospitals. These specialist pox hospitals took different forms in different regions of Europe. In the German lands, for example, confraternities and city councils were active in financing small institutions that offered specialized forms of treatment for the disease. After the Reformation, and the consequent dissolution of confraternities that had a religious basis, most German pox hospitals came under the supervision of the local authorities – though some hit hard times owing to a lack of proper funding (Jütte, 1996, pp.105–6). Elsewhere, provision of help to those affected by the pox was left to the initiative of private individuals and religious orders. In Italy, there was a degree of hesitation on the part of health boards to take active measures against the pox. A possible explanation for this lack of action is that it reflected both the general feelings of uncertainty surrounding the disease – people thought it might disappear as quickly as it had appeared – and its slow progression, which contrasted with the immediate threat to life posed by the plague (Arrizabalaga *et al.*, 1997). Many Italian hospitals for the sick poor provided good standards of care, but tended to have strict admission policies and often refused admission to those suffering from the pox or other contagious or **chronic** diseases. Even where special wards for syphilitics were created, these would quickly fill up, leaving hundreds of sufferers to their own devices. As you saw in Chapter 4, in the late sixteenth century, the Catholic response to the Reformation led to the establishment of new religious orders and to a new wave of lay devotion. This coincided with the height of the pox epidemic. Sufferers of the pox, for whom obtaining medical treatment by normal means was difficult, became an obvious target for the charitable urges provoked by this increase in piety. The sores and sufferings of the afflicted represented an irresistible call for action as well as a novel vehicle of salvation. Wealthy individuals, in particular, found in them a new arena in which to display their munificence. Money was raised to establish and run special hospitals, which opened across Catholic Italy and came to be known as 'hospitals for the incurables'.

It would be easy, but anachronistic, to describe the German hospitals as publicly funded and the Italian hospitals as privately funded. The dichotomy between private and public with which we are familiar today was not evident in the early modern period. The wealthy families in the Italian cities who gave money to these hospitals were more often than not either part of, or well connected to, the governing elite. It was through these personal links (at one and the same time both public and private) that grants and tax privileges for the new hospitals were established.

So far, I have shown how many of the measures taken to contain contagious diseases revolved around the management of the sick poor, whether by authorities that worried about the spread of contagion or by charitable institutions that provided help and treatment. The provision of health care for the poor, however, was not limited to times of epidemics, and it increasingly became a major component in poor relief schemes in both Catholic and Protestant countries. These were implemented by a range of bodies, including parishes, trade guilds, municipal authorities and religious orders. Medical assistance came in various forms, from outdoor relief (where food and medicine were distributed to the poor in their homes, and physicians and apothecaries were paid to treat them) to hospital care. But in all these schemes, a distinction was always made between the 'deserving' and the 'undeserving' poor. Based on economic as well as moral criteria, this distinction came to play an increasingly important role in the perception, and management, of poverty. The deserving poor included all those who were regarded as victims of their condition. Among these were people of rank who had fallen on hard times as well as skilled artisans and urban labourers, who frequently received the support of the guilds and confraternities to which many of them belonged. They were rigorously distinguished from the undeserving poor, such as beggars, vagrants and prostitutes, who were allegedly to blame for their condition and were regarded with increasing moral loathing and intolerance.

Scholars are agreed that this distinction between the deserving and the undeserving poor became more marked throughout Europe during the course of the seventeenth century. Those categorized as undeserving became the target of increasingly strict policies, which essentially aimed at confining and disciplining them. Keep in mind these developments as I now turn to examine the specific role played by hospitals in the provision of health care to the poor between 1500 and 1800. Examples taken from sixteenth-century Florence, seventeenth-century France and eighteenth-century England will allow me to discuss continuities and changes in their organization, structure and activities.

6.3   Hospitals

For a long time, historians argued that early modern hospitals were filthy, abominable places where the poor simply went to die. This view was modified somewhat in the work of the influential French scholar Michel Foucault (1965), who categorized hospitals as essentially repressive institutions where the poor were confined, if not to die, then to be kept out of sight and forced to work. In both interpretations, medical activities carried out in hospitals before the end of the eighteenth century have been left out of the picture. A number of recent studies, however, have painted a different picture in which the medical activities of early modern hospitals are fully recognized (Jones, 1996b; Kinzelbach, 2001; Park, 1991).

In the Middle Ages, hospitals were run by members of religious orders as shelters for the poor and for those bereft of family support. In addition, they provided short-term accommodation for travellers, pilgrims and the elderly. Sick people were also among the inmates, but the main function of a hospital was to offer food, accommodation and religious comfort rather than medical assistance. By the end of the fifteenth century, this began to change. It is now becoming clear that, from an early date, poor patients voluntarily went to a hospital to undergo some form of medical treatment, and many recovered sufficiently to be discharged. Starting in northern and central Italy, hospitals began to take on a more therapeutic function, and this model rapidly spread to other parts of Europe.

Exercise

Now read 'Healing the poor: hospitals in Renaissance Florence' (Source Book 1, Reading 6.4) and then answer the following questions:

1   Who were the patients of the hospitals of Santa Maria Nuova (Figure 6.4) and San Paolo?

2   What do these categories of patients tell us about health care in early sixteenth-century Florence?

Discussion

1   By analysing the admission records of the two hospitals, Katharine Park makes a distinction between male and female patients and argues that the majority of the

male patients were suffering from **acute** diseases, which though serious, were often curable. The most frequent diagnosis was 'fever', followed by skin conditions and then wounds and fractures. The time they spent in hospital was relatively short and the rate of mortality low. These hospitals did not care for chronically ill men or for those with contagious diseases (though patients with the pox were admitted). By contrast, records from Santa Maria Nuova suggest that women tended to stay longer – some even for several years. This indicates that, in contrast to the male patients, the female patients were not suffering from acute diseases.

2   On this evidence, Park concludes that, as early as the beginning of the sixteenth century, these hospitals were providing free medical care to a specific category of men – labourers, who constituted the bulk of the workforce of Renaissance Florence. The health of these workers was crucial to the urban economy, and institutions such as Santa Maria Nuova and San Paolo made sure that sick or injured labourers received the care and treatment needed for them to recover quickly. For women, the situation seems to have been different. This was probably the result of contemporary demographic trends, in particular the fact that Florence contained many poor widows, who were economically vulnerable and subject to chronic, rather than acute, illnesses. In the case of women, therefore, the hospital functioned as a hospice as well as a medical institution. Overall, Park stresses that the main goal of these institutions was not to confine or repress the poor, but to offer help, including medical treatment, to those who could not otherwise afford it. At the same time, such activities had a specific political function, as they met the economic needs of a city whose wealth depended on artisans and labourers.

Other evidence used by Park to argue for the medical nature of the care provided in these Florentine hospitals is the range of medical practitioners employed in them. These included surgeons, apothecaries and even physicians of renown. Many Italian hospitals offered a wide range of medical posts, and were regarded by surgeons and physicians as good places to start, and to consolidate, their careers.

Of what did the medical care provided in hospitals consist? An appropriate diet was the most important element in any contemporary medical treatment; money spent on food thus often constitutes the largest sum in a hospital account book of this period, though ingredients to make drugs were also regularly purchased. Early modern hospitals often had well-equipped pharmacies, where drugs were prepared and stored, and which sometimes specialized in the preparation of specific drugs. For example, the pharmacy at the Santo Spirito hospital in Rome achieved widespread fame in the late seventeenth century for its manufacture of a drug based on chinchona bark, which originated from South America and was extensively employed in cases of fever. Although physicians might devote some attention to the humoral make-up of their hospital patients, it is likely that they standardized their treatments, including the drugs they prescribed, much more than they did in the case of their private patients.

From the late sixteenth century onwards, there was a general trend towards hospital specialization. The most common type of hospital was that which provided

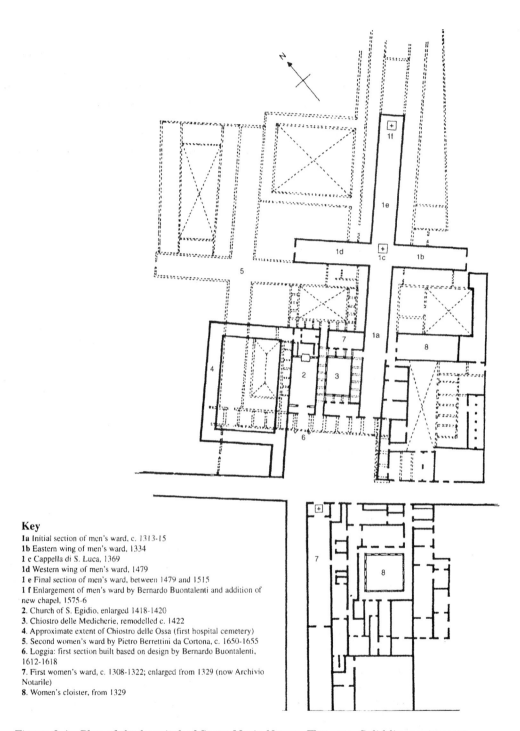

Key

1a Initial section of men's ward, c. 1313-15
1b Eastern wing of men's ward, 1334
1 c Cappella di S. Luca, 1369
1d Western wing of men's ward, 1479
1 e Final section of men's ward, between 1479 and 1515
1 f Enlargement of men's ward by Bernardo Buontalenti and addition of new chapel, 1575-6
2. Church of S. Egidio, enlarged 1418-1420
3. Chiostro delle Medicherie, remodelled c. 1422
4. Approximate extent of Chiostro delle Ossa (first hospital cemetery)
5. Second women's ward by Pietro Berrettini da Cortona, c. 1650-1655
6. Loggia: first section built based on design by Bernardo Buontalenti, 1612-1618
7. First women's ward, c. 1308-1322; enlarged from 1329 (now Archivio Notarile)
8. Women's cloister, from 1329

Figure 6.4   Plan of the hospital of Santa Maria Nuova, Florence. Solid lines represent construction *c*.1500. In the later buildings, notice that both the male and the female wards form the shape of a cross; the male ward has a chapel in the middle. (The female ward was originally built on the other side of the road.) The hospital also incorporated a church, several courtyards and a cemetery. Reproduced from Henderson (2001), p.193

care to poor people who were suffering from acute and curable diseases. Then, as you have seen, there were the more specialized institutions that catered for those who had contagious diseases such as the plague and the pox. Finally, there were those new institutions for the chronically disabled and other categories of social and moral outcasts who either would not or could not work. In France, for example, roughly two hundred of these institutions, called *hôpitaux-généraux*, were established in the late seventeenth and eighteenth centuries as part of a major reorganization, and concentration, of poor relief. In them, vagrants, prostitutes, beggars and the insane, as well as gypsies and members of religious minorities, were confined and subjected to intense moral and religious re-education, a substantial part of which included forced labour (Brockliss and Jones, 1997, pp.678–88; Jütte, 1994). Though some inmates were sick, and doctors made regular visits to these establishments, they were not really intended to provide medical care. Instead, they combined the functions of a workhouse with those of a home for the elderly, the disabled and the chronically sick. At the same time, institutions more specifically dedicated to providing medical care for acute and non-contagious illnesses retained their old name of *hôtels-dieu*. Of course, such a distinction between institutions was not achieved overnight, neither was it equally implemented across Europe, and hospitals that did not have a strict admission policy remained common throughout the early modern period.

Exercise

Now read 'Caring for the sick poor: St Bartholomew's Hospital, London (1653)' (Source Book 1, Reading 6.5) and then answer the following questions:

1 Why were the governors discontented?

2 What kind of hospital was St Bartholomew's becoming?

Discussion

1 From the hospital minutes it emerges that, traditionally, patients who could walk were given money to go out and buy their own food rather than having their meals provided by the hospital. However, instead of purchasing 'good' food, as the governors intended, the minutes indicate that they either saved the money or spent it on 'bad' food and beer. This was not acceptable to the governors, who therefore decided to impose stricter controls.

2 That the hospital had traditionally handed out money testifies to the fact that it functioned as part of a broader scheme of poor relief. By the middle of the seventeenth century, however, concern for the inmates' health combined with moral unease about bad 'habits', had led the governors to call for tougher rules. Instead of just supplying inmates with the means to live, the hospital was becoming increasingly focused on providing them with medical treatment (in this case in the form of food, but food was often a substantial part of therapy), and on enforcing a stricter code of discipline and conduct.

The extract is from the minutes of the Board of Governors, so we can take it as a faithful description of the arguments the governors put forward. On the other hand, governors had their own agenda and, in their discussions, they might have exaggerated the patients' behaviour to justify the imposition of stricter regulations. It would be interesting to contrast this source with patients' accounts of life in the hospital, but, as I discuss later, to reconstruct the perspective of early modern hospital patients is very difficult.

Body and soul

You might be tempted to think that as medical activities intensified in hospitals, their original religious mission receded. This is, however, far from the case (Henderson, 2001). Until at least the mid-eighteenth century, hospitals remained places for the cure of the soul as well as of the body. The Christian significance of bearing suffering and physical misery was evoked regularly in both Protestant and Catholic hospitals, where religious services or masses were held daily. You saw in Chapter 4 that, in Catholic countries, part of the response to the Reformation was the founding of new religious orders, uniquely devoted to the care of the sick. Such religious nursing orders placed particular emphasis on the spiritual functions of a hospital – on helping patients to die free from sin, so that they might enter heaven, and therefore on ensuring they made a final confession and took the sacraments. How did the members of such religious nursing orders relate to the medical staff – surgeons, apothecaries, physicians – who worked alongside them in hospitals? Research carried out by the historian Colin Jones on various French hospitals in the seventeenth and eighteenth centuries has revealed a very interesting picture. He has shown, for example, the wide range of activities carried out by the members of the Daughters of Charity, a religious nursing order established in Paris in 1633. In addition to providing spiritual comfort and attending to patients' physical needs, the nuns also carried out various medical tasks. For example, they prepared drugs – they sometimes ran the hospital pharmacies – and might also perform minor surgical operations (Plate 8). As a rule, late seventeenth- and eighteenth-century doctors spent little time with each patient, and 'for the rest of the day, sisters of charity filled the vacuum in hospital medical services'. Members of the order were trained at their mother houses according to the principles of the learned medical tradition and 'were often viewed as providing a more appropriate form of medical care than formally qualified practitioners' (Jones, 1996b, pp.66, 67). Of course, they were also guided by their firm religious convictions. This often meant that they sought to exclude those tainted by sin, for example syphilitics and prostitutes.

Although religious nursing orders such as the Daughters of Charity took an active role in the provision of medical treatment, their concerns increasingly differed from those of physicians. In the eighteenth century, for example, physicians began to see hospitals as sites of medical teaching. Medical students attended bedside lectures, observed patients and attended the post-mortem dissections that their teachers, the hospital physicians, were increasingly keen to carry out. Jones shows that, in the French hospitals he studied, one area in particular led to frequent clashes between the nursing sisters and the doctors. The sisters persisted in regarding the patients' souls, as well as their bodies, as the focus of their concern, and so objected to the doctors performing post-mortems on those who had died.

Physicians finally succeeded in dominating hospital life in the nineteenth century. Until that time, however, they were just one group among many – including nurses, benefactors and administrators – who both cooperated and competed with each other in the day-to-day running of the hospital.

Charity, medicine and the wealth of a nation

The **voluntary hospital** movement, a pre-eminently British institution, vividly illustrates the many purposes that hospitals continued to serve in the eighteenth century. Voluntary hospitals were based on the principle that private individuals freely contributed towards the hospital's foundation and running costs. In return for this financial commitment, subscribers enjoyed the right to be involved in hospital affairs. They were allowed to put forward a certain number of people for admission as patients, who were then entitled to receive medical care free of charge. If their donation was above a certain amount, subscribers also acquired the right to be appointed to the hospital's board of governors. Although humanitarian and religious concerns certainly played their part in this philanthropic movement, the more tangible benefits are clear to see. Being a subscriber allowed people with means – including members of the newly emerging middle classes, who had made their money from the expansion of trade in this period – to exercise patronage over grateful beneficiaries while at the same time it provided them with valuable opportunities to network with other benefactors, many of whom were rich and powerful. Since the late Middle Ages, hospitals had been associated with such individuals. The voluntary hospital movement of the eighteenth century thus extended membership of these institutions to more people than ever before. During the course of the eighteenth century, almost forty new voluntary hospitals were founded in Britain (Woodward, 1974) (Figure 6.5).

An important consequence of the fact that the admission of patients to such hospitals was dependent upon a patron's recommendation was that the patient's credentials and conduct were susceptible to close scrutiny. While the deserving poor could get all the help they needed, the undeserving poor and those who faked illness to obtain free bed and board were more easily detected, and this minimized the risks of wasting resources on those deemed unworthy of medical assistance.

Since the late seventeenth century, political philosophers and advisers had argued that the prosperity of a country depended on its having a large and active population. The size of the population became a measure of a country's strength. Building on such theories, in the eighteenth century, work came to be regarded as the key component in a country's affluence. This had important implications for attitudes towards poor relief. A rigorous work ethic was promoted at all levels and, while workhouses were established to put the healthy but feckless poor to work, hospitals were increasingly expected to restore to health those in the workforce who had succumbed to acute, but curable, diseases. To maintain, improve and restore the health of the workforce acquired an economic and political significance, even if in Britain, unlike other major European countries such as France and the German lands, the initiative remained primarily in private hands, with the government, on a local or national level, playing no part in the process.

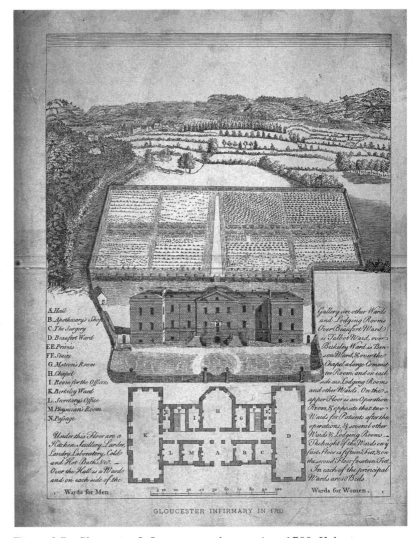

The labels on the engraving read:

A. Hall
B. Apothecary's Shop
C. The Surgery
D. Beaufort Ward
E.E. Privies
F.F. Stairs
G. Matron's Room
H. Chapel
I. Room for the Officers
K. Berkeley Ward
L. Secretary's Office
M. Physician's Room
N. Passage

Under this Floor are a Kitchen, Scullery, Larder, Landry, Laboratory, Cold and Hot Baths &c. — Over the Hall is a Ward, and on each side of the

Wards for Men

Gallery are other Wards and Lodging Rooms. Over Beaufort Ward is Talbot Ward, over Berkeley Ward is Benson Ward, & over the Chapel a large Committee Room, and on each side are Lodging Rooms and other Wards. On the upper Floor is an Operation Room, & opposite that two Wards for Patients after the operations, & several other Wards & Lodging Rooms. The height of the Wards on ye first Floor is fifteen feet, & on the second Floor fourteen Feet. In each of the principal Wards are 13 Beds.

Wards for Women.

GLOUCESTER INFIRMARY IN 1760

Figure 6.5 Gloucester Infirmary, wood engraving, 1760. Voluntary hospitals such as this were often designed by well-known architects. Gloucester Infirmary was designed to resemble a great country-house of the period – notice the extensive park surrounding it. Wellcome Library, London

Exercise

Now read 'The establishment of the county hospital at Winchester (1736)' (Source Book 1, Reading 6.6) and then answer the following questions:

1   According to this document, what were the main benefits to the community in investing in this charitable new enterprise?

2   How, in the opinion of the document's author, were the poor likely to benefit from admission to the new hospital?

1　The main advantage of donating to a voluntary hospital was that it fostered economic rationality. Unlike 'random' charity, where donations were wasted for the lack of clear and well-planned goals, voluntary hospitals offered the possibility of judicious and economically sound generosity. By gathering needy people in one place, it was possible to make the most of the money while reducing the risks of mismanagement, which, according to this account, was a common problem in other charitable schemes. The presence of medical personnel guaranteed that fakes would be unmasked, and donors were reassured that their money would be spent only on those who deserved it. Moreover, by caring for a sick family member, hospitals allowed the rest of the family to carry on being industrious and productive. While the physical cure of patients contributed to the growth of the population ('a means of increasing the number of the People'), the moral and spiritual reform of the poor was an additional element in the fight against idleness.

2　The admission of poor people to hospital, where they could be provided with food and medicine on site, was seen as a major advantage over giving them money. The phrase 'the Evils that are common to the Poor' was an implicit reference to the misuse of money by the poor (to buy alcohol or unwholesome food) – a problem that also concerned the governors of St Bartholomew's, in Reading 6.5. The author also argued that, by employing university-trained physicians or licensed practitioners, hospitals prevented poor people from falling into the clutches of quacks and gave them the opportunity to undergo 'medical education'. In addition, the poor were subjected to moral and religious edification, and removed from the presence of 'bad examples'. Finally, feelings of gratitude to their superiors were reinforced.

Voluntary hospitals clearly formed an integral part of social policy in the eighteenth century, alongside workhouses, outdoor medical assistance in the form of medical dispensaries, and alms distribution through parishes and Poor Law authorities. Importantly, the presence of such hospitals relieved parishes of the burden of caring for the sick, making it easier for them to focus on the needs of orphans and old people. In the booming eighteenth-century British economy, the call to rationalize charity sounded particularly well in the ears of benefactors increasingly used to optimizing their investments (Porter, 1989). At the same time, we should not underestimate the religious and moral commitment of those who subscribed to voluntary hospitals, for whom self-interest and Christian philanthropy often went hand in hand (Fissell, 1992).

The poor as patients

So far, I have discussed hospitals from several different perspectives, but that of one important group is still missing: the patients. Because patients' accounts of hospital life in the early modern period are notoriously thin on the ground, historians have turned to other sources. These include hospital registers, which became more detailed and accurate in the eighteenth century, and the notebooks of medical students, who, as you have seen, were increasingly attracted to hospitals

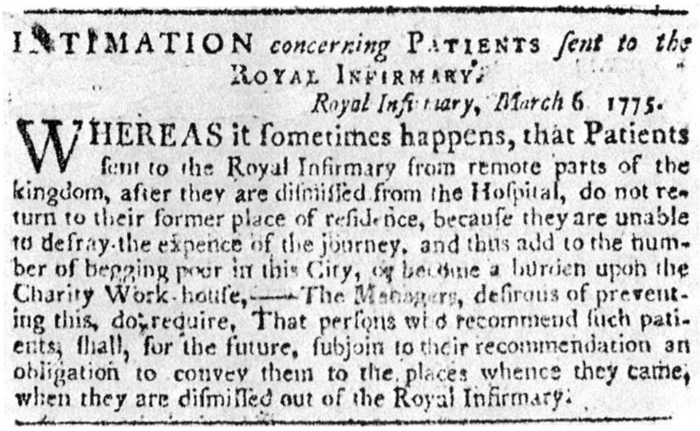

INTIMATION *concerning* **PATIENTS** *sent to the*
ROYAL INFIRMARY.
Royal Infirmary, March 6. 1775.

WHEREAS it sometimes happens, that Patients
sent to the Royal Infirmary from remote parts of the
kingdom, after they are dismissed from the Hospital, do not return to their former place of residence, because they are unable
to defray the expence of the journey, and thus add to the number of begging poor in this City, or become a burden upon the
Charity Work-house,——The Managers, desirous of preventing this, do require, That persons who recommend such patients, shall, for the future, subjoin to their recommendation an
obligation to convey them to the places whence they came,
when they are dismissed out of the Royal Infirmary.

Figure 6.6   When patients were discharged from voluntary hospitals, they often
lacked the money to return to the place from which they had come, and consequently
added to the number of beggars in the city. To reduce the burden on local
workhouses, the governing body of the Edinburgh Royal Infirmary decided to ask
sponsors also to pay for the cost of returning to their own homes the patients they
had recommended for admission. Advertisement from the *Edinburgh Evening
Courant*, 8 March 1775. Reproduced from Risse (1986), p.83

for on-the-job training. Both types of document have been extensively used to
throw light on the daily routine of patients and the treatment they received. Here I
draw extensively on the work of the historian Guenter Risse (1999) in relation to
the Edinburgh Royal Infirmary.

The Royal Infirmary – a voluntary hospital – opened in Edinburgh in the 1740s. It
was housed in an entirely new, four-storey building, and replaced a much smaller
hospital, which had been founded in 1729. The building comprised a central
admissions room, several separate wards, lodging for the nurses, a kitchen and a
pharmacy, as well as an amphitheatre, which was used for lectures, surgery and
religious services. The city was prosperous and donations were generous: in
addition to donations from a wide range of private benefactors, the hospital
received money from the city guilds and the church (Figure 6.6). The hospital also
had the full backing of the local college of physicians and of the university medical
faculty. Edinburgh was fast becoming one of the most important and lively centres
of medical education in the British Isles. The construction of this large hospital
improved the teaching facilities and helped young physicians to expand their skills.

Exercise

Now read 'The medicalisation of the hospital in Enlightenment Edinburgh,
1750–1800: the case of Janet Williamson (1772)' (Source Book 1, Reading 6.7)
and then answer the following questions:

1   What took place during the admission process?

2   Why was Professor Cullen interested in Janet Williamson's case?

3   What treatment did Janet receive?

1   Janet Williamson was a servant who had little or no family in Edinburgh. Feeling unwell, she applied to the infirmary for help. Admission was a two-stage process and took place in a purpose-built room. First, a patient had to prove that he or she was worthy of assistance. Janet presumably had a letter of recommendation which testified that she had a sponsor and therefore was deserving of admission; however, the name of her patron is not recorded. Risse suggests that her master may have contributed to the hospital's Servants' Fund. The second step was a medical check. The physician had to verify that she really was sick – faking an illness was a practice abhorred by the governors. The medical check also determined whether her symptoms matched the range of diseases that the hospital was prepared to treat. The hospital's policy was to avoid admitting patients who were suffering from incurable or contagious diseases. Two points worth noting are the entirely secular nature of the admission process and the complexity of the record-keeping.

2   Professor William Cullen, who taught medicine at the university, was also in charge of the teaching ward at the infirmary. Janet was suffering from fever, and was admitted during a period in which Cullen was preparing a series of lectures on this disease. Cullen was keen to select interesting cases to present to his students, and so Janet was admitted to the teaching ward, where his lectures took place.

3   Janet was seen by Cullen, who took her pulse and prescribed bloodletting, emetics, enemas – still among the most popular medical procedures – and a special diet. A nurse looked after her, especially when she was delirious, and gave her regular **fomentations** of the legs and feet. Bloodletting was carried out by medical students. To treat Janet's cough, Cullen prescribed an **expectorant**, and he also ordered a blister to be raised on her back. Blistering was a time-honoured remedy to stimulate the body's reaction to a fever, but Cullen offered a new explanation for its efficacy. The treatment that Janet received seems to have been extremely thorough, and was probably no different from that which Cullen offered to his wealthy private clients.

So, the reason we know so much about Janet Williamson is because Cullen used the details of her case as teaching material, basing his lectures on the medical notes of patients in the ward register. However, this is probably the closest we can ever hope to get to the actual experience of patients in an eighteenth-century hospital. Even Risse, who investigated this subject in great depth, was forced to admit that many of his conclusions were the fruit of guesswork.

As the century drew to an end, and physicians gained the upper hand in hospitals, the use of patients as teaching material became normal practice, and the relationship between medicine and poverty took a new turn. Historians have argued that, in the nineteenth century, hospital patients – a group of people who usually had no family connections or means of support – became the object of growing medical experimentation. Fundamental changes in medical knowledge and practice took place in hospitals, including new ways of examining patients and regular post-mortem dissections, which in turn led to the establishment of a new discipline: pathological anatomy. These changes have been hailed as among the most important medical advances of their time, and it was the bodies of the hospitalized poor that made them possible (Risse, 1999, pp.329–31).

6.4 Public health in the eighteenth century: the Habsburg territories and the German lands

As fundamental institutions for the provision of care, hospitals are part of the history of health policies. Yet, as you saw from the measures taken to fight the plague, policies relating to health could also include attempts on the part of the authorities to intervene in other areas. For example, some anti-plague measures involved efforts to control the environment and to regulate trades and commerce. In the eighteenth century, the fiercest epidemics were in decline, but diseases such as smallpox were becoming endemic. A change can be detected across Europe, whereby in addition to policies that focused on the needs of local communities, national governments also concerned themselves with the health and welfare of the population at large. In some places, for example in the territories ruled by the Habsburg dynasty, and in the German lands, specific political conditions made it possible for comprehensive health policies to be designed, even if these were not always implemented. In this section, I shall take a brief look at these developments.

The connection between health and environment is discussed in more detail in Chapter 11.

As the economies of most European countries steadily expanded, there arose a new belief in the possibility that the conditions of humankind could be improved by the implementation of rational measures. Constant progress and amelioration were now regarded as the key features of human history. Under the influence of the movement known as the Enlightenment, some political authorities started to adopt policies based on these optimistic premises. One of the main focuses of state intervention was health, since, as you have already seen, a growing and an active population was regarded as the most important contributory factor to a country's economic and political strength.

Under the rule of Maria Theresa (1740–80) and her son Joseph II (1780–90), the vast territories that constituted the Habsburg Empire became one of the laboratories of 'enlightened despotism', a political project based on the Enlightenment creed. It was characterized by the confidence that an absolutist and centralized political power could act in the best interest of the population by introducing – sometimes imposing – a series of political and social reforms that were inspired by the new ideas. **Absolute states**, such as those of the Habsburgs, were paternalistic – that is, they tended to regard their subjects, especially those of the lower classes, as if they needed looking after in all aspects of their lives. Such regimes therefore gave their subjects strict guidelines and rules to follow. Improvements in the sphere of health might be achieved in many ways, including programmes of public hygiene and control over the environment, housing and water supply. Increasingly, the state also claimed that areas traditionally left to personal or cultural choice (such as marriage or pregnancy) were of public and political concern and thus susceptible to regulation. (It was proposed, for example, that people with abnormalities or diseases should be prevented from getting married.)

You may remember that physicians were not asked to sit on the health boards of the early modern Italian states; their role was mainly confined to giving advice. In the eighteenth century, 'medicine experienced nearly a quantum leap in the range of its mission' (Risse, 1992, p.172), as doctors became increasingly sought after as experts and advisers. Thus, the image of the physician as a legislator – that is, someone who oversaw or contributed to the making of law – became popular. Together with political philosophers, physicians in the Habsburg territories and the German lands made an important contribution to the formation of a system that came to be known as 'medical police'. This comprised 'the creation of systematic medical policy and its implementation through administrative regulation' (Rosen, 1974, p.138). Physicians found in an absolutist state the best ally in their efforts to broaden their fields of competence.

It was in the work of the Austrian physician Johann Peter Frank (1745–1821), in particular his *System einer vollständigen medicinischen Polizey* [A Complete System of Medical Police] (1779–1826), that state intervention on health issues was most thoroughly and strenuously advanced. Among the topics he discussed were the promotion of marriage (including the proposal of a bachelor tax); support for childbearing (for example by offering financial help to poor mothers); the supervision of children's education (including regulations concerning school buildings, and their ventilation and heating); and public hygiene (including control over such aspects as food production, the disposal of rubbish, and street cleaning).

With the proliferation of ideas such as these, the figure of the *physicus* (an official who had responsibility for public health issues) acquired new importance in the German-speaking lands. Since the Middle Ages, German urban authorities, like Italian ones, had traditionally appointed a 'city physician' who would accomplish a range of tasks, including caring for the poor, giving expert testimony at court, monitoring public hygiene and providing advice in time of epidemics. In the eighteenth century, new regulations insisted that each administrative district (composed of a main city and its rural surroundings) should have a *physicus*, whose duties included the gathering of medical information about diseases (both animal and human), the collection of statistics relating to births and deaths, and the assumption of overall control over the whole range of healing practices (often deemed as 'superstitious') in the community. The revitalization of this medical office has traditionally been interpreted as evidence of the success of reformist, centralized and 'modern' political regimes in Enlightenment German lands. However, the ideal of the centralized bureaucratic state did not really develop in the German lands until the mid-nineteenth century. Recent research has shown that in the eighteenth-century German state, the role of the *physicus* was in fact constrained by a complex web of competing authorities and vested interests – local communities, notables, physicians, other practitioners and representatives of the state (Lindemann, 1996). It was in this intricate and multilayered social and political system, rather than in an ideal 'enlightened' political arena, that health policies were formulated and implemented.

The organization and practice of health care in the eighteenth century is discussed in Chapter 13.

That things were more complicated than previously thought is true even for the authoritative plan of Frank himself. It remained influential and was regarded as a model by all those concerned with health policy, but in practice it was implemented only on a limited scale. Moreover, his detailed scheme was the outcome of very specific economic and social conditions. When the industrialization process posed new challenges to both the people's health and the public response to them, it quickly became outdated.

6.5 Conclusion

Well before the modern state as we know it today took shape, political powers have paid attention to what have come to be known as public health issues. In the early modern period, the focus of their intervention was mainly on the prevention and the containment of plague epidemics. Sophisticated measures were routinely implemented, and these were based on the contemporary understanding of the causes of the disease, including the link between poverty, sin and plague. Health policies increasingly became the object of political concern and proved highly attractive to those governments that wished to extend control over every aspect of the lives of their subjects, particularly in the absolutist regimes of seventeenth- and eighteenth-century Europe. This was especially the case in the eighteenth century, when social and political commentators, inspired by economic concerns as well as by the humanitarian aspirations of the Enlightenment, demonstrated the benefits of a healthy and expanding population.

This emphasis on the 'modern-looking' aspects of early modern approaches to public health and welfare should not obscure the fact that, when confronted with the problem of how to make sense of the diseases of the past, including their prevention and cure, we still need to engage with the moral and religious codes of belief and practice that fundamentally shaped this earlier world. The case of the pox is particularly illuminating. Charity remained the key factor in the provision of health care over the centuries, though the motives for, and practice of, charitable giving changed over time. Private benefactors and religious orders interacted in various ways with the political authorities, and the best way to appreciate this is to look at the changing role of hospitals in this period. The history of hospitals is a thriving field of scholarly endeavour, and much is now known about their organization and finances, as well as the various purposes they served. Historians have unearthed a great deal of information about who worked in them, how the different personnel interacted, and what patients gained from the experience, though recovery of the patient's perspective remains elusive.

Finally, I have highlighted the role played by medical experts in the provision of health to communities. For much of the early modern period, they were forced to work alongside a host of other 'experts', including administrators and other interested parties. By the end of the eighteenth century, however, their status was much enhanced, their advice widely sought, and their control of medical space, particularly the hospital, secured. The way was now clear for the emergence of a new and more powerful medical profession in the nineteenth century.

References

Arrizabalaga, J., Henderson, J. and French, R. (1997) *The Great Pox: The French Disease in Renaissance Europe*, New Haven and London: Yale University Press.

Brockliss, L. and Jones, C. (1997) *The Medical World of Early Modern France*, Oxford: Clarendon Press.

Cipolla, C. (1981) *Fighting the Plague in Seventeenth-Century Italy*, Madison, WI and London: University of Wisconsin Press.

Cook, H. (1989) 'Policing the health of London: the College of Physicians and the early Stuart monarchy', *Social History of Medicine*, vol.2, pp.1–33.

Cunningham, A. (1992) 'Transforming plague: the laboratory and the identity of infectious disease' in A. Cunningham and P. Williams (eds) *The Laboratory Revolution in Medicine*, Cambridge: Cambridge University Press, pp.209–44.

Cunningham, A.R. and Grell, O.P. (2000) *The Four Horsemen of the Apocalypse: Religion, War, Famine and Death in Reformation Europe*, Cambridge: Cambridge University Press.

Eamon, W. (1998) 'Cannibalism and contagion: framing syphilis in Counter-Reformation Italy', *Early Science and Medicine*, vol.3, pp.1–31.

Fissell, M.E. (1992) 'Charity universal? Institutions and moral reform in eighteenth-century Bristol' in L. Davison, T. Hitchcock, T. Keim and R. Shoemaker (eds) *Stilling the Grumbling Hive: The Response to Social and Economic Problems in England, 1689–1750*, Stroud: Alan Sutton, pp.121–44.

Foucault, M. (1965) *Madness and Civilization: A History of Insanity in the Age of Reason*, translated by R. Howard, New York: Pantheon Books.

Gilman, S.L. (1988) *Disease and Representation: Images of Illness from Madness to Aids*, Ithaca and London: Cornell University Press.

Henderson, J. (2001) 'Healing the body and saving the soul: hospitals in Renaissance Florence', *Renaissance Studies*, vol.15, pp.188–216.

Jones, C. (1996a) 'Plague and its metaphors in early modern France', *Representations*, vol.53, pp.97–127.

Jones, C. (1996b) 'The construction of the hospital patient in early modern France' in N. Finzsch and R. Jütte (eds) *Institutions of Confinement: Hospitals, Asylums, and Prisons in Western Europe and North America, 1500–1950*, Cambridge: Cambridge University Press, pp.55–74.

Jütte, R. (1994) *Poverty and Deviance in Early Modern Europe*, Cambridge: Cambridge University Press.

Jütte, R. (1996) 'Syphilis and confinement: hospitals in early modern Germany' in N. Finzsch and R. Jütte (eds) *Institutions of Confinement: Hospitals, Asylums, and Prisons in Western Europe and North America, 1500–1950*, Cambridge: Cambridge University Press, pp.97–115.

Kinzelbach, A. (2001) 'Hospitals, medicine, and society: southern German imperial towns in the sixteenth century', *Renaissance Studies*, vol.15, pp.217–28.

Lindemann, M. (1996) *Health and Healing in Eighteenth-Century Germany*, Baltimore: Johns Hopkins University Press.

Nutton, V. (1990) 'The reception of Fracastoro's theory of contagion: the seed that fell among thorns?', *Osiris*, vol.6, pp.196–234.

Park, K. (1991) 'Healing the poor: hospitals and medical assistance in Renaissance Florence' in J. Barry and C. Jones (eds) *Medicine and Charity before the Welfare State*, London: Routledge, pp.26–45.

Porter, R. (1989) 'The gift relation: philanthropy and provincial hospitals in eighteenth-century England' in L. Granshaw and R. Porter (eds) *The Hospital in History*, London and New York: Routledge, pp.149–78.

Pullan, B. (1992) 'Plague and perceptions of the poor in early modern Italy' in T. Ranger and P. Slack (eds) *Epidemics and Ideas: Essays in the Historical Perception of Pestilence*, Cambridge: Cambridge University Press, pp.101–23.

Risse, G.B. (1986) *Hospital Life in Enlightenment Scotland*, Cambridge: Cambridge University Press.

Risse, G.B. (1992) 'Medicine in the age of Enlightenment' in A. Wear (ed.) *Medicine in Society*, Cambridge: Cambridge University Press, pp.149–95.

Risse, G.B. (1999) *Mending Bodies, Saving Souls: A History of Hospitals*, Oxford: Oxford University Press.

Rosen, G. (1974) *From Medical Police to Social Medicine: Essays on the History of Health Care*, New York: Science History Publications.

Slack, P. (1985) *The Impact of Plague in Tudor and Stuart England*, London: Routledge & Kegan Paul.

Wear, A. (2000) *Knowledge and Practice in English Medicine, 1550–1680*, Cambridge: Cambridge University Press.

Woodward, J. (1974) *To Do the Sick No Harm: A Study of the British Voluntary Hospital System to 1875*, London: Routledge & Kegan Paul.

Source Book readings

C.M. Cipolla, *Fighting the Plague in Seventeenth-Century Italy*, Madison, WI and London: University of Wisconsin Press, 1981, pp.51–64 (Reading 6.1).

P. Slack, *The Impact of Plague in Tudor and Stuart England*, London: Routledge & Kegan Paul, 1985, pp.295–307 (Reading 6.2).

S. Bradwell, *Physick for the Sicknesse, Commonly Called the Plague*, London: Benjamin Fisher, 1636, pp.5–11 (Reading 6.3).

K. Park, 'Healing the poor: hospitals and medical assistance in Renaissance Florence' in J. Barry and C. Jones (eds) *Medicine and Charity before the Welfare State*, London: Routledge, 1991, pp.31–9 (Reading 6.4).

Minutes of the Meeting of the Board of Governors for St Bartholomew's Hospital, London, 3 January 1653; St Bartholomew's Hospital Archives, Ha 1/5 [Minute Book, 1647–1665], fols 88v–89r (Reading 6.5).

'An account of the establishment of the county hospital at Winchester' in J. Woodward, *To Do the Sick No Harm: A Study of the British Voluntary Hospital System to 1875*, London: Routledge & Kegan Paul, 1974, Appendix 2, pp.149–52 (Reading 6.6).

G.B. Risse, *Mending Bodies, Saving Souls: A History of Hospitals*, Oxford: Oxford University Press, 1999, pp.231–51 (Reading 6.7).

7

Old and New Models of the Body

Silvia De Renzi

Objectives

When you have completed this chapter you should be able to:

* identify the various changes that took place in anatomical and physiological knowledge between 1600 and 1800;

* explain the persistence of holistic notions of the body;

* assess the complex interaction between medical theory and practice;

* describe how medical knowledge was a resource for, and was shaped by, broader cultural perceptions of the body.

7.1   Introduction

In Chapters 4 and 5, you read about the challenge issued by Paracelsus and his followers to the Galenic medical tradition and the Aristotelian natural philosophy that underpinned it. New ideas made some inroads, but the works of Aristotle and Galen continued to provide the foundations of medical instruction in the universities of seventeenth-century Europe as well as the framework within which most learned physicians practised their art. Paracelsus' bold and radical vision of a new medical system, which owed much to a mystical image of the cosmos and its relationship to the human body, was rejected by the medical elite. There were some gains, however: for example, the widespread adoption of remedies obtained from metals by chemical procedures, some of which were integrated into mainstream medical practice.

Paracelsus and his followers may not have succeeded in overturning medical orthodoxy, but scholars agree that their promotion of chemistry in the service of medicine helped pave the way for a series of further and increasingly formidable challenges. By the beginning of the eighteenth century, the Aristotelian system of natural philosophy was finally replaced by new approaches to nature culminating in the mathematical model of the universe associated with Isaac Newton (1642–1727). However, the process of change was much slower and more gradual than the sudden event implied in the term 'scientific revolution' – a term that is widely used by historians to describe this period of transformation, but that has become increasingly controversial.

A key feature of this new approach to nature was its rejection of the four Aristotelian elements. Causation in the natural world, and by implication in the human body, was no longer seen as the product of alterations in the qualities associated with the elements, but was rather explained by recourse to the notion of matter in motion. Following the pioneering work of, among others, René Descartes (1596–1650), matter was now held to consist of particles or atoms, the movement of which produced all action and causation in nature. Unlike Aristotle's elements and qualities, movement could be measured. By 1700, observation, including the deployment of the recently invented microscope, and mathematics, including the use of measuring instruments, provided the key to a new understanding of nature.

In this chapter, I discuss five new 'models of the body' (that is, ways of understanding and representing it), which came into vogue between 1600 and 1800. The five models are based on:

- the discovery of the circulation of the blood by William Harvey in the late 1620s;

- the notion of the body as a machine, as proposed by Descartes in the 1630s;

- the idea that the body was a compound of glands, following studies by Marcello Malpighi (1628–94) in the 1660s;

- the theory that the body could be expressed in mathematical terms, as explored by Newtonian physicians in the first decades of the eighteenth century;

- theories about the nervous system and the 'sensible' body, as propounded by Albrecht von Haller (1708–77) and enthusiastically adopted by many eminent Scottish philosophers and physicians in the mid- to late eighteenth century.

In traditional accounts, these figures and their innovative theories, based on observation and experiment, have been widely celebrated as exemplary manifestations of medical and scientific progress. However, historians of medicine have recently questioned this interpretation for several reasons.

First, many scholars have suggested that the impact of the new theories on the actual practice of medicine was minimal. By the end of the eighteenth century, educated physicians may have learned to describe the body and its activities in increasingly minute anatomical detail, but to cure diseases they continued to prescribe centuries-old remedies such as purges and bloodletting. Moreover, the different parts of the body were regarded as being interconnected; physicians therefore continued to minister to the whole body, and to restore its overall balance, rather than to focus on the cure of its defective parts. Not surprisingly, the question arises as to why physicians who embraced the new theories remained so conservative in their medical practice.

Second, the new theories, which were often accompanied by major anatomical investigations, certainly introduced new concepts and drew the attention of physicians to organs and bodily functions that in the Galenic tradition had received less consideration. But historians are increasingly interested in understanding not just how new theories were proposed, but also to what extent they circulated in society at large, and how far they affected lay people's perception of their bodies, health and sickness. The holistic perception of the body – according to which health and disease depended on an individual's lifestyle and biography, including his or her emotional and spiritual life – was not really challenged by the new theories. To a large extent, the newer, learned models of the body which were taught to university students ran alongside older and perhaps more popular and better understood models.

Finally, historians are increasingly dissatisfied with an account that explains medical theories as primarily the product of philosophical and scientific innovation. Instead, they are more interested in understanding how the new medical and scientific theories were intertwined with broader social and political assumptions about nature and the social order. The models that guided a physician's understanding of the functions of the body are no longer regarded as the outcome of abstract and value-free sets of ideas. Medical theories and representations, or models, of the body are produced at specific times, are shaped by broader social, religious and/or political assumptions, and are often mobilized for purposes other than medical ones – for example, to provide 'scientific' authority for social and political projects. What then, we might ask, were the dominant social and political values that helped to shape the production and reception of new concepts of the body in seventeenth- and eighteenth-century Europe?

With these questions in mind, I explore the five models mentioned above. Rather than just focusing on the technicalities of the medical theories and concepts involved, or assessing how 'innovative' were the investigations on which they rested, I am interested in showing how these models were received by the medical community, to what extent they affected medical practice and also how they circulated outside the medical arena.

7.2   Harvey and the circulation of the blood

In Chapter 3, Sachiko Kusukawa discussed the importance of bloodletting in Renaissance medical practice and showed how the groundbreaking anatomical investigations of Vesalius were rooted in the heated debates surrounding this form of medical intervention. Padua, where Vesalius had taught, remained one of the major centres of medical and anatomical research long after he had left. It was here that Realdo Colombo (d.1559), one of Vesalius' pupils, started the extensive animal **vivisection** that led him to challenge Galen and claim that blood moves from the right to the left ventricle of the heart via the lungs.

Fabricius' 'little doors' are discussed in Chapter 3.

While studying medicine in Padua, the Englishman William Harvey became familiar with Colombo's observations and the anatomical investigations of other Italian physicians, including Fabricius, who had detected 'little doors' (*ostiola*) in the veins. Back in London in 1602, Harvey started a successful medical practice and continued to perform regular dissections. In his investigations, he focused on the heart, which, following Aristotle, he regarded as the body's chief organ. From this starting point, how did Harvey arrive at his audacious conclusion that the blood circulates around the body?

Before discussing this further, let me briefly recap on how Galen explained the production and function of the blood. According to Galen, the body contained two kinds of blood: venous and arterial. The venous blood was produced in the liver from digested food; its prime function was to nourish each part of the body via the system of veins. Some of the venous blood reached the left ventricle of the heart, where it mixed with the *pneuma*, spirits extracted from the air in the lungs, to produce the arterial blood. The arterial blood endowed the body with vitality by means of the arteries – a system of vessels entirely independent of the veins. Both the venous and the arterial blood were 'used up' by the body and had to be constantly replenished, the former in the liver, the latter in the heart.

See Chapters 1 and 3 for discussions of Galen's understanding of blood flow.

Galen also believed that the heart was not involved in moving the blood through the arteries, but that the arteries 'sucked in' blood from the heart, as the heart itself sucked in the venous blood. He thus understood the active phase of the heart's motion to be when it was dilated, or expanded, and did not believe that the heart expelled blood with any great force. (In fact, we now know that the heart contracts with some force to expel blood.) For Galen, therefore, the pulse that could be felt in the arteries was an indication that they too were expanding and contracting, to disperse blood to all parts of the body.

Harvey's experiments led him to question three major features of the Galenic system:

- the idea that the blood was 'used up' by the body and had to be constantly replenished;

- the theory that the heart's main function was to mix the *pneuma* (coming from the lungs) with the venous blood to produce the arterial blood;

- the belief that when the heart dilates, the arteries, which are continuous with the heart, also dilate, and actively 'suck in' and disperse the blood.

A passionate believer in first-hand experience and direct observation, Harvey performed innumerable vivisections on all sorts of animals, concentrating on the movements of the heart. He was struck by the great quantity of arterial blood that left the heart and doubted that it could all be used up by the body. Since the blood vessels did not burst, he naturally wondered where all the blood went. Focusing on the 'little doors' of the veins described by Fabricius, Harvey argued that their structure and position could be accounted for only if their function was to direct blood back to the heart. If the blood returned to the heart, Harvey reasoned, then instead of being constantly produced, the same blood must be used again and again: in other words, it must circulate. To prove his point, he needed to show that the veins and arteries were interconnected – as indeed they are, by the network of what we now call **capillaries**. However, Harvey was working with magnifying lenses that did not allow him to detect these fine structures. Since his predilection for observation could not be satisfied, in his *Exercitatio Anatomica de Motu Cordis et Sanguinis* [Anatomical Exercise on the Movement of the Heart and Blood] (1628) he described a series of experiments by which he could demonstrate that the blood flows out from the heart via the arteries, passes in some way to the veins, and then flows back to the heart again (Figure 7.1). To understand the results of these experiments, you need to know that in the arm, the arteries lie deeper than the veins. By using a very tight ligature, or cord, it is possible to stop blood passing through both veins and arteries. If the ligature is loosened slightly, blood can pass through the arteries, but not the veins. Harvey therefore tied a ligature very tightly around the upper arm, so that no arterial blood could flow

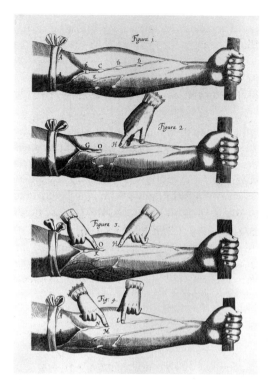

Figure 7.1   Four diagrams from Harvey's *Exercitatio Anatomica de Motu Cordis et Sanguinis*, 1628.
'Figure 1' shows an arm prepared for bloodletting – i.e. with a ligature tightly bound around it to make the veins swell – with letters marking the position of the valves. In 'Figure 2', a finger presses on valve *H*. The section of the vein below valve *H* (i.e. nearer to the heart) is shown to be empty of blood until the next valve along, valve *O*. The blood does not flow back through valve *O*, to fill the vein. In 'Figure 3', one finger presses on valve *H*, stopping the flow towards valve *O*, while another tries to push the blood from below valve *O* towards valve *H* (i.e. towards the periphery). The section of the vein between *O* and *H*, however, remains empty; this must be because the valves are stopping the blood from flowing in this direction. 'Figure 4' shows a section of the vein emptied of blood (labelled *M*) between valve *L* and valve *N*. As long as the finger keeps pressing on valve *L*, the section stays empty. When the finger is raised, however, the vein fills with blood. Harvey's experiment clearly proves that the valves in the veins ensure that the blood flows around the body in one direction only, from the periphery to the heart.
Wellcome Library, London

beyond it to reach the hand. The veins in the arm appeared normal. However, when the ligature was loosened slightly, so that the blood flowed in the arteries but not in the veins, the veins swelled. This could happen only if there were one continuous system of vessels, with the veins and arteries interconnected, and the blood returning from the periphery to the heart. In a further series of experiments, again based on extensive observations, Harvey demonstrated that the blood passed into the lungs, where it was cooled and filtered, and then returned once again to the heart to complete the cycle.

Partly by projecting backwards onto Harvey attitudes that only later came to characterize anatomists' research, scholars for a long time regarded the discovery of the blood's circulation as a striking example of the 'modern' way of thinking, and Harvey as a hero of the scientific revolution. But a more historically sensitive reading of Harvey's works has made scholars more cautious.

Exercise

Now read 'William Harvey and the discovery of the circulation of the blood' (Source Book 1, Reading 7.1).

1   How does Andrew Cunningham explain Harvey's specific interest in the heart?

2   In what sense was the discovery of the circulation a by-product of Harvey's wider research programme?

1   Having been trained in Padua, a major site of Aristotelian natural philosophy, Harvey set out to pursue an essentially Aristotelian inquiry. This led him to focus on the structure and function of a specific organ – the heart – in a range of animals, not just in humans: anatomy rather than medicine was the aim of his investigations. According to Aristotle, the heart was the most important organ: the source of life, growth and sustenance. Yet, in his extensive investigations, Harvey's teacher, Fabricius, had not dealt specifically with the heart. It therefore made sense for him to complete his teacher's work. But Cunningham also indicates, though the argument is just sketched, that it was Harvey's staunch royalism that directed him towards the study of the heart. According to Cunningham, Harvey's anatomical project was driven by old-fashioned principles very similar to those driving his political allegiances.

2   Cunningham stresses that Harvey did not set out with any preconceived intention either to test or to demonstrate a hypothetical circulation of the blood (as in our modern understanding of the scientific method). He was mainly interested in understanding the basic functioning of the heart, and it was only gradually and slowly that he started to think of the circulation as a way to explain a number of issues, such as the presence of valves and the quantity of blood.

Cunningham's intention is not to deny how innovative and far-reaching Harvey's conclusions were, but to understand the philosophical and political framework within which he carried out his observations and experiments. From the reading it is clear that Harvey's model of the body was a completely Aristotelian one. Here, for example, is Harvey's explanation of digestion and excretion:

> For this reason just as the food *designed* to nourish the parts is partly conveyed to them by the digestive *faculty* and partly *attracted* to them and partly seeks them *spontaneously*, so the excrements partly seek a way out, partly sink down to wherever there is a way out and are in part *attracted* and in part expelled ... Just as it is in the world so is it in the *microcosm*, all things are *moved of their own accord to their proper place*.
>
> (quoted in Brown, 1977, p.34; my emphasis)

Following Aristotle, Harvey held that all things in the world move 'of their own accord to their proper place'. In other words, according to a general law of nature, things try to reach their predesignated place. This also applies to the body, revealingly defined by Harvey as the 'microcosm' ('little world'). So, for example, food is 'designed' to nourish the bodily parts; this is its main aim. It follows that food naturally tends to go towards the parts that require nourishment, and that these parts, in turn, naturally 'attract' it. Similarly, because the nature of the excreta is to be expelled, they are attracted towards the bottom of the body and 'seek' a way out. Different parts of the body are endowed with special powers, or 'faculties', and do different things according to what they are designed to do – that is, according to their intrinsic nature.

Despite its debt to Aristotelianism, Harvey's discovery of the circulation of the blood set in motion a series of anatomical investigations that would fundamentally change the map of the body. Consider the liver, which in the Galenic tradition transformed digested food into blood. Harvey showed that venous blood does not flow from the liver towards the extremities, but moves from the periphery back to the heart. Blood is not formed in the liver, but reaches it just as it does any other part of the body. Lively discussions about the actual function of the liver multiplied among Harvey's followers, who carried out extensive anatomical investigations of this organ. The idea that the liver functions as a filter, separating **bile** from the blood, gradually prevailed, though how exactly this separation took place remained controversial for a long time. Another topic that attracted the interest of scholars was the function of the blood. If the blood was constantly circulating, there seemed to be no time for it to be absorbed by the body. How, then, was the body nourished? Was the nutritive function taken on by other fluids? As to the blood, what was it made of? And what was its function? It was to answer questions such as these that anatomists continued to dissect and vivisect hundreds of animals and even tried to transfuse blood from a sheep into a man.

The notion of blood incessantly circulating in the veins and arteries captured the imagination of writers and provided them with an effective metaphor to describe non-medical phenomena. Commenting in 1706 on the booming British economy, the writer Daniel Defoe wrote:

> Manufactures and Trade are in this Nation like the Blood in the Body, they subsist by their Circulation; if once that Motion ceases, is inverted, or otherwise interrupted, it stagnates and corrupts, or breaks out in Torrents beyond its ordinary Course, and these prove infallibly mortal, and incurably contagious to the Life of the Creature.
>
> (1938, p.15)

As to medical practice, the discovery of the blood's circulation certainly had the potential to make meaningless sixteenth-century debates on the location of bloodletting. Some, indeed, expressed the fear that the principles upon which this medical procedure was based might be undermined. Few of those who endorsed the circulation, however, rejected the benefit of bloodletting, while notions of stagnation, corruption and the balance of humours remained the bedrock of medical treatment.

To give you a better sense of how traditional the model of the body at the centre of Harvey's research was, I turn now to consider the work of the Frenchman René Descartes, who knew, and approved of, Harvey's discovery, but whose search for a new philosophical system led him to formulate an extraordinarily original, controversial and very different model of the body.

7.3   The mechanical body

In opposition to most Aristotelian-trained Christian natural philosophers, who believed that the immaterial and immortal soul was the organizing principle of life, Descartes argued that body and soul were completely separate entities. The body was pure matter and the soul, which was possessed by humans only, was nothing but immaterial thought. In his *De Homine* [On Man] (1662) (published in French in 1664 as *Traité de l'homme* [Treatise of Man]), Descartes examined one by one the main physiological processes, including the blood's circulation and sensation (Figure 7.2), and argued that they could all be explained according to the same principles – that is, by the laws regulating the movement of inanimate matter.

Exercise

Now read 'The mechanical body: Descartes on digestion' (Source Book I, Reading 7.2), an extract from his *Traité de l'homme*.

I   How did Descartes describe the process of digestion, and in what way did his description differ from that of Harvey?

2   What image did Descartes use to represent the body and what for him was the body's main living principle?

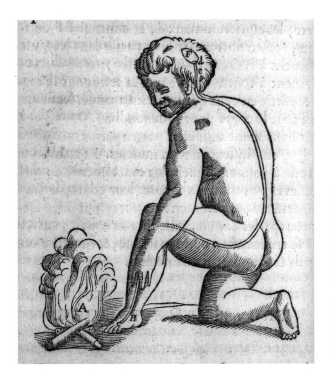

Figure 7.2   This is one of the pictures which illustrated Descartes's mechanical explanation of the muscular reaction to sensation – in this case, the sensation of burning. Particles of the fire, *A*, hit the skin of the foot, *B*, and pull the little thread, *c*, which reaches the inner brain. Thread *c* opens the exit of the short conduit, *de*, allowing the animal spirits in the cavity, *F*, to flow in the opposite direction and act on the muscles, which withdraw the foot from the fire. From Descartes, *Traité de l'homme*, 1664. Wellcome Library, London

1   Descartes represented digestion as a process centred on the movement of food particles through a series of channels. Unlike Harvey, who had invoked the principle that everything in nature moved of its own accord towards its natural place, Descartes argued for a much more local cause of this movement – the mechanical agitation of the stomach, which shook up the particles and heated them. Another key factor was the size of the food particles and the shape of the fibres of the stomach. Descartes explained that the coarser particles were expelled, but that the smallest particles could pass through certain minute holes. The different size of the food particles was the sole cause of their different trajectories. Digestion could therefore be explained as a sequence of local causes and effects which were exactly those regulating any kind of matter in motion. For Descartes, food in the stomach behaved precisely as did flour in a sack.

2   Descartes's pervasive image of the body was that of a mechanical device – a clock, or a more complicated self-moving automaton, both of which were popular in mid-seventeenth-century France. For him, the living principle in the human body was not the soul, but the heat constantly produced in the heart, which generated and communicated movement to all its parts.

Though he never denied the existence of the immaterial soul or of God, many of his contemporaries argued that Descartes's views must ultimately lead to materialism and atheism. The vivid image of an automaton, which he used to describe the body, stirred much controversy (Figure 7.3). Descartes's coherent model of the body nonetheless became enormously influential and was the first real alternative to Aristotelian and Galenic physiology on the one hand, and to the radical spiritualist overtones of Paracelsian and Helmontian medicine on the other. Here, for example, is what the English physician George Castle wrote a few years after the publication of Descartes's treatise:

> It is not, I think, to be question'd, that a man is as Mechanically made as a Watch, or any other Automaton; and that his motions, (the regularity of which we call Health) are perform'd by Springs, Wheels, and Engines, not much differing ... from those pieces of Clock-work, which are to be seen at every Puppet-play ... He ... who considers these works of Art, and compares with them the subtil contrivances of Nature, will certainly rest better satisfied in the Mechanical account of the operations, and diseases of an Animal, than in the *Ens Pagoicum, Cagastricum, Illiastrum, Archaeus* ... and a thousand such conjuring unintelligible words of the Chymists.
>
> (1667, pp.5–6)

Descartes was a philosopher, not a physician, and he pursued anatomical investigations on a limited scale. One of his followers was the Italian mathematician Giovanni Alfonso Borelli (1608–79), who provided an entirely mechanical explanation of bodily movement (Figure 7.4). But Descartes also stirred a great interest among physicians, some of whom strongly believed that dissection was an indispensable step towards making sense of how the 'body machine' worked.

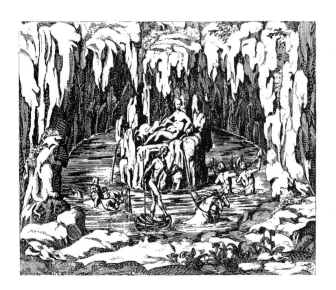

Figure 7.3 Automated garden figures in the grottoes of the royal gardens at Saint-Germain-en-Laye. From an engraving in Salomon de Caus, *Les raisons des forces mouvantes avec diverses machines tant utilles que plaisantes ausquelles sont adjoints plusieurs desseings de grotes et fontaines* [Explanation of Forces of Motion, with Different Machines, Both Useful and Amusing, to which are Joined Several Designs of Grotto and Fountain], 1615. Descartes was very interested in automata, and described the human body in terms of these popular mechanical devices. Reproduced from Descartes (1972)

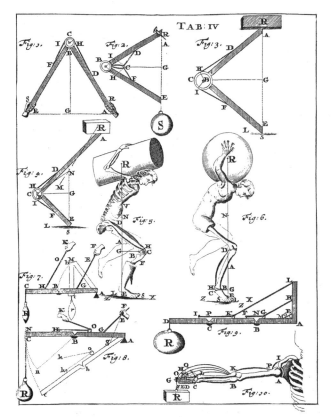

Figure 7.4 Demonstration of joints as a system of levers, from Borelli, *De Motu Animalium* [On the Motion of Animals], 1685. This diagram shows how Borelli reduced the movements of the knee and the hand to a system of pulleys and levers, which he described by means of geometrical drawings. Wellcome Library, London

7.4   Glands everywhere: the body according to Malpighi

One of the leading anatomists of the time was Marcello Malpighi. After a period spent teaching medicine in various Italian universities, in 1666 Malpighi settled in Bologna, where he obtained the chair of practical medicine. As well as carrying out anatomical dissections on a massive scale, he cultivated international relationships. One of these was with the Royal Society in London, which at that time was promoting a vast programme of research into natural phenomena.

Malpighi was familiar with Descartes's mechanical model, and he also knew that the recently invented microscope could help him put that model on firmer observational ground. Magnifying lenses had been used in investigations into nature since the beginning of the seventeenth century. As different types of microscope were made available over the next hundred years, anatomists increasingly turned their attention to the fine rather than the gross structure of the body. The latter had been the focus of Vesalius' studies, but the new natural philosophy based on particles and their movements, combined with the increasing availability of the microscope, led scholars and anatomists to explore the minute structures of the body in order to see how these might throw light on a range of bodily functions (Figure 7.5). The scale of their investigation changed dramatically. The engravings and woodcuts with which they illustrated their publications allowed many others to see the previously hidden structure of the body and its fluids.

By employing a series of sophisticated preparation techniques, including boiling and dyeing sections of flesh before placing them under the microscope, Malpighi was able to see and describe the finest features of the body's structure; he observed, for example, the tiny vessels connecting the veins and the arteries, which Harvey had been unable to see and which now provided visual evidence of the circulation of the blood. In particular, Malpighi's attention was caught by what he defined as the glandular structure of most organs. One of the main questions that puzzled anatomists and physicians in the seventeenth century was how bodily fluids, such as saliva, urine and semen, were produced. According to Galen, semen was the product of a process of concoction in the blood which took place in the testes, and urine was formed when the kidneys' special faculty extracted superfluous **serum** from the blood. However, those scholars who had rejected the existence of faculties had to look elsewhere to understand the functioning of the body. In 1666, Malpighi published *De Viscerum Structura* [On the Structure of the Viscera], in which he reported his observations on the liver, brain cortex, spleen and kidneys. Here and in other works, he argued that, when properly observed, most organs showed a complex glandular structure that resembled a bunch of grapes. Furthermore, they all produced excretions: the liver produced bile, the brain produced nerve fluid and the kidneys produced urine. The blood was constituted of particles of different shapes and sizes and as it passed through the various glands, these particles were differently filtered. The end result was the various bodily fluids. When the blood entered the kidneys, for example, the particles whose shape and size matched those of the pores of the kidney entered them and became urine; the other particles kept moving. In his explanation of the mechanism of physiological processes, Malpighi was following Descartes; the

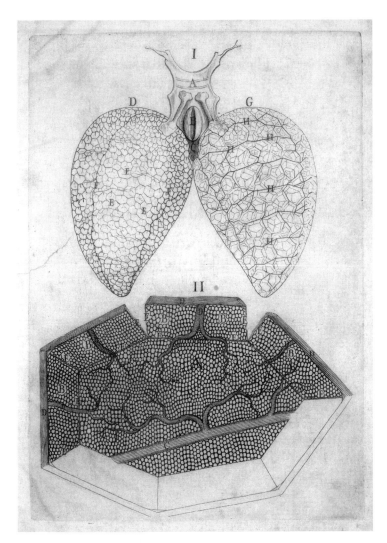

Figure 7.5 Engraving of the lungs in Malpighi's *Opera Omnia* [Complete Works], 1686. Malpighi studied the lungs intensively. The top image shows the lungs of a frog; the bottom image shows a portion of the lung as viewed with the recently invented microscope. By using the microscope, Malpighi was able to show the network of interconnected capillaries in the lungs, which provided proof of the circulation of the blood. Wellcome Library, London

particles were separated off simply because of their size and shape, not because of any quality or property with which they were endowed. More precisely, most of the body's physiology could be explained in terms of a filtering process, which was constantly carried out by the glandular organs. For Malpighi, the gland was the 'archetypal machine' (Giglioni, 1997, p.152). Looking for the fundamental structure of the body, Malpighi found it in the gland, which he described as 'the workshop' of nature, a powerful image confirming his mechanical approach to the body. A meticulous microscopist, he acknowledged that some of the most minute activities of nature would always escape the human senses. Much could be turned into visual display, but not everything.

Malpighi was highly regarded both in Italy and abroad; contemporaries perceived him as one of those who were fundamentally changing the traditional view of the living body. Not everyone, however, appreciated his investigations. Girolamo Sbaraglia, professor of anatomy and medicine in Bologna and a member of the city's college of physicians, launched a fierce attack on Malpighi, who, in turn, replied with a passionate defence. Exploring their argument helps us to consider the fraught relationship between anatomy and medical practice at this time.

Exercise

Now read 'Debating the medical benefits of the new anatomy: Girolamo Sbaraglia versus Marcello Malpighi' (Source Book 1, Reading 7.3). (Extract (i) is Sbaraglia's attack; extract (ii) is Malpighi's defence.)

1   What was Sbaraglia's main accusation?

2   Which authorities did he rally to support his view?

3   How did Malpighi defend his position?

Discussion

1   Sbaraglia said that three main kinds of anatomical investigation were carried out by physicians of his time: finer anatomy, plant anatomy and comparative anatomy. However, all these subtle investigations contributed little to the actual practice of medicine. Microscopic study of the various organs of the body did not provide any new cures. To know the most minute structure of the liver did not lead to an increased understanding of its function or provide solutions when it stopped working. For Sbaraglia, knowledge of effective therapy through experience rather than what he perceived as the pedantic mastering of anatomy remained the core of medical practice.

2   You may have noticed that Sbaraglia praised Galen (an obvious authority for a conservative physician), but also referred to the discoveries of 'modern' anatomists such as Eustachio and Harvey, whose works he clearly knew, though he argued that they had not improved medical practice. He also quoted van Helmont as one who paid attention to the therapeutic side of practice rather than anatomy.

3   Malpighi saw the study of anatomy as an integral part of medical practice, which for him was not just about prescribing remedies, but also about understanding the causes of disease. Knowledge of the anatomical structure of the healthy body allowed the physician to understand what could go wrong. The main assumption was that nature worked consistently and that humans could develop the skill to understand how the body functioned. They could do this by observing nature and also by constructing models and machines that worked in the same way as the body, and made visible what remained hidden. Remedies could then be prescribed not just on the basis that they had worked on a previous occasion, but because the physician understood rationally how they could restore health.

In defending the importance of anatomy, Malpighi was very assertive. Indeed, in many of his medical cases he used his anatomical discoveries to throw light on the causes of diseases. But what therapies did he recommend to his patients?

Continuity and change in medical practice

Malpighi was a busy physician and wrote hundreds of letters of consultation to his patients, who were mainly members of the wealthier families of Bologna. Here, for example, was his advice to a noblewoman in 1676, who was suffering from what he described as a debilitating abdominal discharge:

> I advise her to continue with the cow serum, reducing the dose to [six] ounces, and if her stomach refuses it, she could take a broth made with winnowed barley and pumpkin seeds. I am sending some tincture of coral. Should she want it, she may take four drops in a broth two or three times a day between meals, in the hope that this might strengthen the bowels and sweeten the humours. I am also enclosing some packets of powder of crab eye and *terra sigillata*. These should be [ground up and] mixed with food, as is done with pearls ... If her symptoms persist, she should continue with what I have previously prescribed ... that is, serum in the morning, deer horn, either alone or mixed with **bezoar**, and the cordials already prescribed. I have nothing further to add.
>
> (Malpighi, 1988–92, vol.1, p.21; my translation)

Coral and crab eye were hardly new remedies, but Malpighi routinely resorted to centuries-old drugs like these, and also recommended procedures such as bloodletting and purges, the linchpins of the most time-honoured medical practice. How could the mechanical model of the body, here focused on the filtering process performed by glands, coexist with features of the old medical tradition? Could it be that the same actions were endowed with different meanings? Let us try to untie this complex knot.

On one level, sweetening the humours, strengthening the bowels, purging the blood and purifying the viscera were Malpighi's goals, just as they were the goals of any other physician of the time. Like his arch-enemy Sbaraglia, Malpighi believed that traditional remedies worked. In this respect, then, Sbaraglia was right: the new anatomical investigations were bringing nothing new to medical practice. However, unlike most of his conservative colleagues, Malpighi offered a wholly mechanistic account of how these remedies worked. For example, he pointed out the blatant contradiction in the use of milk to treat fevers. Milk, argued Malpighi, had always been regarded as a hot substance and yet it was prescribed to cure a condition that resulted from abnormal heat in the body. This went against the Galenic assumption that opposite cured opposite. He did not deny that milk and substances derived from it, such as butter, were effective in fighting fever; however, he claimed that this was due to the fact that, by clinging to the blood particles that were fermenting, they prevented further fermentation. While he continued to prescribe old remedies, therefore, Malpighi was reformulating 'the theoretical justification of standard therapies. It is in this reformulation, rather than in actual therapies, that we can locate the novelty of his work' (Bertoloni Meli, 1997, p.35).

Malpighi's example has two important implications for the historian of medicine. The first is that the same act – prescribing coral or milk, say – possessed different meanings for different practitioners, depending on the model of the body favoured by each, though they all expected to obtain the same result. The second is that the coexistence of different understandings of the same action is even more important if we take patients into account. Of course, it is difficult to talk of patients as a homogeneous group, and evidence about what patients in seventeenth-century Bologna thought is scarce, though not completely absent. It is reasonable to speculate that Malpighi's patients held a fundamentally Galenic view of the causes of sickness, and regarded the main goal of medical treatment as the restoration of the balance of the humours. To this they probably added a strong belief in the possibility that supernatural intervention could restore health (Pomata, 1999). Thus, when they turned to a physician, patients expected him to recommend and administer traditional therapies such as bloodletting or emetics, regardless of his mechanical explanations and anatomical investigations. In the importance he placed on the relationship between doctor and patient, therefore, Malpighi was no different from any other practising physician. In his anatomical investigations, he might have changed the way the body was viewed, but, despite Sbaraglia's accusations, as a doctor he did nothing to jeopardize the relationship of trust he had with his patients.

This complex state of affairs was typical of the relationship between medical theory and medical practice in the period between the mid-seventeenth and the mid-eighteenth centuries, not just in Italy, but across Europe. Medical theory was in flux: the main tenets of Galenism were being challenged by ever more sophisticated anatomical investigations and replaced by innovative chemical and mechanical theories. Medical debates flourished. If the common ground was that the body was a machine, disagreement might arise over more detailed explanations of how the machine worked or what caused a disease. Influential physicians and teachers such as Hermann Boerhaave, whose works became the gospel for generations of students who flocked to Leiden to attend his lectures, revised Descartes's model by claiming that the body was a hydraulic system rather than a clockwork one, and that it was the constant circulation of blood and other fluids through the vessels that kept the body healthy. This circulation followed the laws of hydrodynamics. Whenever a blockage was created and the normal blood flow was altered, with a consequent increase in pressure, disease might occur. For example, the ubiquitous and devastating fevers could now be put down to friction between solid and fluid bodily parts caused by blockage of the vessels (Risse, 1992, pp.158–9). Other physicians argued that the chemical composition of bodily fluids was also important, and that substances such as salts were responsible for alterations in the blood which could bring about stagnation and ultimately result in diseases. These differences were not trivial, and generated animated discussions, but a combination of mechanical and chemical principles remained the dominant idiom for thinking about physiology well into the eighteenth century.

Without belittling the importance of these debates, historians now emphasize the apparent continuity that characterized contemporary medical practice. If we look at therapeutics, it is impossible to deny the extraordinary resilience of the traditional remedies associated with humoral medicine, even after the major tenets of Galenic physiology had been completely undermined and rejected. Like Malpighi, Boerhaave too continued to prescribe bloodletting and purges, although, when he was teaching, he explained their efficacy in terms of the positive effect they had on the flow, volume and pressure of the blood rather than their ability to evacuate putrid matter. Consequently, the mechanical and hydraulic model of the body did not replace, but rather coexisted with, the older notion – shared by patients – of a healthy body in which humours were required to flow freely, and stagnation, when it occurred, had to be removed to restore balance. The consistency with which physicians, regardless of their philosophical orientation, recommended bloodletting and evacuation in order to regain health was clearly reassuring to their patients.

Chapter 8 provides a more detailed discussion of patients' perspectives.

To explore a further example of this complex situation, I now turn to consider the medical investigations and practice of a group of eighteenth-century physicians who made great use of the work of the renowned natural philosopher Isaac Newton. By the end of the seventeenth century, Newton had put forward a completely mathematical explanation of major natural phenomena, including a strictly mathematical account of the attraction between bodies – the law of gravity. Following Newton's lead, these physicians tried to put medical knowledge on a truly quantitative basis, and even promoted the use of measuring instruments.

7.5   The body expressed in numbers

According to humoral medicine, the body naturally rid itself of accumulating pollutants and corrupt matter through urine, stools and sweat. Revising and expanding these principles, the professor of medicine in Padua, Sanctorius Sanctorius (1561–1636), argued in his *De Statica Medicina* [On Medical Statics] (1614) that health was the result of a balance between ingested food and the excreta. These included perspiration, which was made up not only of the visible sweat, but also of an imperceptible moisture excreted through the pores of the skin. Sanctorius argued that the quantity of food taken in should be proportionate to the amount of liquid perspired. The only way to monitor both visible and invisible perspiration was by weighing one's body regularly. Sanctorius designed a special weighing chair, which he himself used for many years to carry out his investigations (Figure 7.6).

Sanctorius combined traditional ideas about excretion and health with a new interest in mechanical devices and precise, minute calculation. *De Statica Medicina* achieved some success, but it was as a result of the popularization of Newton's mathematical approach to nature that Sanctorius' ideas underwent further development in the work of a number of British physicians. For example, James Keill (1673–1719), a successful practitioner in Northampton, and the physician Bryan Robinson (1680–1754), carried out long trials and diligently recorded on a daily basis their weight and what they had eaten, drunk and evacuated. Robinson even tried to collect data from different countries, to show the

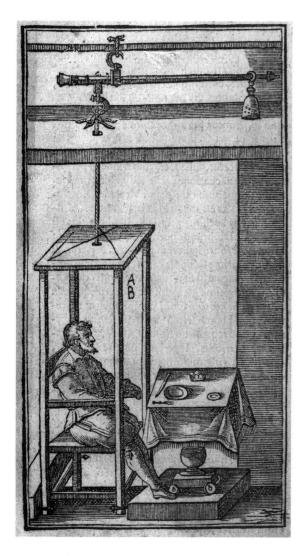

Figure 7.6   Sanctorius in his weighing chair, 1626. This picture was included in one of Sanctorius' books to illustrate the importance and feasibility of monitoring changes in one's weight in relation to food intake and daily excretion. Wellcome Library, London

effect of climate on the rate of bodily excretion (Dacome, 2001, p.481). In their publications, both men included tables charting the precise numerical changes that the body had undergone. This was certainly an unprecedented way of representing the body.

Self-monitoring gradually acquired popularity beyond the circle of Newtonian physicians and became the latest fad in booming eighteenth-century England. Lay people, especially wealthy men with no experience of hunger, took up weighing themselves. Scales tended to be kept in public places, such as the fashionable London coffee shops, where it was possible to step on them after sacks of tea or sugar had been weighed. Some started to record their weight in their diaries (Rogers, 1993).

Both the physicians' trials and the new vogue for weighing are tangible evidence of the growing conviction that the body could be expressed in mathematical terms: it could be measured, precise calculations of physiological processes could be made, tables could be compiled. Scales complemented other devices such as the barometer, one of the first scientific instruments used by experimental philosophers, which had become part of the furniture of wealthy households by the middle of the eighteenth century (Golinski, 1999). Meanwhile, other aspects of the body's physiology had started to be investigated with the help of mathematical laws. In the 1730s, the Englishman Stephen Hales (1677–1761) measured the force and speed at which the blood circulates, while Keill had earlier tried to establish the impulsive force of the human heart with the help of hydraulic principles (Brown, 1987). It might seem reasonable to conclude that all this measuring was bound to change the way the body was treated in medical practice. However, the mathematical approach pursued by physicians working in Newton's shadow did not radically transform the overall approach to medical practice. On the contrary, acts such as weighing were seamlessly incorporated into the centuries-old approach to health and sickness which emphasized the importance of diet and regimen (Dacome, 2001, p.490).

The trajectory of a successful physician

An interesting example of how the mathematical approach to the body by no means meant the demise of older perceptions can be found in the career and writings of George Cheyne (1671–1743). A Scot who moved to London and joined the Newtonian circle of physicians, in the 1720s Cheyne became one of the most popular and successful practitioners in England. He remained a prolific author throughout his life, and the following extracts from three of his works – published many years apart – reveal the ideas he embraced at different periods.

Exercise

Now read 'New theories, old cures: the Newtonian medicine of George Cheyne' (Source Book 1, Reading 7.4). Note the language used in the different extracts, and consider which model of the body is at work in each.

Discussion

The mathematical formulae and the equation in extract (i) show that in discussing his theory of fevers Cheyne was embracing a quantitative, Newtonian approach to the body. The shape and size of the blood vessels are considered, along with the velocity of the blood, to calculate how the circulation of the fluids has been reduced by obstruction. The model of the body here is an entirely mathematical one: the language of numbers is used to understand and explain the body's functioning. Extract (ii) is written in an entirely descriptive mode. The vocabulary is rich: notice the variety of words used to define the qualities of the sulphur – 'tenacity', 'ropiness' 'elasticity' – and its activities – 'cleanses', 'imbibes', 'retains', 'carries ... out', 'softens', 'smooths', 'defends'. The effectiveness of sulphur is described in terms of a 'story', in which the 'good' substance protects the body against 'bad' substances ('their efficacy in destroying the mischief of all saline particles'; 'sheaths and defends'). This extract employs mechanical and chemical concepts: gout is understood to result from salts that clog the blood vessels. Some chemical concepts are mentioned – 'saline particles', 'soap', 'acid salt', 'diluent', 'oily parts' – but the language is much less specialized than in extract (i). No mathematical formula is used to explain the phenomena causing the disease, for example. Extract (iii) contains even fewer technical terms ('sharpness in your blood', 'obstructed glands', 'paroxysms', 'chyle'), and the prose is generally very accessible. This is a model of a body whose physiology and main problems can be described in simple, well-established terms: obstruction, weak perspiration, laxity of bowels, or too frequent childbearing.

In writing the first treatise in 1701, Cheyne was addressing the community of his fellow Newtonian physicians; he therefore assumed that they all could follow and appreciate his mastery of mathematical formulae. But in the 1710s, after a personal and spiritual crisis, he abandoned theoretical and mathematical speculation and started to regard health as fundamentally shaped by moral restraint and spiritual search (Guerrini, 2000). Instead of writing academic books, Cheyne now devoted himself to medical practice and the production of popular treatises in which he provided a growing readership with advice on how to live a healthy, controlled and long life. By deploring overindulgence in eating and drinking, Cheyne showed a good understanding of the habits of the wealthy men and women who constituted his potential clients. The style of the second extract, and even more that of the letter, was designed to appeal to educated people who had no specific medical or mathematical knowledge. Cheyne was writing to instruct and encourage them at both the medical and the moral level. It was perhaps his wholehearted commitment that explains his continuous success. Patients such as the Countess of Huntingdon might well have approved of and shared in his confidence that good health depended as much on the control of an individual's spiritual and emotional life as it did on a skilfully and individually tailored regimen.

Cheyne's dissatisfaction with mathematics and his appreciation of the spiritual dimension of health were quite extreme. However, as you will see in the next section, they were in tune with an increasing discontent – which spread through Europe – with the reductionism implied in purely mechanical accounts of the body. And Cheyne's success as a practitioner is evidence of the strength and popularity of the centuries-old holistic notion of the body. It is little wonder that regimen and attention to the interactions of body and soul remained the main focus of medical practice in the eighteenth century.

7.6 The power of patients

Of course, eighteenth-century physiology was no longer Galenic. No one would have objected to the idea that the blood circulates around the body, while the fine structure of major organs such as the brain, the kidneys and the liver was common knowledge among medical students and probably not unknown to some learned patients. As the focus of anatomical and physiological investigations, the body was now cut up and subjected to a variety of experiments much more often than before: several magnificently illustrated anatomical atlases were produced in the late seventeenth century and throughout the eighteenth century. In the centres for medical teaching that multiplied across Europe, professors taught generations of students a plethora of competing physiological and pathological theories. Some of these theories, called 'vitalistic', took to task the exclusively mechanical model and invoked a unique principle that sustained life, the complexity of which could not be reduced to the laws regulating inanimate matter; others eclectically combined elements from different systems (Risse, 1992, pp.161–7). Often complicated and all-embracing, these theories followed each other in rapid succession; scholars have traditionally stressed their short life and quick turnover, and suggested that a certain sterility underpinned medical knowledge in the eighteenth century.

A thought-provoking interpretation of the most striking feature of eighteenth-century medicine, namely the coexistence of a plethora of new medical theories alongside an older, holistic tradition of healing, was proposed by the sociologist Nicholas Jewson in a seminal article published in 1974.

Exercise

Now read 'Medical knowledge, patronage and its impact on practice in eighteenth-century England', an extract from Jewson's article (Source Book 1, Reading 7.5).

1   Identify the main outlines of Jewson's argument.

2   On what grounds might you wish either to criticize or to moderate his conclusions?

Discussion

1   Jewson argued that the complex social status enjoyed by learned medical practitioners in eighteenth-century England provides the key to understanding the ebb and flow of competing medical theories as well as the lack of true innovation in medical practice at this time. On the one hand, the physician's university education placed him quite high in the social hierarchy. Those who were not members of the nobility or gentry (that is, the majority), could nonetheless adopt the taste and manners of the aristocratic classes whom they sought both to cure and to emulate. On the other hand, because they depended professionally on their clients – wealthy patients were their chief source of income and determined the success or failure of their careers – physicians had to win their trust and meet their expectations. Familiarity with the latest medical theories might boost a physician's credibility and intellectual authority, but it was the patient's need for an effective therapy that set the tone of the medical encounter. Although new physiological systems rapidly followed each other, they all shared the same assumptions, which were also the basis of lay patients' understanding of health and sickness. Under these constraints, medical innovation was never likely to occur, while ancient conceptions of disease simply continued to reappear under a new guise.

2   Jewson's theory is open to criticism on a number of grounds. First, it presupposes an oversimplified image of the nature and variety of eighteenth-century medical encounters. Completely absent from his account are patients

from different social backgrounds, whose relations with medical practitioners, although less frequent, did exist and might throw a different light on physicians' careers and social aspirations. Second, it is noticeable that Jewson does not engage with the content of any of the various medical theories he evokes; his claim about the lack of innovation in eighteenth-century medicine is anachronistic, as it judges the eighteenth century by standards of scientific change that developed a century later. And third, he uses the very specific social conditions of English physicians to explain the proliferation of medical theories, which was actually a phenomenon characteristic of other European countries as well.

Jewson's model nonetheless has been praised by historians of medicine for providing a framework for further research on the interactions between physicians and patients (for example, Porter, 1985). After Jewson's article appeared, historians increasingly began to take into account the patients' perspective, not just to make sense of medical encounters, but also to understand how medical knowledge was produced and disseminated. Jewson's approach constituted a direct challenge to traditional thinking on this subject, providing as it did an interesting attempt to ground medical knowledge in its social context.

Exercise

With Jewson's model in mind, reread extract (iii) of Reading 7.4. What does this tell us about the social interaction between Cheyne and his patient?

Discussion

It is clear that the letter was written after a face-to-face encounter between doctor and patient had taken place, during which the patient had narrated her troubles. Cheyne's attitude towards his patient is best described as deferential, almost obsequious ('having had the honour of ... conversation with your ladyship'). Like many of his colleagues, Cheyne put every effort into gaining and retaining his patients' trust: pleasing them and doing what they expected was the most obvious way of achieving prosperity.

An approach that similarly looks into the social and political context in which medical knowledge was produced has been taken to explain the success of other medical theories and associated models of the body that proliferated in this period. One of these, which became all the rage in the late eighteenth century, claimed the pre-eminence of the nervous system.

7.7 The sensible body

For centuries, and well into the early modern period, sense experience, including seeing, hearing and touching, as well as bodily movement, had been explained according to the precepts of Galenic physiology – that is, as the result of the action of animal spirits flowing along the nerves between the brain and the periphery. Nerves were understood as hollow ducts that distributed animal spirits to sustain sensation and motion. In his groundbreaking model of the body as a machine, Descartes retained elements of this theory, though his emphasis on mechanical principles altered the Galenic understanding of nerves and muscles. His work also encouraged others to pursue further research into the notion of animal spirits and the anatomy of nerves, muscles and brain in order to account for movement and sensation. In the second half of the seventeenth century, the structure of the nerves and the brain became the object of minute exploration. The Englishman Thomas Willis, for example, claimed that different parts of the brain performed different tasks and argued that the muscles contracted as the result of a chemical reaction occurring in the animal spirits. Gradually, the notion of animal spirits came to be replaced with that of a 'nerve fluid', which was consistent with the hydraulic model of the body prevailing at the time. The nerve fluid was conceived by some, including Boerhaave, as the subtle and highly mobile secretion of the brain, which was widely thought to act like a gland. Sensation was due to the impact of external stimuli on the sentient extremities (skin, eyes, ears) and was transmitted by this fluid back to the brain.

The nature of this nervous fluid remained, however, a controversial topic in medical and scientific circles. Following Newton, many argued that the nerves were solid (not hollow), and that sensation and motion were the result of the vibrations (not the flow) of an ethereal medium – that is, an imperceptible, subtle and very elastic fluid, which was diffused throughout the universe, including animal and human bodies. Throughout the eighteenth century, physicians and philosophers argued over these different models, and sometimes combined them, for example by retaining the idea of the glandular function of the brain but conceiving of nervous transmission as a vibration rather than a flow (Jackson, 1970).

A major change in making sense of how the nerves worked occurred when, after extensive physiological experiments, which involved cutting and stimulating the nerves of hundreds of animals, the Swiss anatomist Albrecht von Haller argued that the nerve fibres possessed an intrinsic and exclusive quality, which he called 'sensibility' (Figure 7.7). This quality, the capacity of the nerves to perceive outside stimuli, was located in their inner core. Tissues that possessed a rich network of nerves, such as the skin, also possessed sensibility to a high degree. Muscles too had a reactive property – they contracted in reaction to stimuli. Haller characterized this property as 'irritability'. Published in 1752, Haller's findings were enormously influential and led to a major reorientation in medical theory. For example, they shaped the thinking of Scottish anatomists, such as Alexander Monro II (1733–1817) (Figure 7.8), and of the renowned professor of medicine at Edinburgh University, William Cullen, whom you met in Chapter 6.

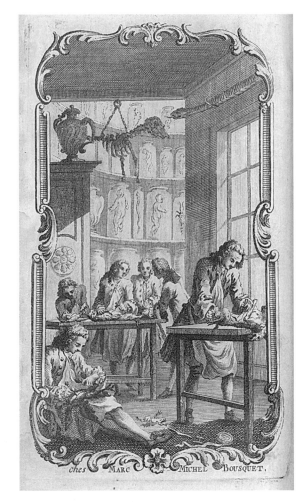

Figure 7.7   This is the engraved frontispiece of Haller's *Mémoires sur la nature sensible et irritable des parties du corps animal* [Treatises on the Sensitive and Irritable Nature of Parts of the Animal Body], 1756–60, in which he discussed the results of his investigations on the physiology of nerves and muscles. Vivisection on animals, as is shown taking place here, was a staple procedure of the research. Note also the collection of foetuses preserved in jars and the hanging skeleton. Often, the spaces used for natural investigations doubled their function as museums. Medizinhistorisches Institut, Bern

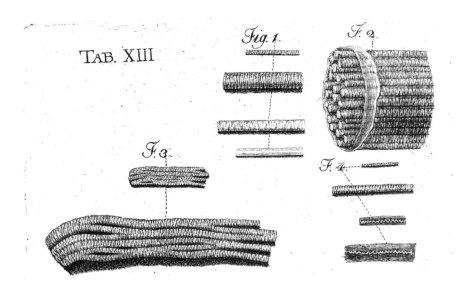

Figure 7.8   Human nerves, from Monro's *Observations on the Structure and Functions of the Nervous System*, 1783. Wellcome Library, London

In the physiological model Cullen taught to his Edinburgh students, he described the body as a complex and highly integrated mechanism composed of solid organs, nervous system and fluids. While the proper functioning of each part was crucial to health, in Cullen's view it was in the nervous system that the 'generative source of life lay' (Stott, 1987, p.133). He regarded sensibility and irritability as the most important qualities in an individual. For Cullen, sensibility was the capacity of nerves to receive sensation and transmit will: different people showed different degrees of sensibility. Irritability was a kind of nervous power possessed by the muscles and was quite distinct from their vigour. In fact, irritability and muscle strength were to be found in inverse relation to one another, so that a very strong person would also be prone to torpor, and a debilitated person would have a high degree of irritability. Health was now characterized by a balance between nerves' sensibility and muscles' irritability, while disease was the result of the deficiency or excess of these qualities. A certain degree of 'excitement' in the body was required for the nerves to transmit the impulses necessary to ensure bodily functions, but outside agents could either stimulate or depress this 'excitement'. Remedies would either bring it back or reduce its excess. In locating the ultimate cause of disease in alterations of the nervous system, Cullen sneered at the importance traditionally attached to the fluids and their affections: 'When I was first acquainted with Physic, I found Physicians reasoned very boldly, they spoke of thickening or thinning the blood with as much clearness as a Scotch maid would speak of making pottage thicker or thinner' (quoted in Stott, 1987, p.139). It was to the nervous system that physicians were now advised to direct their medical treatment.

Cullen's extensive correspondence with his wealthy patients provides numerous examples of the way in which he applied these new theories to his medical practice:

> Your nervous system, originally weak, has received some shocks and your complaint is entirely from disordered nerves affecting both mind and body ... You have got into a very relaxed state of nerves ... I suspect your constitution originally has been strong but intemperance has been especially to blame and your first step is to avoid this for the future.
>
> (quoted in Risse, 1993, p.149)

If most patients continued to perceive diseases as the product of a blockage of the humours or extremes of heat or cold, some were gradually convinced that nerves were to blame: 'Dr. Gem, Physician to ye Embassy, has exerted all his skills and knowledge ... I have no Fever at present, I have head-Ache, and Indigestion, & I have lately been convinc'd that I have Nerves' (quoted in Porter and Porter, 1988, p.70). As a result of the shift from a hydraulic to a nervous model of the body, the notion of sensibility gained great popularity.

One of the media that helped to popularize the importance of nerves and the concept of sensibility was to be found outside medical encounters, in a new and extremely successful literary genre, the 'novel of sentiment'. Writers such as Samuel Richardson, Laurence Sterne and Henry Mackenzie, who were familiar with the current medico-physiological debate, openly drew on these notions and made their characters' sensibility and response to external events the driving force of their writing (Barker-Benfield, 1992, pp.15–36). By adopting the language of

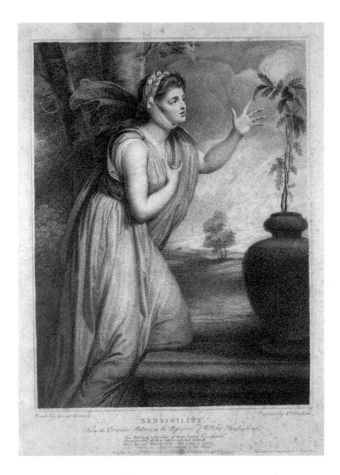

Figure 7.9　Richard Earlom, stipple engraving after George Romney, *Sensibility*, 1789. Unsurprisingly, the personification of sensibility in this picture is a young woman, whose bodily language expresses her heightened feelings, here anguish. Historians have argued that the emergence of sensibility brought about a certain feminization of social customs. Wellcome Library, London

physiology as the tool with which to explore the emotional adventures of their heroes and, especially, their heroines, these writers contributed to circulating the idea that 'delicacy of feeling' and 'a high sensibility' should be regarded as the quintessential qualities of a human being (Figure 7.9). Not only were characters and plot now built around sentiments, but readers were also meant to respond with heightened 'feeling' to what they read. Never before had physiology so directly shaped literature, and never before had literature served medicine so well.

Exercise

Now read 'The popularisation of the new medical theories in the eighteenth century: the novels of Laurence Sterne' (Source Book 1, Reading 7.6). Make a note of the various physiological concepts which, albeit expressed with much irony, pepper Sterne's writing.

Discussion

Extract (i) is a hymn to sensibility, which is praised for being not only the source of our feelings as individuals and a sort of divine presence in human beings, but also the basis for social bonding. It is because we feel that we are able to go beyond ourselves and act with compassion.

In extract (ii), the question of the origin of intelligence and the site and function of the soul in relation to the body is discussed with reference to the theories of famous philosophers such as Descartes and anatomists such as Bartholinus. In making fun of some of these theories – for example, by comparing the activity of the soul to that of a 'tad-pole' – Sterne assumes that his readers are at least conversant with discussions on the structure of the brain and the cerebellum, the intricacy of nerves and the location of the soul. Moreover, Tristram's father, a man deeply involved in these debates, who even proposes his own theory, was presumably a familiar character to contemporary readers. They would regard issues such as the source of intelligence, wit and memory as plausible topics of conversation between gentlemen with no specific scientific or medical expertise, though how it was conducted might stir a smile.

Through novels, a growing readership familiarized themselves with a whole set of expressions and concepts based on the 'sensible' body, which they might then apply to their own bodies, health and feelings. Despite Sterne's reference to the sensibility of the 'roughest peasant', sensibility was increasingly regarded as an attribute confined to those whose nervous apparatus was well developed. As opposed to coarseness, delicacy became a valued quality, which, though it might imply a tendency to develop nervous disorders, was generally perceived as socially positive.

To explain the success of this new model of the body, particularly in England and Scotland, Christopher Lawrence has looked at its broader social and political implications and argued that it served well a specific political and ideological project first proposed by eighteenth-century Scottish philosophers and politicians:

> The nervous system gained importance in Scotland not only from the physiological side of the bridge but from the philosophical side also. In the second quarter of the century Scottish philosophy turned from reason to feeling, both as the basis of morals, and as the mainspring of action. On this foundation was developed a sophisticated theory of society and history, as well as a school of sentimental novel-writing ... Scottish social thinkers discerned a relation between social life and the quality of sensibility. History was a process involving a gradual refinement of feeling.
>
> (Lawrence, 1979, pp.28–9)

The social implications of such thinking – found, for example, in the writings of such leading authors of the Scottish Enlightenment as David Hume (1711–76) and Adam Smith (1723–90) – were clear. Uncivilized populations and the labouring poor were regarded as devoid of sensibility, their skin, muscles and nerves being different from those of refined people. At the medical level, they were thus unlikely to develop nervous conditions. It is not surprising then that we find a clear distinction between the needs of different patients in Cullen's practice. Stomach problems, menstrual disorders, colic, **hysteria** and gout were the chronic ailments that characteristically afflicted his wealthy, private patients. In such cases, the best solution was to restore the balance of the nervous system through exercise, diet and the appropriate degree of stimulation. By contrast, poor, hard-working people could not afford to be as fussy about their health as the wealthy; nor could society in general, as Cullen explained:

> Happily their manner of life and even their hardships are the best means of preserving their health. It is true that this is not universal and many men are doomed to employments more or less directly pernicious to health, but it is necessary for the good of the whole society, and the only compensation the society can make to them is the taking the greatest care of them, in disease and old age.
>
> (quoted in Stott, 1987, p.140)

Thus, political thought and medical theories successfully interacted in providing 'rational' justification for contemporary social hierarchy.

Finally, we might ask, what impact did the model of the sensible body have on therapy? Once again, the picture is a mixed one. As studies in electricity grew in the 1740s and 1750s, a link between nervous excitement and the regenerative and therapeutic value of electrical force was established. Machines generating shocks were devised and applied to cure a range of illnesses, including hysteria and paralysis. By acquiring one of these machines in 1750, the Edinburgh Infirmary made electric shock therapy available to the sick poor. As one physician observed, servants through 'continual intercourse with people of decent manners' acquired a 'delicacy of body and sensibility of mind' similar to that displayed by their employers (Risse, 1988, pp.11, 15). However, following initial interest, learned physicians across Europe tended to become sceptical about the benefits of electrical therapy, which subsequently became the preserve of the numerous non-learned medical practitioners who thrived in the commercial economy of the late eighteenth century. Cullen did recommend electric shock treatment, but his favourite remedies to strengthen or relax the nerves were still diet, exercise, change of air and taking the waters. You may remember from Chapter 6 that to treat the servant Janet, Cullen prescribed the tried and tested procedures of applying fomentations, bloodletting and blistering. True, the rationale for these treatments had changed; by their use, Cullen was seeking to stimulate the nervous system, not purge the body. But for most of his patients, the notion of disease as the result of extreme hot or cold, humoral imbalance, impeded evacuations and blockage of the free flow of fluids still held true. Like Malpighi's milk and butter, Cullen's blisters and emetics were at one and the same time both innovative and traditional.

7.8   Conclusion

In the seventeenth and eighteenth centuries, a series of innovative models of the body was produced, from the mechanical to the mathematical to the sensible. As groundbreaking anatomical investigation and physiological experimentation were carried out, the map of the body changed, and different parts (vessels, glands, nerves) acquired visibility and became the focus of much research. New atlases and images of the body were produced to help students grasp the object of their study. We cannot dismiss the importance of these changes within medicine, nor their complex relationship with broader transformations in contemporary culture and society. Indeed, in this chapter you have encountered some examples of the way in which both new tools such as the microscope and social and political concerns affected the production and the reception of new medical knowledge.

The construction of these diverse models of the body, however, represents only half of the story. When contrasted with the dramatic changes that occurred in nineteenth-century medicine – for example, the development of cell theory – the various models of the body I have discussed in this chapter look very similar. This is apparent in the negligible change they brought to medical practice and the minimal impact they had on patients' expectations. As medical theories ebbed and flowed, the centuries-old holistic view of health and sickness survived almost intact in patients' narratives. For the vast majority, the body remained a system of closely interconnected parts, composed largely of vessels through which fluids moved and accumulated, causing imbalance and putrefaction. Disease, far from being located in one organ, was still thought to be the product of corrupt matter which travelled around the body and was able to affect any part of it. Such a holistic understanding was perfectly compatible with all the new medical theories, however different they were on the surface and in the eyes of their most partisan adherents. And it was this understanding, and the expectations it generated in the sick, which continued to set the agenda for most medical practitioners well beyond 1800.

References

Barker-Benfield, G.J. (1992) *The Culture of Sensibility: Sex and Society in Eighteenth-Century Britain*, Chicago and London: University of Chicago Press.

Bertoloni Meli, D. (1997) 'The new anatomy of Marcello Malpighi' in D. Bertoloni Meli (ed.) *Marcello Malpighi: Anatomist and Physician*, Florence: Leo Olschki, pp.21–62.

Brown, T.M. (1977) 'Physiology and the mechanical philosophy in mid-seventeenth century England', *Bulletin of the History of Medicine*, vol.51, pp.25–54.

Brown, T.M. (1987) 'Medicine in the shadow of the *Principia*', *Journal of the History of Ideas*, vol.48, pp.629–48.

Castle, G. (1667) *The Chymical Galenist*, London: Sarah Griffin for Henry Twyford.

Dacome, L. (2001) 'Living with the chair: private excreta, collective health and medical authority in the eighteenth century', *History of Science*, vol.39, pp.467–500.

Defoe, D. [1706] (1938) *Review*, facsimile edition, with an introduction by A.W. Secord, vol.IX, New York: Columbia University Press.

Descartes, R. [1662] (1972) *Treatise of Man*, ed. by T.S. Hall, Cambridge: Harvard University Press.

Giglioni, G. (1997) 'The machines of the body and the operations of the soul in Marcello Malpighi's anatomy' in D. Bertoloni Meli (ed.) *Marcello Malpighi: Anatomist and Physician*, Florence: Leo Olschki, pp.149–74.

Golinski, J. (1999) 'Barometers of change: meteorological instruments as machines of Enlightenment' in W. Clark, J. Golinski and S. Schaffer (eds) *The Sciences in Enlightened Europe*, Chicago: Chicago University Press, pp.69–93.

Guerrini, A. (2000) *Obesity and Depression in the Enlightenment: The Life and Times of George Cheyne*, Norman: University of Oklahoma Press.

Jackson, S.W. (1970) 'Force and kindred notions in eighteenth-century neurophysiology and medical psychology', *Bulletin of the History of Medicine*, vol.44, pp.397–410, 539–54.

Lawrence, C. (1979) 'The nervous system and society in the Scottish Enlightenment' in B. Barnes and S. Shapin (eds) *Natural Order: Historical Studies of Scientific Culture*, Beverly Hills and London: Sage, pp.19–40.

Malpighi, M. (1988–92) *Consulti*, ed. by G. Plessi and R.A. Bernabeo, 3 vols, Bologna: Istituto per la Storia dell'Università di Bologna.

Pomata, G. (1999) 'Practising between earth and heaven: women healers in seventeenth-century Bologna', *Dynamis*, vol.19, pp.119–43.

Porter, R. (ed.) (1985) *Patients and Practitioners: Lay Perceptions of Medicine in Pre-Industrial Society*, Cambridge: Cambridge University Press.

Porter, R. and Porter, D. (1988) *In Sickness and in Health: The British Experience 1650–1850*, London: Fourth Estate.

Risse, G. (1988) 'Hysteria at the Edinburgh Infirmary: the construction and treatment of a disease, 1770–1800', *Medical History*, vol.32, pp.1–22.

Risse, G. (1992) 'Medicine in the age of Enlightenment' in A. Wear (ed.) *Medicine in Society: Historical Essays*, Cambridge: Cambridge University Press, pp.149–95.

Risse, G. (1993) 'Cullen as a clinician' in A. Doig, J.P.S. Ferguson, I.A. Milne and R. Passmore (eds) *William Cullen and the Eighteenth Century Medical World: A Bicentenary Exhibition and Symposium Arranged by the Royal College of Physicians in Edinburgh in 1990*, Edinburgh: Edinburgh University Press, pp.133–51.

Rogers, P. (1993) 'Fat is a fictional issue: the novel and the rise of weight-watching' in M. Mulvey Roberts and R. Porter (eds) *Literature and Medicine during the Eighteenth Century*, London: Routledge, pp.168–87.

Stott, R. (1987) 'Health and virtue: or, how to keep out of harm's way: lectures on pathology and therapeutics by William Cullen c.1770', *Medical History*, vol.31, pp.123–42.

Source Book readings

A. Cunningham, 'William Harvey: the discovery of the circulation of the blood' in R. Porter (ed.) *Man Masters Nature: Twenty-Five Centuries of Science*, London: BBC Books, 1987, pp.68–76 (Reading 7.1).

R. Descartes, *Treatise of Man*, ed. and translated by T. Steel Hall, Cambridge: Harvard University Press, 1972, pp.5–8, 113 (Reading 7.2).

H. B. Adelmann, *Marcello Malpighi and the Evolution of Embryology*, 5 vols, Ithaca: Cornell University Press, 1966, vol.1, pp.559–62, 570–1, 575 (Reading 7.3).

G. Cheyne: *A New Theory of Continual Fevers* in T.M. Brown, 'Medicine in the shadow of the *Principia*', *Journal of the History of Ideas*, 1987, vol.48, pp.634–5; *An Essay of the True Nature and Due Method of Treating the Gout*, London: G. Strahan & H. Hammond, 1722, pp.38–9; *The Letters of Dr. George Cheyne to the Countess of Huntingdon*, ed. by C. Mullett, San Marino: Huntington Library, 1940, pp.54–6 (Reading 7.4).

N.D. Jewson, 'Medical knowledge and the patronage system in eighteenth-century England', *Sociology*, 1974, vol.8, pp.369–83 (Reading 7.5).

L. Sterne: *A Sentimental Journey and Other Writings*, ed. by T. Keymer, London: Everyman/J.M. Dent, 1994, pp.95–9; *The Life and Opinions of Tristram Shandy, Gentleman*, ed. by I. Campbell Ross, Oxford: Clarendon Press, 1983, pp.117–19 (Reading 7.6).

8

Women and Medicine

Silvia De Renzi

Objectives

When you have completed this chapter you should be able to:

- outline the contribution of medical knowledge to the understanding of differences between the sexes in the early modern period;

- analyse the model of the body underpinning female patients' accounts of their health and illnesses;

- compare and contrast early modern theories of generation;

- describe how competence over childbirth and the female body was transformed during the early modern period and assess different historical explanations of this change.

8.1 Introduction

In the course of this volume, you have encountered some of the different ways in which early modern medical practitioners conceptualized and treated the body. However, up to now, no attention has been paid to differences between the sexes, and how these were understood in the past. It may seem that sex differences – that is, the anatomical and physiological differences between the female and the male body – are constant and universal: of course men and women in the early modern period were biologically different, as they are today. Nonetheless, as the preceding chapters have shown, the body has a history (Porter, 1991). Perceptions and understandings of its anatomy and physiology change over time – and are shaped by the wider social context and prevailing cultural values. Sex specificity is no exception. Though often presented as a 'timeless' reality, it has been the subject of intense investigation and redefinition. Historians are now exploring past understandings of sex differences and how they were used to establish **gender** roles; this research usually goes under such headings as **'women's history'** and 'gender history' (Scott, 1991). Scholars are keen to investigate how roles were defined and perpetuated in the legal, religious, philosophical and cultural domains (Wiesner, 2000). Medicine is obviously an important area of inquiry, as medical knowledge has always provided some of the most authoritative ideas and practices with respect to allegedly 'natural' differences. One important issue is how, in exploring this important aspect of anatomy, physicians were expressing as well as shaping contemporary values and cultural assumptions about gender roles.

Among the fruits of historical studies of gender, women and medicine is a growing interest in the experience of women as patients as well as medical practitioners, two themes that figure prominently in this chapter. I begin in Section 8.2, however, by exploring how definitions of the female body in the Aristotelian–Galenic tradition were discussed and reworked in the early modern period. You will see how debates on the female body inevitably involved discussing the male body too, as they tended to be defined in relation to each other. One of the most disputed topics was the function of the female body in the process of generation; Galen had disagreed with Aristotle about this, and the debate between opposing schools of thought remained lively in the early modern period. In Section 8.3, I discuss competing accounts of generation, as well as the broader social repercussions of such controversies. I then go on in Section 8.4 to discuss the role of women in medical practice by focusing on midwives, to whom women turned when pregnant, but also when suffering from a range of female diseases. The old-fashioned, doctor-centred, history of medicine tended to portray the early modern midwife as well intentioned, but often ignorant and dangerous. Recent research, however, has undermined this view. I also look at the way in which the traditional authority of women in this sphere was increasingly eroded in the eighteenth century as man-midwives began to assert their primacy in the field of pregnancy and birth. This change offers an interesting insight into the broader processes at work in medicine in this period, when the learned physician was increasingly expanding his competence and authority over many aspects of people's lives.

8.2 A different body?

The humoral body is discussed in Chapter 1.

According to Galen, everyone was characterized by a distinctive temperament, which was the result of their particular combination of humours and the four main qualities of hot, cold, dry and wet. Certain categories of people, however, were thought to share a similar combination of qualities; for example, owing to the natural process of ageing, elderly people tended to be dry and cold; children, on the other hand, were full of vital spirits, and so tended to be hot and moist. Similarly, the Galenic tradition explained differences between the sexes in terms of a fundamental difference in the balance of the qualities: women were perceived as colder and more moist than men. This was due to an intrinsic deficiency of heat in the female body, which could account for a range of phenomena, from the internal location of the female sexual organs, to women's regular discharge of blood through menstruation, and from their relative lack of body hair to their higher-pitched voices. The female body was constantly compared with what was regarded as the model of physiological perfection – the male body – and found wanting. For example, although Galen thought that women contributed to conception by producing a kind of semen (from the Latin *semen*, meaning 'seed'), he claimed that overall this was of an inferior quality and less active than the male variety. Outside the Galenic tradition, the physical and intellectual inferiority of women was stated with even more vigour by Aristotelian natural philosophers. The Aristotelian tradition, which claimed that women were defective creatures who possessed a weak intellectual capacity, remained authoritative throughout the Middle Ages and the early modern period, and helped to justify the inferior social and legal status of women. On the topic of generation, for example, Aristotelian theorists denied the existence of female semen and restricted the female contribution to the provision of brute and passive matter in the form of menstrual blood. The issue of women's nature, however, remained controversial: a broad range of different positions, from highly misogynistic claims to proto-feminist stances, found expression in the works of both male and female writers of the early modern period. The view that both sexes were equally important in procreation, and that each sex was perfect in its own terms, gained some popularity in the Renaissance, especially among physicians (Maclean, 1980, pp.29–46). However, this variety of opinions did not lead to any significant social transformation in the position of women. Although early modern society was not the monolithic patriarchal system that has sometimes been described, overall there is a general consensus that things 'got worse for women over the course of the seventeenth and eighteenth centuries ... the picture [was] one of fewer options and declining status for the female sex' (Fissell, 1995, p.444).

The American scholar Thomas Laqueur controversially argued that, when properly examined, the Aristotelian and the Galenic views on differences between the sexes were much more similar than was previously thought. The two schools of thought shared a model of sex difference that was fundamentally different from the one with which we are familiar today (Laqueur, 1990). Laqueur referred to the modern view – that is, that the sexes are anatomically and physiologically incommensurable – as the 'two-sex model'. In Laqueur's argument, what was dominant until the eighteenth century was a 'one-sex model'. In such a model, the two sexes were not regarded as anatomically irreconcilable but as points on a continuum. Male and female sexual organs were fundamentally analogous – that is, they shared the same essential structure and differed only in their bodily location. Laqueur based his argument on various pieces of evidence, including the representation of female organs in early modern anatomical literature and contemporary beliefs about the possibility of sexual metamorphosis.

In most Renaissance anatomical literature, including Vesalius' *De Humani Corporis Fabrica* (1543), the female organs were usually described as a version of the male organs, but located inside rather than outside the body. In addition to explicit statements such as 'the neck of the uterus is like the penis, and its receptacle with testicles and vessels is like the scrotum' (Jacopo Berengario da Carpi, quoted in Laqueur, 1990, p.79), accompanying illustrations underlined the point. Again and again, images such as that in Figure 8.1 were reproduced in anatomical works and reinforced the idea among their readers, usually medical students, of a link between the male and female genital organs. The original model was obviously the male body, but the two sexes were perceived as related by a fundamental law of homology, in which the female organs were not regarded as different in kind, structure and function, but simply as a version of the male organs. How should we explain the extraordinary persistence of this representation, and what does it tell us about the assumptions driving anatomists' investigations? Clearly, what was at stake here was not a lack of observational skills, since the Renaissance was a time when great pride was taken in accurate anatomical investigations, usually performed in trumpeted defiance of old authorities. Laqueur proposed to interpret this persistence as evidence of the great power of the traditional one-sex model, which was still effectively guiding the minds and eyes of anatomists, despite their avowed challenge to Galen.

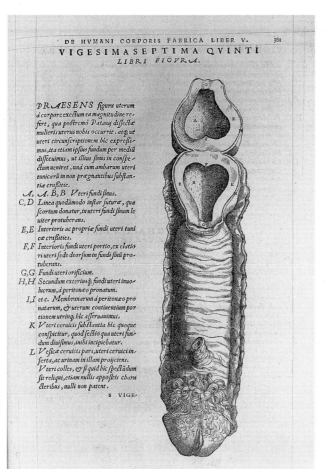

Figure 8.1   The uterus as a penis in Vesalius' *De Humani Corporis Fabrica*. Wellcome Library, London

Furthermore, in the early modern period it was widely believed that individuals who had been born female could, at some point in their lives, simply transform into men. This was explained as follows. A lack of bodily heat during pregnancy could result in the foetus not completing its development in the womb. Consequently, the genitalia remained inside the body, and the baby was born female. An excess of heat, typically around the time of puberty, could cause the internal organs to be pushed outside the body, thus resulting in the sexual transformation of a woman into a man. Such cases were widely debated in the medical literature and Laqueur argued that belief in this occurrence was possible only in a framework that regarded the difference between the male and the female body as a matter of degree (that is, relative to the amounts of moisture and heat in the body) rather than of kind. Woman was thus regarded 'as a lesser version of man along a vertical axis of infinite gradations' and not as irreconcilably distinct from man (Laqueur 1990, p.148). Other phenomena, for example the possibility that some men, as a result of an unusually cold and moist temperament, could produce milk in their breasts, caught the attention of early modern physicians and natural philosophers, and were debated at length. Lactating, which to us is one of the most distinctive properties of the female body, was understood in the Galenic framework to occur when blood was transformed into milk through a process of concoction that was favoured by a certain combination of bodily qualities. This generally happened in female bodies, but the possibility that it could also occur in men was not ruled out.

So, once again, no incommensurable differences set men and women apart, although it was understood that the male body was the standard of perfection: for example, the metamorphosis of men into women was considered highly improbable, because nature always worked to achieve perfection.

According to Laqueur, the two-sex model with which we are familiar came to replace the one-sex model only in the eighteenth century, when for a variety of reasons social distinctions (not only between men and women but also between men) started to be explained on the basis of allegedly fundamental biological differences. As the social disadvantage of black people was accounted for in terms of supposedly natural racial differences – for example, anatomists and natural philosophers argued that black people had coarser nerves and smaller brains – so women's confinement to the domestic sphere was also justified in terms of anatomical and physiological differences – for example, their larger pelvis and weaker nerves. An obsession with ranking spread in the eighteenth century. Now women were described as completely distinct from men, and, as Laqueur put it, 'as an altogether different creature along a horizontal axis whose middle ground was largely empty' (Laqueur, 1990, p.148).

Not everyone agrees with Laqueur's theory. Historians have argued that in describing the one-sex model as dominant until the eighteenth century, Laqueur overlooked important differences between competing traditions which cannot be conflated. However stimulating it may have been, his theory was a reductive one and could not account for the popularity of the position traditionally associated with Aristotelian theorists, for whom

> women's sexual function was in no way parallel to men's. Women were essentially incubators; they provided a place for the fetus to develop and the matter to nourish it, while male semen contributed the formal principle or soul ... Woman [was] thus the perfect antithesis of the male ... [A] more complete reading of the sources shows that there never was a one-sex model in Laqueur's sense.
>
> (Park and Nye, 1991, p.54)

Laqueur's theory is nonetheless thought-provoking, and has stimulated innovative research on how sex differences were perceived in the past. Historians have taken up the challenge and have explored how bodily properties and functions, which we now regard as uniquely female, were understood somewhat differently in the past. An example is the work of Gianna Pomata on menstruation (Pomata, 1992; see Pomata, 2001, for an edited English translation).

Fluids flowing in the body: the benefits of menstruation

In Chapter 7, I discussed William Harvey's discovery of the blood's circulation and its paramount importance for anatomical and medical knowledge. Inevitably, this discovery led physicians to rethink a number of tenets of established medical

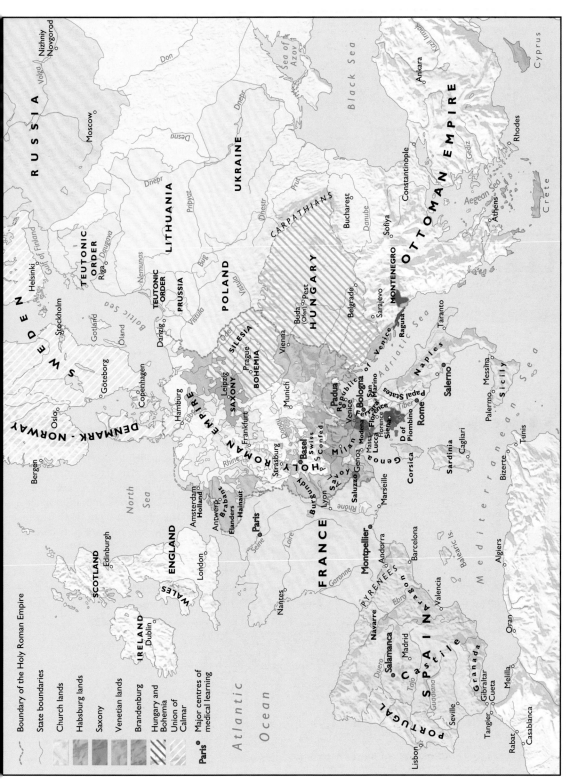

Key (legend):

— Boundary of the Holy Roman Empire
— State boundaries
Church lands
Habsburg lands
Saxony
Venetian lands
Brandenburg
Hungary and Bohemia
Union of Calmar

● Paris   Major centres of medical learning

Plate 1   Europe, c.1500

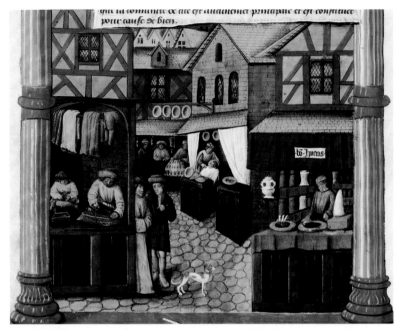

Plate 2 Street scene from a fifteenth-century manuscript, *Le Livre du Gouvernement des Princes*. The sign above the apothecary's shop on the right reads 'Bo[n].[H]Ippocras' ('Good Hippocrates'). Next door, a barber-surgeon shaves a customer; note the bleeding basins hanging from the pole. Bibliothèque Nationale de France, Paris

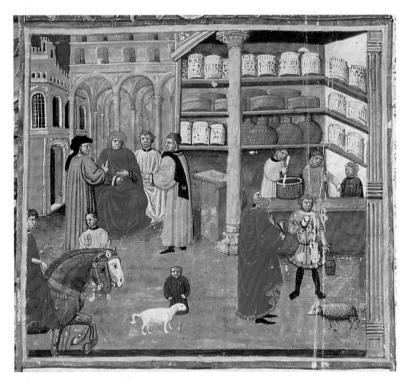

Plate 3 Apothecary's shop, from a fifteenth-century manuscript of Avicenna's *Canon*. The patient on the right holds a urine flask in a basket, for examination by the physician. On the left, the physician appears to be in conference with other doctors. Codex 2197, fol.492a–38b, detail. Biblioteca Universitaria, Bologna

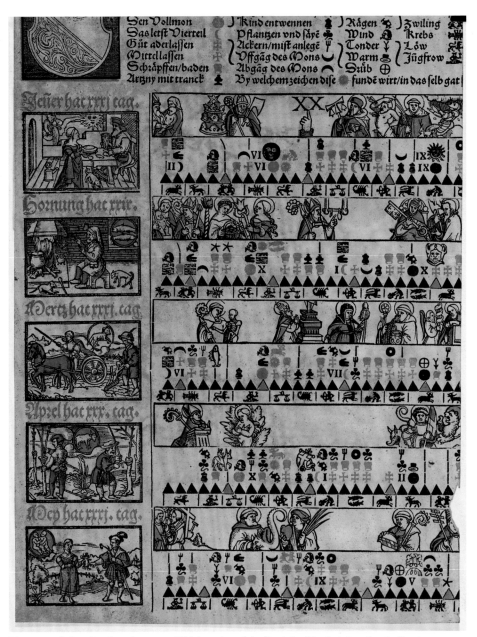

Plate 4   Calendar for the year 1544, printed in Zurich. Black triangles indicate working days, and red triangles holidays. Saints' days are marked with images of the relevant saints and their attributes: e.g. 20 January shows St Sebastian with his arrows (top row, third from the right). Beneath these triangles are the signs of the zodiac in which the moon will be located; above them, the phases of the moon are indicated in circles or crescents. Above the triangles, too, are signs giving medical information. A vertical line with a horizontal bar across it indicates a good day for bloodletting; a line with two bars indicates a particularly good day. A red cup-shaped symbol indicates a good day for bathing; these tend to coincide with good bloodletting days. A black clover-shaped mark indicates a good day for gathering herbs. Badische Landesbibliothek, Karlsruhe

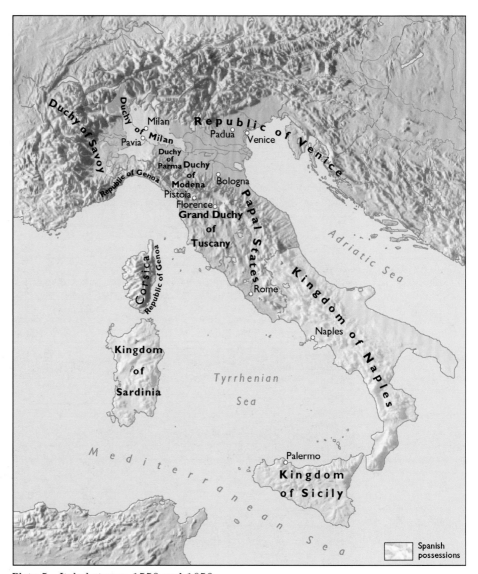

Plate 5   Italy between 1550 and 1650

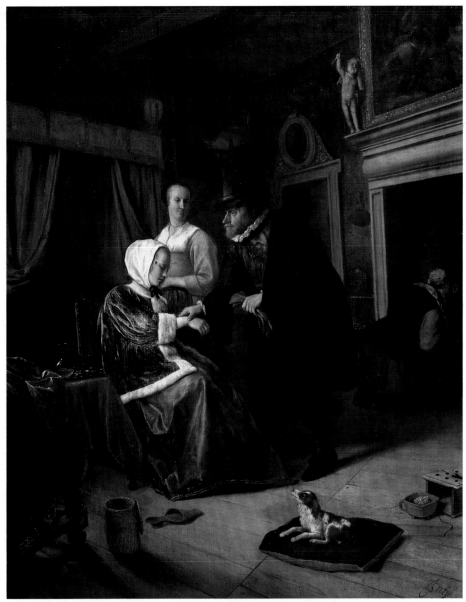

Plate 6   Jan Steen, *The Doctor's Visit*, *c*.1663–5. This is one of several genre paintings (paintings depicting subjects drawn from everyday life) in which Steen depicted an encounter between a doctor and a patient. Although not necessarily painted from real life, the picture indicates what the sickroom in a rich household may have looked like: notice the large bed and rich furnishings; the expensive and warm clothes worn by the sick woman; the presence of the two maids. The flask on the table may contain urine. The physician, who is shown in the act of taking the patient's pulse, is wearing a hat and holding his gloves. Why Steen chose to portray the doctor in this way is open to interpretation. It may represent an implicit criticism of the behaviour of busy physicians, or it may be accepted practice. Royal Cabinet of Paintings, Mauritshuis, The Hague

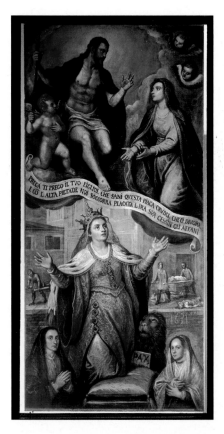

Plate 7   Domenico Tintoretto, *Venice Imploring the Virgin, Who Intercedes with Christ to Stop the Plague*, Church of San Francesco della Vigna, Venice, 1631. Venice is personified by the woman in the centre of the painting, with upraised arms, who is begging the Virgin Mary to intercede with Christ. The cartouche reads: 'We beg you to implore your son to heal this cruel scourge which is devouring us, and to help us with his great piety. May his wrath be satisfied and our sorrow end.' Christ is shown, holding a sword, at the top left. Note the plague scene in the background, showing corpses being carried away. The two women kneeling at the bottom are the patrons who commissioned the painting. Photo: Osvaldo Böhm

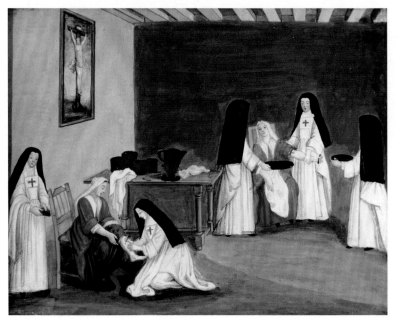

Plate 8   Nuns sometimes carried out medical procedures such as bloodletting, an activity usually left to barber-surgeons. This painting, attributed to Madeleine de Boulogne, may be an idealized representation, but it indicates that this type of medical intervention was regarded as an appropriate activity for the sisters who nursed hospital patients. The Art Archive/Musée de l'abbaye de Port-Royal-des-Champs, Magny des Hameaux/Dagli Orti

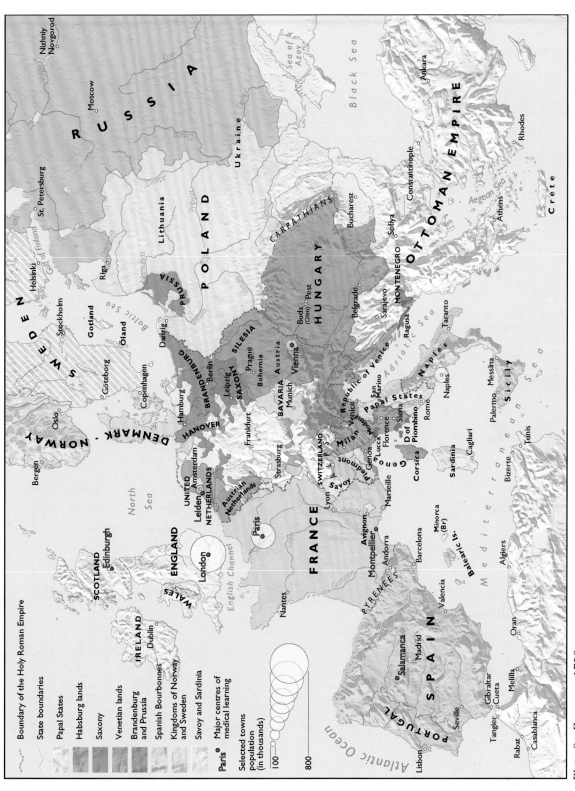

Legend

	Boundary of the Holy Roman Empire
	State boundaries
	Papal States
	Habsburg lands
	Saxony
	Venetian lands
	Brandenburg and Prussia
	Spanish Bourbonnes
	Kingdoms of Norway and Sweden
	Savoy and Sardinia

Paris● Major centres of medical learning

Selected towns
population
(in thousands)

100
800

Plate 9 Europe *c*.1750

Map labels

RUSSIA
Nizhniy Novgorod
Moscow
Volga
Don
Sea of Azov
Black Sea
Desna
Dnepr
Ukraine
Dnepr
Pripyat
Neman
St. Petersburg
Gulf of Finland
Helsinki
SWEDEN
Stockholm
Gotland
Öland
Baltic Sea
Riga
LITHUANIA
POLAND
PRUSSIA
Danzig
Vistula
CARPATHIANS
HUNGARY
Bucharest
Belgrade
Sarajevo
MONTENEGRO
Ragusa
Sofiya
OTTOMAN EMPIRE
Ankara
Constantinople
Aegean Sea
Athens
Rhodes
Crete
NORWAY
Oslo
Bergen
DENMARK
Copenhagen
Göteborg
Hamburg
HANOVER
BRANDENBURG
Berlin
SILESIA
SAXONY
Leipzig
Prague
Bohemia
Austria
Vienna
Buda (Ofen) Pest
Pesth
BAVARIA
Munich
Frankfurt
Strasburg
UNITED NETHERLANDS
Leiden
Amsterdam
Austrian Netherlands
Rhine
SWITZERLAND
ALPS
Republic of Venice
Venice
Milan
Mantua
San Marino
Papal States
Siena
Florence
D. of Piombino
Rome
Lucca
Genoa
Piedmont
Savoy
Lyon
Rhône
Marseille
Corsica
Sardinia
Cagliari
Naples
NAPLES
Taranto
Messina
Palermo
SICILY
Bizerta
Tunis
Mediterranean Sea
FRANCE
Paris
Seine
Loire
Nantes
Garonne
Avignon
Montpellier
Andorra
PYRENEES
Barcelona
Minorca (Br)
Balearic Is.
Algiers
SPAIN
Madrid
Salamanca
Valencia
Seville
Gibraltar
Cueta
Melilla
Oran
Tangier
Rabat
Casablanca
PORTUGAL
Lisbon
Atlantic Ocean
North Sea
English Channel
ENGLAND
London
WALES
SCOTLAND
Edinburgh
IRELAND
Dublin
Adriatic Sea

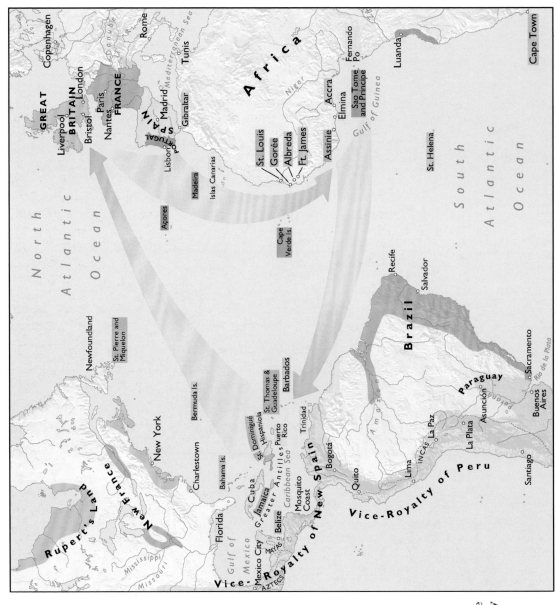

Plate 10 The new world, Atlantic and Africa, c.1650. Black African slaves were transported to the Americas by European ships, which also exported goods to the growing colonies across the Atlantic. The trade was largely funded by the profits of the colonial plantation owners, who exported valuable goods such as cotton, tobacco and sugar on the return leg across the Atlantic

belief, including the purpose of blood. However, other major assumptions of the Galenic tradition remained unchallenged – for example, the therapeutic benefits of bloodletting and the fact that what happened to blood was different in men and in women.

According to Galen, liquefied food, or 'chyle', was transformed into blood. In the male body, some of the blood underwent a further transformation to become semen; because the female body had less innate heat than that of the male, this process produced an inferior type of semen. In women, however, blood served other functions, which related to childbearing. It was used to nourish the foetus and some of it was also transformed into milk. Because of these extra functions, blood was believed to be more abundant in women than in men. But if a woman did not bear a child, the extra blood had to be disposed of, and this was the reason why women menstruated. Following this assumption, some medieval anatomical drawings even represented an extra vein in the female body through which the menstrual blood supposedly flowed (Pomata, 1992, pp.71–2). This account of the 'female purges' was based on, and confirmed once again, the notion of women's inferiority in relation to male perfection: in this case, their inability to transform blood into good semen and their consequent need to evacuate its excess. There is abundant evidence that in the past, as well as in other cultures, menstrual blood has been generally associated with notions of impurity and danger, and various forms of monthly segregation of women seem to have been practised. In the early modern period, religious and medical treatises, both learned and popular, often reinforced the belief that menstrual blood was impure and poisonous, and various taboos about the polluted condition of a bleeding woman were strong (Crawford, 1981). However, within the medical tradition, another perspective on menstruation was also tenable.

You have already seen that bloodletting was regarded as the best remedy against plethora (excessive blood) and was a linchpin of medical practice; however, Galen advocated the greater benefit of spontaneous discharges of blood. Among the natural ways of avoiding plethora, Galen counted menstruation. Indeed, in his work on bloodletting, he claimed that menstruation was one of the most effective ways in which nature kept a body healthy (Pomata, 1992, p.80). If a woman regularly menstruated, she was protected from a range of common diseases. On the other hand, when menstruation did not occur, a woman experienced discomfort and, in the long run, illnesses of various kinds. For once, the normal functioning of the female body was considered exemplary: with regard to the fundamental issue of keeping the body in a healthy balance, it set the standard.

You may be puzzled to discover that the same learned medical tradition that supported the view of an intrinsically weak and inferior female body could also offer the resources from which to draw the opposite conclusion. It was precisely this richness, though, that made the Galenic tradition a long-lasting and at the same time flexible framework, within which different interpretations could coexist. Historians are now keen to reconstruct this variety of positions and to recapture lines of thought and topics of reflection that were discarded in subsequent periods or lost in earlier scholarship on 'Galenism'. Menstruation is one such theme.

Pomata shows how female bleeding came to be seen as the model by which other spontaneous methods of ridding the body of excessive blood, for example the phenomenon of bleeding haemorrhoids, were understood. However surprising it may appear today, in the early modern period haemorrhoids were often discussed as though they were a sort of male menstruation. The following passage from a German medical publication of the 1680s is a case in point:

> The nobleman Felix Rauschart ... of sanguine and melancholic complexion, experienced for the first time a bleeding from the haemorrhoids when he was a student of 20. Since then, nature has repeated it regularly every month ... It is worth noting that when the haemorrhoids are irregular, as to the time or the amount, his natural faculties are disturbed and weakened; and he suffers from obstruction in the abdomen, breathing difficulties, inflammation of the hypochondrium with weakness in the body and soul. And every time the flux comes back, these symptoms disappear.
>
> (quoted in Pomata, 1992, p.60; my translation)

The comparison to a woman's period is here implicit, but unmistakable. You may have noted the reference to the monthly cycle of the man's bleeding, the healing nature of it and the symptoms that accompanied any alteration of the periodical flow. Discussions of cases such as this appear again and again in medical literature well into the eighteenth century, including in the biographical writings of physicians themselves. This has led Pomata to argue that the female body was the lens through which the male body was perceived and conceptualized. And menstruation, which to us now is the clearest sign of adult womanhood, could be perceived in an altogether different way, as a bridge connecting the sexes. No better example can be given of the cultural and historical relativity whereby sexual specificity is perceived and of the fundamental role played by medical knowledge in this process.

In the following passage, which is a medical case presented by an Italian physician in the mid-1650s, another interesting element emerges:

> A certain builder periodically bleeds from his leg; an external varicose vein spontaneously breaks and blood runs out until it closes by itself without the application of any remedy. If he were a woman, I, and with me any other doctor, would be certain that this is the way she expels her purges.
>
> (quoted in Pomata, 1992, p.60; my translation)

What we would now explain as an annoying and potentially serious problem in the peripheral circulation, was understood as an indication of good health. The regularity with which the bleeding started and stopped signalled that nature was doing its job properly, though in this case the route of superfluous blood was not the haemorrhoid vein, but a leg vein. For the physician, the only thing to do was to make sure that this channel remained open and fully functioning. In addition to haemorrhoids, different kinds of bleeding, including nosebleeds and bleeding ulcers, were conceived as a natural response to plethora. This is surprising, but even more disconcerting is what the physician says about the possibility that a woman could menstruate through a vein in her leg. Where did he get this idea from?

The 'alternative route' of menstruation was a centuries-old concept described by both Hippocrates and Galen, and cases of unusual menstruation were routinely discussed in early modern medical treatises. Blood was understood to accumulate in a woman's womb and, if it was not used to nourish a foetus, it was discharged through the female genitals. If, for any reason, an obstruction occurred in a woman's blood vessels, then menstrual blood could take a different route and be expelled from other orifices. These could include the nipples, the eyes and the nose, but also small ulcers; furthermore, menstrual blood could be expelled mixed in urine or vomit. To understand this phenomenon of the 'alternative route' of menstruation, bear in mind the fundamental holism of the medical tradition. Well into the eighteenth century, both medical practitioners, including learned physicians, and patients, perceived the living body as fundamentally interconnected; where we see clear boundaries between different organs and systems, contemporaries saw parts of a whole in constant relation to each other. As a consequence, it was believed that bodily fluids could flow in different directions and that orifices could have multiple functions. Despite important changes in anatomical knowledge, medical practice continued to be based on these widespread and time-honoured assumptions (Duden, 1991, pp.126–7). Another important conviction shared by medical practitioners and patients alike was that the body had an innate ability to cure itself. It was widely believed that, if the obstruction of one part of the body had caused a dangerous stagnation of fluids, an innate healing force might initiate flow in another direction, and lead to expulsion of the **morbific** matter or the excess blood through alternative orifices, abcesses and wounds. As the case of the builder shows, this was by no means unique to the female body. However, Pomata argues that 'the menstruating female body was seen as a therapeutical model, as the prototype of the healing force of nature' (Pomata, 1992, p.83; my translation). The female and the male bodies were analogous, but now the paradigm of the analogy was the female body. Although the exemplary nature of the female physiology was widely shared, its impact on other areas of women's life was limited, and it probably had little or no effect on broader cultural and social perceptions of women.

So far I have been looking at notions of male and female bodies in the learned literature, but, as you know from previous chapters, historians are also increasingly keen to explore how patients made sense of their health and illness. One of the first works to engage with this topic was *The Woman beneath the Skin*, a groundbreaking study by the feminist historian Barbara Duden, first published in 1987 (Duden, 1991). Duden was particularly interested in reconstructing how early modern women understood and described their bodies. She based her study on the casebook of Johann Storch (1681–1751), a German physician, who mostly attended female patients. By careful reading of Storch's notes, Duden tried to recapture both his medical knowledge of women and his patients' views of their bodies.

Now read 'Female complaints: the flux' (Source Book 1, Reading 8.1).

1 What was a 'flux' according to the women and how did it manifest itself?

2 Were there obvious disagreements between the physician and his patients?

1 'Flux' was an umbrella term used by the women to describe a variety of bodily experiences. It was used to account for the sensation of matter flowing in or outside the body, but also to describe the uncomfortable feeling of matter stuck inside the body and stagnating; the flux was perceived as a sign of good health, but, when it did not flow, also as one of the main causes of discomfort and disease (for example, one of the women complained of a sudden attack of flux in the chest area, which had allegedly caused a speech impediment). The 'inner flux' was healthy as long as it did not dry up, kept moving and was regularly discharged, giving way to an 'outer flux'. The flux could be evacuated as pus, blood or other matter, which flowed through a number of different orifices, including the eyes and the nipples; these evacuations were mostly perceived as healthy.

2 By and large, Storch shared his patients' interpretation of the functioning of their bodies, especially about the need to keep the fluids moving inside the body and to help them come out regularly. Like the women, he was concerned that the flux could be driven back inside the body, where it might cause harm; consequently, he prescribed remedies that helped to 'redirect' the flow of fluids and expel them. Storch did not, however, trust home-made remedies, which the women probably self-prescribed.

Storch and his patients clearly shared a concept of the female body that was very different from the one now dominant in western societies. Duden's main aim is to recapture female voices, and the overwhelming majority of her sources relate to Storch's female patients. However, in so far as Storch's casebook presents cases of male patients, it provides us with further evidence that, in the eighteenth century, male and female physiology was understood in an interestingly 'analogous' way. For example, Storch discussed bleeding from various parts of men's bodies as though this phenomenon was equivalent to women's purges; like menstruation, male bleeding could be dangerously interrupted by various kinds of distress. He also noted the phenomenon of men and boys lactating and reported 'documented experience' of men using their milk to feed children (Duden, 1991, p.117).

Laqueur, Pomata and Duden all deal with important issues relating to gender and medicine. By looking at a wide range of sources, from pictorial representations to learned treatises and more popular accounts of health and disease, they show that what constitutes a male or a female body is culturally and historically specific, rather than a timeless fact. As Duden writes:

There is an extraordinary range of possible ways in which culture can link sexual identity to corporeality, and interpret corporeality as a sign for the difference between man and woman. No morphological element nor any process such as the flow of semen or the monthly bleeding has been seen at all times and everywhere as unique to a specific gender ... Gender is in the eye of the observer. ... [At the time of Storch] biology was not yet the science of the body polarized by its sexual characteristics.

(Duden, 1991, pp.117–18)

Of course, one counter-argument is that everywhere and in all periods only women have babies. In biological terms, this is undeniable, but even conception, pregnancy and birth can be subject to historical investigations that show the different ways in which these events were understood and experienced. What we now call 'reproduction' has been understood and experienced differently in the past. For a start, it was only towards the end of the eighteenth century that the word 'reproduction' began to replace other expressions, including 'generation' and 'procreation' (Jordanova, 1995). Today, a woman can find out whether she is pregnant in a couple of minutes by taking a simple urine test. If the result is positive, she is offered a number of sophisticated tests which even allow her to 'see' her child. Specialist doctors and midwives regularly monitor the growth of the foetus and keep a check on the health of mother and baby; when it is time for the baby to be delivered, in most western countries this procedure usually takes place in a hospital. The medicalization of pregnancy is one of the most obvious outcomes of the expansion of medical knowledge and authority in our society. But what happened in the early modern period? Who then were the 'experts' on pregnancy? How were conception and pregnancy understood? How did early modern Europeans visualize the foetus? Who was in charge at the moment of delivery? The period between 1500 and 1800 saw a number of substantial changes in all these areas.

8.3 Questions of generation

In early modern England, once a woman was married she gave birth, on average, to a child every two years, or, if she sent her child out to nurse, every year (Crawford, 1990, p.15). It is reasonable to assume that, with some variations, this pattern of fertility was common in the rest of Europe. Women tried to have some control over their fertility and resorted to various contraceptive methods, including herbal remedies that induced abortion. Because of the high mortality rate in childbirth, anxiety and fears associated with pregnancy were a frequent cause of emotional distress in women. A pregnancy also had an extraordinary social importance, both in wealthy families, where the birth of a child meant the prolongation of the dynasty, and in poor families or for single mothers, for whom a child was often a financial or moral burden. However frequent and important a pregnancy was in the life of a woman, it was a phenomenon surrounded by uncertainty. For a start, it was very difficult to detect.

Chapter 9 contains a discussion of mental disorders in relation to women.

Establishing pregnancy

Women felt certain they were pregnant only when they could feel the baby moving inside them: until then, signs and indications were regarded as unreliable and fallacious (Duden, 1991, pp.157–70; Gélis, 1991, pp.46–92; Pollock, 1990). Sources such as diaries and autobiographies show that women tended to consider a missed period a strong indication of pregnancy. However, they were also aware that the lack of menstruation could be caused by a range of other conditions, including physical illness or emotional upset. Obstruction of the menses, as you have seen, could indicate a stagnation or blockage inside the body that required removal. A sudden bleeding following lack of menstruation could therefore be interpreted as evidence that a potentially dangerous blockage had been overcome, and not, as we would interpret it now, as an early miscarriage.

One of the alleged causes of blockage was the formation of fleshy and hard matter inside the womb, which was known as a 'mole'. A mole could have various origins, from clotted menstrual blood that had not been properly discharged to semen that had been retained inside the uterus and had hardened, to the remnant of a dead foetus or of the thick fluids surrounding it. Such formations were routinely discussed in the medical literature. Whatever its cause, the received view was that a mole would sooner or later block the normal flow of menstruation. While this could be misinterpreted as a sign of pregnancy, when the mole was expelled, regular bleeding would be restored. There was no way a woman, even the most experienced midwife, could differentiate between a mole and the growth of a foetus until the stage at which the baby began to move.

Other common signs of pregnancy listed in the popular advice manuals on pregnancy and female health were enlargement of the breasts, a closed cervix, which a midwife might feel during internal examination, swollen veins in the neck or unusual cravings (Pollock, 1990, p.43). Another traditional test for pregnancy was to immerse a needle in the woman's urine; the appearance of red spots on the needle signalled that she was pregnant. Physicians, however, felt ill at ease with the widespread use of **uroscopy** by non-learned practitioners, and argued that it was of no use in determining pregnancy.

Physicians' use of bodily signs in diagnosis is discussed in Chapter 2.

Medical semiotics was the basis of the learned physicians' practice and was regarded as an important professional trademark. With regard to pregnancy, the medical literature unanimously emphasized the difficulties involved in detecting the condition. The duration of pregnancy was also a controversial topic, and one that was discussed extensively. Medical interest in these issues was augmented by their legal implications. Doctors and midwives were frequently asked to give their expert testimony at court in paternity disputes, when it was crucial to establish the date of conception. Physicians, however, tended to debate these issues mainly in theoretical terms. Until the eighteenth century, pregnancy and childbirth were by unanimous consent the province of women; male doctors, regardless of their reputation, were largely excluded from this area of medical practice. For a male practitioner to carry out an internal examination of a female patient was taboo, and physicians agreed that on a number of issues relating to the female body, women were the main source of knowledge. They at least could rely on the experience and lore handed down through the generations, either informally or through the widely read advice literature for midwives and would-be mothers.

If detecting whether a woman was pregnant was a controversial topic, even more controversial was the process by which a foetus was formed. Between 1650 and 1750, the topic of generation provoked intense research, and engendered major disputes among physicians, anatomists and natural philosophers.

Seeds, eggs and the pleasures of procreation

Generation was one of the subjects on which Galen had departed from Aristotle, and it remained controversial in the early modern period. According to Aristotle, conception occurred as a result of the male seed acting upon menstrual blood in the womb (Figure 8.2). The female contribution to the process was the menstrual blood; this was thought to consist of passive matter only, as opposed to the male contribution – the active principle inherent in the male seed. The action of the male seed was 'formal' – that is, it provided the organizing principle that guided the formation of the embryo. Aristotle likened this process to that of a craftsman fashioning an object out of a piece of wood. The male seed was comparable to the

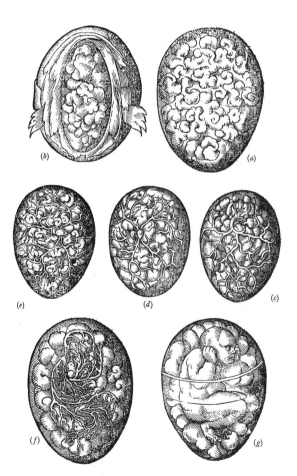

Figure 8.2 Illustrations from Jacob Rueff, *De Conceptu et Generatione Hominis*, 1554. Rueff (1500–58) was a Zurich surgeon. His book on conception and generation was first published in German for a broad audience, including midwives and pregnant women, and then in Latin for a narrower readership. This sequence illustrates Aristotle's concept of the formation of the embryo. In Rueff's book, the pictures appeared on different pages; they were arranged in this sequence by the medical historian Charles Singer (1876–1960): (a) and (b) the coagulum of semen and menstrual blood in the uterus and the formation of membranes; (c) to (e) the formation of blood vessels and of organs; (f) and (g) the vessels outlining the body and the fully formed foetus. Reproduced from Needham (1959)

craftsman's art, because it supplied the formal organizing principle; as passive matter, the female blood was comparable to the wood. In Aristotle's explanation, the craftsman contributes the idea, which sets in motion a change in the matter, but he does not bring anything material to the process, or therefore to the finished object (Roger, 1997, p.49).

By contrast, Galen argued that conception was the result of the reception, mixing, heating and stimulation of the male and female seeds in the uterus. This view rested on the important assumption that women produce seed, which, though of a weaker nature than the male seed, contribute to the formation of the embryo. Menstrual blood provided the foetus with nourishment. Galen linked the production of the female seed to the woman's experience of pleasure during sexual intercourse. For him, female orgasm was a necessary condition for conception, and, as many early modern handbooks on marital life explained, it was a husband's duty to make sure that this happened, especially if he wanted offspring (McLaren, 1985). In theories of generation, then, a major rift divided Galenists and Aristotelians. However, within each camp, too, controversies might arise as to the interpretation of specific aspects of the two theories: for example, how the foetus was nourished during pregnancy, or the order in which organs were formed. Many scholars also tried to reconcile the two main theories.

The increase in anatomical investigation following Vesalius led to more accurate descriptions of the female genital apparatus in humans and in mammals, including the discovery of what are now called the Fallopian tubes by the sixteenth-century Paduan anatomist Gabriele Fallopia. At the same time, investigations into the formation of the embryo in animals provided material for comparative studies. One of the scholars most active in this kind of research was Hieronymous Fabricius of Aquapendente, whom you encountered in Chapter 3 as Harvey's professor at the University of Padua. Fabricius' understanding of generation was shaped by the notion of 'faculties', which, as you may remember from Chapter 7, also permeated Harvey's discussion of digestion. Here is how Fabricius describes the formation of the chicken:

> Under the effect of the generative faculty, the parts of the chicken, which at first did not exist, are produced, and the egg changes thus into the chicken's body ... This procreation is accomplished through a commutation and a conformation of substance. It is thus a transformative faculty and a formative faculty that are the causes of these actions. The first faculty, called the [transformative], is purely natural and acts without awareness, through the action of heat, coldness, wetness and dryness ... But the second faculty, called formative, which differentiates the homogeneous parts and graces them with a suitable shape, with a proper size, and with an appropriate placement and congruent number, is far more noble than the first, and endowed with very great wisdom ... And in fact, once the eye has been engendered by the alterative faculty, it must be placed in the head, and not in the heel, given a spherical shape and not cubic or other, the number established, which is not one, nor three, nor more.
>
> (quoted in Roger, 1997, p.59)

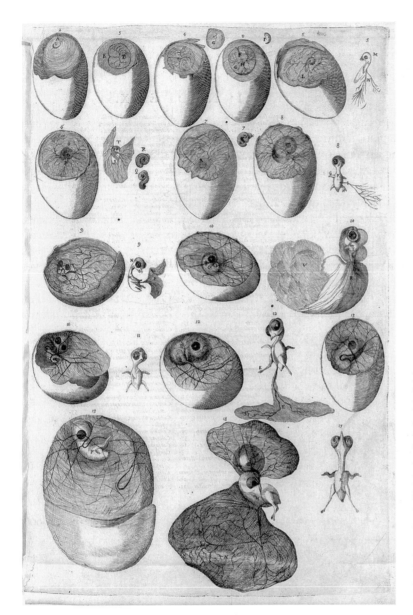

Figure 8.3   Sequence showing the formation of a chicken, from Fabricius, *De Formatione Ovi et Pulli* [On the Formation of the Egg and the Chicken], 1621. This is one of seven engraved tables that accompanied Fabricius' treatise. Notice how numbers are used to identify the different stages. The chicken is always shown both inside and outside the egg, so it can be seen from a different angle and further details can be appreciated. Wellcome Library, London

This extract shows that Fabricius regarded the various faculties as responsible for the emergence of the diverse and highly organized parts of a chicken from an undifferentiated mass (Figure 8.3). Cold, heat and wetness all acted on the matter, but it was thanks to an inner force contained in the semen that a perfectly formed foetus gradually emerged, one organ after another, and each one in the right place, until the final shape was achieved. The theory according to which something that 'at first did not exist' (in the words of Fabricius) gradually took shape as distinctive parts emerged from initial undifferentiated matter was called 'epigenesis'. It was within this framework that scholars, regardless of whether they were of the Galenic or the Aristotelian camp, discussed generation until the middle decades of the seventeenth century.

Generation remained one of the most exciting topics of research in the second half of the seventeenth century, when, thanks to countless dissections and microscopic observations, a series of important discoveries were made. The existence in egg-laying animals of organs in which the eggs were produced had been known for some time, and these organs had been named 'ovaries' (from the Latin *ovum*, meaning 'egg'). By contrast, female mammals, including humans, were believed to produce seed in organs equivalent to the male testicles. Several scholars were engaged in investigating these female 'testicles', and in 1667 the Danish anatomist Nicolaus Steno (1638–86) argued that they were in fact analogous to the ovaries in egg-laying animals. A few years later, the Dutch physician Régnier de Graaf (1641–73) described **vesicles** that he had detected on the 'testicles', which we now know to be the unfertilized eggs. De Graaf had noted that the number of vesicles in the 'testicles' of a female rabbit corresponded to the number of embryos later seen in the animal's Fallopian tubes and uterus. He thus deduced that they must be comparable to the eggs produced by **oviparous** animals and argued that they too should be called 'eggs' (Roger, 1997, p.223) (Figure 8.4). Another

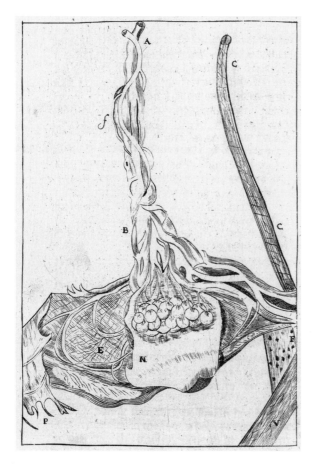

Figure 8.4   The human ovary, from Jan Swammerdam, *Miraculum Naturae Sive Uteri Muliebris Fabrica* [The Wonder of Nature or The Structure of the Female Uterus], 1672. Swammerdam (1637–80) was a Dutch natural philosopher who shared de Graaf's interest in microscopy and the controversy surrounding generation. Notice here the eggs contained in the main cavity of the ovary. Wellcome Library, London

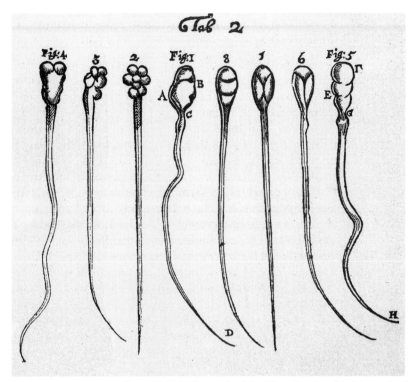

Figure 8.5   Spermatozoa of a rabbit (left, marked 1–4) and a dog (right, marked 5–8). Antoni van Leeuwenhoek presented the results of his microscopic observations of animal sperm in a letter sent in March 1678 to London to be published in the *Philosophical Transactions*, the famous and widely read periodical of the Royal Society. The letter included this drawing. He used microscopes that he built himself and explained that spermatozoa were so small that a 'middle-size grain of fine sand would contain at the least ten thousands'. Wellcome Library, London

momentous discovery made thanks to the microscope was the presence in male semen of minute organisms. These 'animalcules' (which we now call spermatozoa) were detected around the same time by another Dutchman, Antoni van Leeuwenhoek (1632–1723) (Figure 8.5). All these discoveries were controversial and stimulated yet further investigation.

The transparency of the vesicles seen by de Graaf made them difficult to detect, and many contemporaries remained unconvinced of their existence. For those wedded to earlier ideas, the vesicles were not eggs, but a kind of female seed; this meant that the conception and development of the embryo could still be understood in traditional terms – that is, as the action of one seed upon the other, and then as the result of faculties presiding over the formation of the embryo (Roger, 1997, p.232). But for many other scholars, the discovery that **viviparous** animals produced eggs that were equivalent to those produced by oviparous animals, and the detection of animalcules in the male semen, opened up a new way of understanding the whole process of conception.

Minute objects had increasingly been 'discovered' with the aid of the microscope. This encouraged people to believe that fully formed individuals, invisible to the naked eye, might already be present in either the male semen or the female eggs (Gasking, 1967, pp.45–8). The formation of the foetus would thus consist not of the creation of new forms but of an increase in the size and hardness of pre-existing parts (Figure 8.6). This theory, called 'preformationism', gained support towards the end of the seventeenth century and became influential for over a hundred years. For preformationists, the main issue of debate centred on whether this tiny being was located in the female egg or the male semen. The two schools of thought came to be known as 'ovism' and 'animalculism'.

The supporters of ovism claimed that the new individual was contained in the female egg and that the sole purpose of the male seed was to bring about the expansion and enlargement of its parts. As de Graaf put it: 'the male's sperm is nothing other than the vehicle of an extremely volatile animal spirit, which imprints

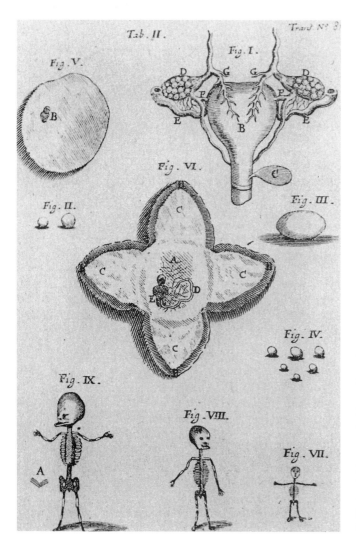

Figure 8.6   The stages of human development, drawings published in *Philosophical Transactions* by Theodore Kerckring, 1672. 'Fig. I' represents the female genitals, including ovaries. 'Fig. II', 'Fig. III', 'Fig. IV' and 'Fig. V' are representations of eggs, both of a cow and of a woman; 'Fig. VI' shows an egg opened a fortnight after conception; 'Fig. VII', 'Fig. VIII' and 'Fig. IX' represent the skeleton of the embryo at three, four and six weeks after conception. Notice that they look like miniature adults. Reproduced from Speert (1973)

a vital contact onto the matter of the embryo, that is the female egg' (quoted in Roger, 1997, p.238). Many, however, did not accept what they perceived as an inappropriate reduction of the male role in generation and, following the position of Leeuwenhoek, argued that it was in each animalcule contained in the male semen that there was a preformed individual, ready to grow. In Leeuwenhoek's words: 'It is the male sperm alone that forms the embryo, and the only contribution that the woman can offer is to receive the sperm and nourish it' (quoted in Roger, 1997, pp.238–9).

The emergence of preformationism did not lead to the demise of epigenesis. Throughout the eighteenth century, the epigenesis–preformationism controversy remained intense, though both theories were revised to accommodate the results of new research, including that of the renowned German physiologist Albrecht von Haller, whom you met in Chapter 7. In the 1750s, Haller's innovative techniques in microscopy allowed him to make visible various parts of the embryo (Gasking, 1967, p.109). Having previously opposed preformationism, Haller now became a strong proponent of it.

These debates dealt with issues of great importance to everyone, but they were highly technical and complex. We might therefore question the extent to which they remained the province of a few, learned scholars or reached a wider audience, and affected how attending physicians, midwives and the lay public perceived generation. Dealing with England, Angus McLaren has argued that changes in the way generation was understood in medical and philosophical circles had significant repercussions for society at large.

Exercise

Now read 'Popular and learned theories of conception in early modern Britain' (Source Book 1, Reading 8.2). In what way does McLaren think that the new scientific embryological literature affected popular beliefs about procreation and sexuality?

Discussion

One of the outcomes of the new embryological theories was the removal of the traditional link between female pleasure and procreation. In the Galenic tradition, which also shaped popular perceptions of sexuality, the production of female seed was generally regarded as linked to pleasure. With the discovery that the female body contained eggs, conception was now understood as a process that could happen regardless of the woman's experience of pleasure during intercourse. This understanding was even more pronounced in the animalculist theory. Although they were different in other respects, in this instance the animalculist and ovist theories produced similar effects. As the theory of the two seeds was gradually replaced among anatomists and physicians, so was a centuries-long body of popular knowledge about female sexuality.

Faced with evidence of a contrast between the early modern celebration of the necessity of female sexual pleasure and the nineteenth-century model of female sexual passivity and restraint, McLaren argues that an important factor in this gradual shift was the growing impact of new theories of generation, which well-informed physicians increasingly endorsed in their writings and medical practice. Of course, physicians were not entirely responsible for a change that other historians have linked to major religious, moral and economic transformations, including the rise in the eighteenth century of a new middle class striving to distinguish itself from the lower orders. A strict sexual morality, rigidly applied to women, certainly became one of the most valued marks of class distinction. But, in McLaren's view, 'doctors ... contributed to the effort made on a variety of fronts by the middle classes to elaborate new social and sexual roles to differentiate their enlightened lives from the unthinking, hedonistic existences of both the upper and lower orders' (1985, p.340). You may have noticed that McLaren acknowledges some form of 'resistance' to the new rules, still evident in nineteenth-century physicians' complaints about the persistence of the opinion, which they now found 'vulgar', that pleasure was necessary for conception. Indeed, he makes it clear that the traditional view of female sexuality, which had circulated for centuries, did not disappear overnight, but tended to be increasingly associated with social and moral impropriety.

One question that remains unanswered by McLaren concerns the nature of the various channels through which medical theories of generation reached a lay audience. We might assume that candidates for this role were the increasingly popular manuals of midwifery and advice literature on sexual matters. In eighteenth-century England, the rise of a commercial society and the boom of the printing industry created a mass market for works of this kind (Porter, 1992). However, sex manuals provided practical advice as to how one might achieve a prolific sex life or a happy pregnancy, and reference in them to current anatomical or physiological theories tended to be limited (Porter, 1984). In a way, this calls into question McLaren's claim about the impact of learned medicine on society and reveals the existence of a broader issue as to how learned ideas and lay knowledge interacted in the eighteenth century. It is becoming increasingly clear that the process whereby medical knowledge of this kind was acquired by lay people did not follow a simple one-way model, in which learned ideas percolated down from above. On the contrary, readers had access to a variety of sources and, by actively selecting or combining the information they needed, they created their own knowledge. While McLaren's overall picture is still thought-provoking, it demands further research as to how, at different times and in different social groups, theories of generation became part of popular perceptions of sex and procreation (Crawford, 1994).

The combination of medical and social changes that gave rise to a new sexual role for women has been invoked to explain another transformation in the relationship between women and medicine, which was particularly evident in late eighteenth-century England. Throughout the early modern period, childbirth was predominantly a social rather than a medical event, and one that had long been firmly in the hands of women and midwives. By the end of the eighteenth century, this exclusively female experience underwent a major transformation, and man-midwives became a standard presence at the childbirth scene. Historians have offered contrasting explanations for this change.

8.4   Childbirth: from female ceremony to male medical practice

For a long time, historians of medicine have celebrated the 'revolution' that took place in obstetrics in eighteenth-century England. As the traditional story goes, when ignorant midwives fretting around women in labour were finally replaced by male doctors equipped with a proper medical training, and newly designed instruments such as the **forceps**, childbirth was changed for ever and for the better. The use of the forceps, widely employed and popularized by eminent practitioners such as William Smellie (1697–1763), is frequently cited as just one

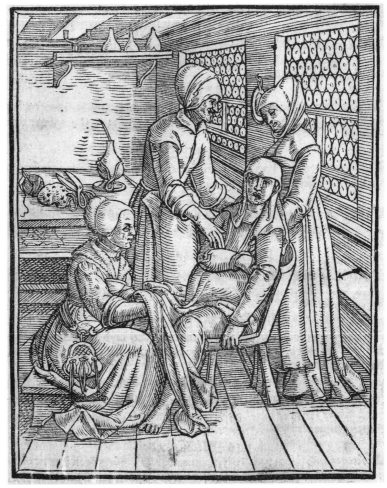

Figure 8.7   Birth scene, from Jacob Rueff, *Ein schön lustig Trostbüchle von dem Empfengknussen und Geburten* (German edition of *De Conceptu et Generatione Hominis*), 1554. Notice the presence of the gossips comforting the woman, and the midwife. Figure 8.8 shows a birthing chair similar to the one in use here. Wellcome Library, London

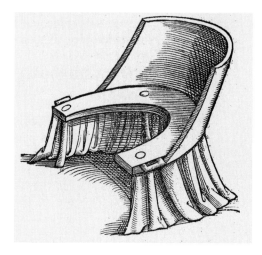

Figure 8.8   Birthing chair, from Jacob Rueff, *De Conceptu et Generatione Hominis*, 1554. Wellcome Library, London

example of the way in which medical practice was beginning to benefit from the new scientific and technological advances of the age (Johnstone, 1952).

In recent years, this tale of the victory of science over superstition and ignorance has become the subject of historical revision. The change that took place in lying-in chambers is now discussed less as a triumph of rationality, and more as an episode in the broader process of medicalization – that is, the expansion of medical authority over all aspects of life.

Within this framework, and inspired by anthropological research on birth in other cultures, scholars have reassessed the history of early modern childbirth and recaptured the dynamics and meanings it possessed for those involved. Adrian Wilson (1995), for example, has explored the lengthy rituals preceding and following birth and claimed that, until the eighteenth century, they represented a cultural heritage shared by all women, regardless of their social origin. Such rituals included the presence of **gossips** (Figure 8.7), the preparation of the lying-in chamber (darkened and closed to men), the swaddling of the baby, the long period of lying-in and the **churching** of the mother (Wilson, 1995, pp.25–30).

In a patriarchal society, Wilson argues, childbirth was one of the few occasions on which women exercised control and a female collective culture held sway. Typically, male practitioners, usually surgeons, were called to the birthing scene only if the baby had died inside the womb. On such occasions, the instruments of the surgeon were required, including the chilling crochet, which was hooked around the head of the dead baby, so that it could be drawn out of the womb (Figure 8.9). A major point in Wilson's argument is that, until the transformation of the eighteenth century, the presence of male practitioners in the lying-in chamber was associated with sorrow and death, not with the exhausting but happy experience of delivering a living baby, which remained the province of women (Figure 8.10).

What do we know about the midwives who supervised this fundamental experience in women's lives? At a time when women were increasingly confined to the domestic sphere and associated with the 'private' side of life, the wide-ranging activities of midwives defied such trends (Wiesner, 1993). One of the few public

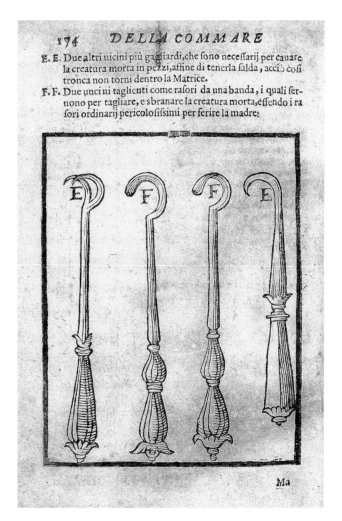

Figure 8.9 A page from Girolamo Mercurio, *Della Commare o Riccoglitrice* [On the Midwife], 1601, showing examples of the crochet, an obstetrical instrument used to draw a dead baby out of the womb. Wellcome Library, London

positions open to women, midwifery enabled them to carry out a variety of duties in the community. Town councils in mainland Europe regularly employed midwives to supervise poor women's deliveries as part of urban health care policies; midwives were also asked to oversee moral standards, and report on the pregnancies of single women; furthermore, they were expected to give expert testimony at court in all those legal cases involving a female body. For example, in alleged infanticides, midwives were asked to inspect the defendant's body and testify as to whether or not she had recently given birth.

And, of course, midwives were busy with their private practice. Often the licence, which in theory they needed in order to practise, simply acknowledged an already well-established activity. Typically, this started with a period of apprenticeship to a senior colleague, often an older relative. In England, the licensing of midwives tended to be in the hands of religious authorities such as bishops, but the attempts of colleges of physicians across Europe to gain control over midwives is well documented. In 1627, an edict of the *protomedico* in Rome established that

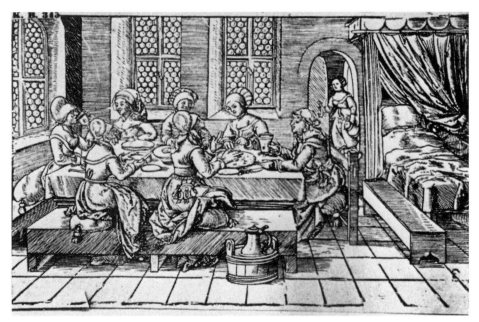

Figure 8.10 Sixteenth-century puerperal feast. Notice the all-female presence at this banquet: the period after the birth was one of celebration for all the women involved. Reproduced from Speert (1973)

women who were caught practising as midwives without the college's permission were liable to prosecution.

Frequently mothers themselves, midwives proudly claimed the advantages of practice over bookish theory. When a series of lectures for midwives was suggested in London in the 1630s, they rejected the proposal and replied: 'those women that desire to learn must be present at the delivery of many women and see the worke and behaviour of such as be skilfull midwifes who will shew and direct them and resolve their doubts' (King, 1995, p.193). The lack of practical training in seventeenth-century medical education can help us understand the midwives' point of view. In the eighteenth century, however, the need for improvement in midwives' anatomical knowledge was recognized by midwives themselves. The midwife Sarah Stone, for example, complained that many of her colleagues did not have the faintest idea about the anatomy of the female pelvis. But she also harshly criticized the ignorance of many male practitioners, who were called in to assist at difficult deliveries and who most of the time appeared to be at a loss (Grundy, 1995, p.139). Faced with extensive evidence of such professional pride, historians have tried to recapture some aspects of the complex dynamics between midwives and male medical practitioners, and of their relationships with female clients.

Midwives in Paris and London

The wife of a surgeon, Louise Bourgeois (1563–1636) (Figure 8.11) undertook midwifery to support her family while her husband was serving on the battlefield. Her rise to fame was astonishingly rapid. Thanks to carefully planned patronage,

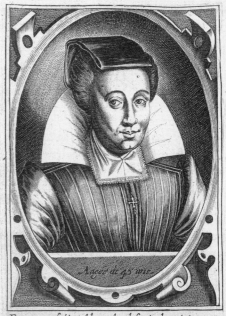

Figure 8.11 Portrait of Louise Bourgeois, from her *Observations diverses sur la sterilité, perte de fruict, foecondité ...*, 1609–26. Note the high velvet collar and golden cross, which distinguished the royal midwife. The velvet cap was usually used by royal nurses. Note also the tranquil and self-confident expression of the sitter. These visual signs point to her elevated status, but also to her use of the portrait to reaffirm and convey her professional confidence. Wellcome Library, London

she found herself in the lying-in chamber of Maria de' Medici, queen of France, at the time of the birth of the dauphin, the future Louis XIII (1610–43), in 1601. This of course boosted Bourgeois's career further and, as she proudly reported, in the 1610s and 1620s she officiated as midwife to the nobility of Paris. She wrote various books, including *Observations diverses sur la sterilité, perte de fruict, foecondité, accouchements et maladies des femmes et enfants nouveaux naiz* [Diverse Observations on Sterility, Loss of Fruit, Fertility, Childbirth Deliveries and the Diseases of Women and Newborn Babies] (1609–26), a three-volume obstetrical textbook. Writing and publishing medical books was quite unusual for a woman in seventeenth-century France, and Bourgeois showed strength and determination to an exceptional degree.

In adopting the media and conventions of learned medicine, Bourgeois was trying to achieve two main goals:

> On the one hand, she established a difference between herself and 'amateurs' or pure empirics, such as priests, totally unqualified 'wise women' and travelling healers. On the other, in adopting theories founded on reason, which belonged in the domain of university-trained physicians, and in perpetuating their medical construction of women to some extent, Bourgeois established her similarity to eminent men, past and present. The value of her book therefore appears to be deliberately acquired from the male culture. If knowledge was power, by using in such a visible, systematic fashion the theories of a much revered tradition, Bourgeois was

signalling her determination to fit, to be part of the intellectual structure of her day. Such a position further allowed her to function successfully in a male world; her approach argues indeed that she was determined to do so. She could not, or did not choose to, project herself as an alternative to male practitioners; for her time she was 'extraordinary', but it was on the terms of those who dominated the medical hierarchy.

(Perkins, 1996, p.51)

Perkins stresses Bourgeois's 'determination to fit'; yet her attitude towards university-trained physicians was to become more complex when, as quickly as she rose, she fell. In 1627, the sister-in-law of the king died after delivering a daughter: Bourgeois had been in attendance and was indirectly accused of malpractice by the surgeons and physicians who performed an autopsy on the princess's body. Bourgeois rejected their conclusions in an apology which, once again, she promptly published. Her line of defence was that the princess had been ill long before the delivery. In Bourgeois's eyes, to blame the princess's death on the midwife's inability to remove a piece of retained placenta without taking into account these deep-seated problems was a serious medical mistake. Moreover, she not only defended herself, but also claimed that the physicians were wrong. This time, her determination did not go down well in the community of male physicians. When a lengthy reply from the doctors appeared, Bourgeois's career was left in tatters.

Exercise

Now read 'A midwife defends her reputation: Louise Bourgeois (1627)' (Source Book 1, Reading 8.3). Extract (i) is taken from Bourgeois's apology; extract (ii) is from the physicians' reply.

1 What is Bourgeois's accusation against the physicians?

2 On what grounds does Bourgeois claim her authority?

3 What is the main accusation in the physicians' reply?

Discussion

1 Bourgeois challenges the way in which the physicians carried out the post-mortem as well as their conclusions. She claims that they neglected to record important aspects of the condition of the princess's body, including the colour and consistency of her organs. By mistaking a part of the uterus for a piece of the placenta, they showed ignorance of the basics of the anatomy of a pregnant woman. Furthermore, they seem to have assumed that a piece of retained placenta would be dangerous, while many other physicians held the opposite view. By pointing out the physicians' mistakes, she places herself on an equal footing with her male colleagues.

2 To attest to her competence and authority, Bourgeois mentions both her long practice as a midwife (thirty-four years in the city and at court) and the books she has published, which she proudly reports to be widely read and

respected. By quoting the works of the surgeon Paul of Aegina and those of the 'modern' anatomist, Fabricius, she also broadcasts her status as a widely read and educated practitioner.

3   The physicians harshly object to Bourgeois's decision to speak aloud and make open her reservations about their handling of the case. Her public challenge to the authority and competence of physicians and surgeons was particularly irritating. Their request that she ought to remain silent for the rest of her life attacked her reputation as a writer. The fact that she had published books was obviously interpreted as further evidence of her unsanctioned trespass into male territory.

Bourgeois's clientele was socially mixed, but it was her royal connections that provided the opportunity for both her fortune and her tribulation. We may wonder how less ambitious midwives sought recognition and built their careers. As in the case of any other medical practitioner, the key element in a midwife's career was the favour she found with her clients. The majority of midwives did not leave as many traces of themselves as did Bourgeois. Is it possible to reconstruct how they built their relationships with women? In the next reading, Doreen Evenden shows how much can be obtained by tapping, and analysing, a range of different, but equally rich, sources.

Exercise

Now read 'The clientele of London midwives in the second half of the seventeenth century' (Source Book 1, Reading 8.4).

1   What are the sources used by Evenden, and how would you characterize her analysis of them?

2   What conclusions does she draw regarding midwives and their clientele in London?

Discussion

1   Evenden's sources are a series of testimonials signed by women endorsing a midwife's application for a licence, and the account book of an anonymous London midwife (Mistress X). Both documents allow her to carry out statistical research and to produce data that she uses to draw a picture of the clientele of an 'average' midwife. You may notice how different this type of historical research is from the biographical approach adopted with respect to Bourgeois, but also how well they complement each other.

2   One of the results of this research is a revision of a number of previous assumptions about early modern midwives. For example, it emerges that midwives could have quite a big 'catchment' area. This contrasts with the traditional picture, which usually limited a midwife's practice to her local parish. At least in an urban setting such as London this was not true, and a midwife's reputation seems to

have been the main criterion for employment. Also, the social origin of her clients appears to have been much more varied and mixed than was previously thought. Even in the eighteenth century, midwives remained popular with wealthy women, evidence used by Evenden to challenge the view that upper-class women, or women who enjoyed freedom of choice, started to turn to male practitioners around 1700.

Men at the birth scene

The growing presence of men at the birth scene in the eighteenth century, even when the delivery was normal, had far-reaching social, cultural and medical consequences. The success and reputation of practitioners such as William Hunter (1718–83), one of the most sought-after man-midwives in late eighteenth-century London, shows that in the metropolis those who could afford it preferred the assistance of a man. So much so that, in upper social circles, to be attended by a man-midwife was now regarded as fashionable. This was certainly a radical break with tradition, and opened up entirely new social and professional paths for male practitioners. It has been claimed that, while this process was particularly evident in English society, other European countries gradually followed suit. However, this was far from a homogeneous, linear and 'inevitable' process. As you have seen in Evenden's discussion, some historians prefer to stress continuity over change, even when discussing England. A range of practices and cultures of childbirth certainly coexisted in continental Europe well into the nineteenth century, with local variations depending on social, cultural and religious conditions. In Catholic Italy, for example, delivering a baby with the help of a female midwife remained the rule until the middle of the nineteenth century, and interesting social dynamics seemed to characterize the event in certain areas. For example, the central figure at the childbirth scene might not be a medical practitioner at all, but the woman's mother-in-law, as children 'belonged' to the husband's family (Filippini, 1990, p.296). Moreover, by the end of the eighteenth century, in various European countries a new interest in midwifery led to the creation of schools and training programmes for midwives rather than to their systematic exclusion from the lying-in chamber (Brockliss and Jones, 1997, pp.740–2; Marland, 1993).

Even those who have focused on midwifery in eighteenth-century England and who agree that here a substantial change did occur, still account for it in very different ways. Some historians have regarded the growing use of the forceps, which allowed practitioners to help the baby out of the womb, as the key factor in securing the success of a new generation of man-midwives. Although the forceps had been invented by Peter Chamberlen (1560–1631) in the seventeenth century, the instrument was redesigned and became widely available a century later. Such technical advancement, which allowed a safer delivery of living babies in difficult conditions, allegedly contributed to the establishment of a new, positive role for male practitioners and paved the way to a more routine entrance for men into the lying-in chamber (Radcliffe, 1967). Recent research, however, has shown that the use of the forceps was controversial, not just among women but also among man-midwives, some of whom, such as Hunter, harboured strong reservations about its use. Hunter himself preferred to build his reputation on a gentler and more 'natural' approach to delivery (Wilson, 1995, pp.175–83). The link between the growth of man-midwives and their use of innovative instruments is not therefore as straightforward as was once supposed. Other historians, such as Edward Shorter (1985), have emphasized that eighteenth-century man-midwives brought about a fundamental change in the approach to normal delivery, as a result of their embracing a new notion of nature initiated by Harvey and fostered by the Enlightenment. Nature had come to be increasingly seen as a benign force; in the case of childbirth, practitioners now agreed that they should follow and help nature rather than interfere with or work against it. An 'anti-interventionist' attitude towards delivery, opposed to the vigorous procedures traditionally applied by midwives to help the woman in labour, spread among man-midwives, and this, according to Shorter, led to a general improvement in childbirth practices.

Wilson has argued that yet another story can be told about this change. In his account, women are the active initiators and not the passive recipients of change.

Exercise

Now read 'The making of the man-midwife: the impact of cultural and social change in Georgian England' (Source Book 1, Reading 8.5). In what sense, according to Wilson, are women perceived as 'active agents who made their own history'?

Discussion

According to Wilson, the reason for the emergence of man-midwives is to be found in a profound social and intellectual change that occurred among eighteenth-century women, including the emergence of a new female culture shared by literate and upper-class women. The success of man-midwives depended on the new demand for social distinction that such women expressed and that they could partly satisfy by making their childbirth a different experience from that of most other women. To call for the expensive service of man-midwives was, then, a sign of social status rather than one of distrust in female midwives. And, while breaking with the centuries-old female culture and practice in which midwives had been pivotal, these women did not abandon a number of other rituals surrounding childbirth, which survived well into the nineteenth century and which man-midwives were forced to accept.

Whereas Shorter is interested in reconstructing the intellectual tradition out of which emerged a 'hands-off' medical approach to childbirth, and sees ideas as the driving force for change, Wilson is more interested in reconstructing a broader social history of the experience. In tune with recent research on the power of wealthy patients in the eighteenth century, he regards women's choice, culture and expectations as shaping obstetrical practice.

8.5   Conclusion

This chapter has taken you through a number of issues surrounding the definition and understanding of the female body and its physiology in the early modern period. Philosophers and theologians had traditionally occupied themselves with the question of the nature and status of women, but since much of the debate was based on an understanding of the specific make-up of the female body, the views of physicians inevitably carried much weight. In the dominant Aristotelian–Galenic medical tradition, definition of the female body was reached by contrast, comparison or analogy with the male body. On the one hand, this tradition offered a range of resources on which to draw, to argue for the intrinsic weakness and inferiority of women. On the other hand, there is evidence that some tenets of Galenic physiology, especially the importance it assigned to nature's own ability to preserve or restore health, led to an explicit appreciation of specific features of the female physiology, in particular menstruation. Generally regarded as a curse and a sign of impurity, menstruation could also be seen to exemplify the idea that nature was designed to rid itself of the dreaded plethora, it thus provided a model that could be applied to understand such phenomena as male bleeding. Together with related ideas, such as those surrounding hermaphroditism or male lactation, early modern medical explanations of menstruation offer valuable evidence that sex differences, like any other anatomical feature, are understood in ever-changing ways, which are historically and culturally specific. Research into topics such as these has formed part of the ongoing attempt of historians, including historians of medicine, to make the body a subject of historical investigation and to reconstruct the different ways in which people understood it in the past.

One of the reasons why the female body was the topic of such intense reflection was the fundamental process of generation. Controversies were fierce. While the Aristotelian tradition granted women a very limited function in procreation, the Galenic theory of the two seeds led to a greater appreciation of the woman's contribution to conception and of female sexuality. As to the growth and development of the embryo, the theory of epigenesis continued to hold sway well into the second half of the seventeenth century, when, following anatomical and microscopic investigations, new theories of generation were developed. Yet even the preformationists were divided as to the respective role of men and women in generation, while controversies surrounding preformationism and epigenesis remained intense in the eighteenth century. Some have claimed that it was the demise of the Galenic two-seed theory, brought about by new anatomical findings, that was ultimately responsible for a fundamental change in the understanding of female sexuality in the nineteenth century. However, the extent to which this new learned attitude succeeded in shaping the perceptions of a broad lay audience is still open to question, and it is likely that different responses emerged in different social groups.

However they framed and understood the process of generation, early modern male physicians were completely excluded from the management of pregnancy and childbirth. These were the remit of female midwives, who were the only practitioners with competence in, and access to, the female body. Historians have started to throw light on their world as well as on the reasons for the change that started to affect childbirth in the eighteenth century. The emergence of man-midwifery has been explained by historians in different ways, but it was certainly instrumental in substantially redrawing centuries-old boundaries of competence over the female body. The culture of childbirth was also fundamentally transformed, though this was a protracted process in which geographical, social and religious variations played a significant part.

References

Brockliss, L. and Jones, C. (1997) *The Medical World of Early Modern France*, Oxford: Clarendon Press.

Crawford, P. (1981) 'Attitudes to menstruation in seventeenth-century England', *Past and Present*, vol.91, pp.47–73.

Crawford, P. (1990) 'The construction and experience of maternity in seventeenth-century England' in V. Fildes (ed.) *Women as Mothers in Pre-Industrial England: Essays in Memory of Dorothy McLaren*, London: Routledge, pp.3–38.

Crawford, P. (1994) 'Sexual knowledge in England, 1500–1750' in R. Porter and M. Teich (eds) *Sexual Knowledge, Sexual Science: The History of Attitudes to Sexuality*, Cambridge: Cambridge University Press, pp.82–106.

Duden, B. (1991) *The Woman beneath the Skin: A Doctor's Patients in Eighteenth-Century Germany*, translated by T. Dunlap, Cambridge and London: Harvard University Press.

Filippini, N. (1990) 'Il medico e la levatrice', *Quaderni Storici*, vol.25, pp.291–7.

Fissell, M. (1995) 'Gender and generation: representing reproduction in early modern England', *Gender and History*, vol.7, pp.433–56.

Gasking, E.B. (1967) *Investigations into Generation, 1651–1828*, London: Hutchinson.

Gélis, J. (1991) *History of Childbirth: Fertility, Pregnancy and Birth in Early Modern Europe*, Cambridge: Polity Press.

Grundy, I. (1995) 'Sarah Stone: Enlightenment midwife' in V. Nutton and R. Porter (eds) *The History of Medical Education in Britain*, Amsterdam: Rodopi, pp.128–44.

Johnstone, R.W. (1952) *William Smellie: The Master of British Midwifery*, Edinburgh: Livingstone.

Jordanova, L. (1995) 'Interrogating the concept of reproduction in the eighteenth century' in F.D. Ginsburg and R. Rapp (eds) *Conceiving the New World Order: The Global Politics of Reproduction*, Berkeley: University of California Press, pp.369–86.

King, H. (1995) '"As if none understood the art that cannot understand Greek": the education of midwives in seventeenth-century England' in V. Nutton and R.

Porter (eds) *The History of Medical Education in Britain*, Amsterdam: Rodopi, pp.184–98.

Laqueur, T. (1990) *Making Sex: Body and Gender from the Greeks to Freud*, Cambridge and London: Harvard University Press.

McLaren, A. (1985) 'The pleasures of procreation: traditional and biomedical theories of conception' in W.F. Bynum and R. Porter (eds) *William Hunter and the Eighteenth-Century Medical World*, Cambridge: Cambridge University Press, pp.323–41.

Maclean, I. (1980) *The Renaissance Notion of Woman: A Study in the Fortunes of Scholasticism and Medical Science in European Intellectual Life*, Cambridge: Cambridge University Press.

Marland, H. (1993) 'The *"burgerlijke"* midwife: the *stadsvroedvrouw* of eighteenth-century Holland' in H. Marland (ed.) *The Art of Midwifery: Early Modern Midwives in Europe*, London: Routledge, pp.192–213.

Needham, J. (1959) *A History of Embryology*, Cambridge: Cambridge University Press.

Park, K. and Nye, R.A. (1991) 'Destiny is anatomy'; review of T. Laqueur, *Making Sex: Body and Gender from the Greeks to Freud*, *The New Republic*, 18 February, pp.53–7.

Perkins, W. (1996) *Midwifery and Medicine in Early Modern France: Louise Bourgeois*, Exeter: University of Exeter Press.

Pollock, L.A. (1990) 'Embarking on a rough passage: the experience of pregnancy in early-modern society' in V. Fildes (ed.) *Women as Mothers in Pre-Industrial England: Essays in Memory of Dorothy McLaren*, London: Routledge, pp.39–67.

Pomata, G. (1992) 'Uomini mestruanti: somiglianza e differenza fra i sessi in Europa in età moderna', *Quaderni Storici*, vol.27, pp.51–103.

Pomata, G. (2001) 'Menstruating men: similarity and difference of the sexes in early modern medicine' in V. Finucci and K. Brownlee (eds) *Generation and Degeneration: Tropes of Reproduction in Literature and History from Antiquity through Early Modern Europe*, Durham and London: Duke University Press, pp.109–52.

Porter, R. (1984) 'Spreading carnal knowledge or selling dirt cheap? Nicolas Venette's *Tableau de l'amour conjugal* in eighteenth century England', *Journal of European Studies*, vol.14, pp.233–55.

Porter, R. (1991) 'History of the body' in P. Burke (ed.) *New Perspectives on Historical Writing*, Cambridge: Polity Press, pp.206–32.

Porter, R. (1992) 'Lay medical knowledge in the eighteenth century: the evidence of the *Gentleman's Magazine*', *Medical History*, vol.29, pp.138–68.

Radcliffe, W. (1967) *Milestones in Midwifery*, Bristol: Wright.

Roger, J. (1997) *The Life Sciences in Eighteenth-Century French Thought*, ed. by K.R. Benson and translated by R. Ellrich, Stanford: Stanford University Press.

Scott, J. (1991) 'Women's history' in P. Burke (ed.) *New Perspectives on Historical Writing*, Cambridge: Polity Press, pp.42–66.

Shorter, E. (1985) 'The management of normal deliveries and the generation of William Hunter' in W.F. Bynum and R. Porter (eds) *William Hunter and the Eighteenth-Century Medical World*, Cambridge: Cambridge University Press, pp.371–83.

Speert, H. (1973) *Iconographia Gyniatrica: A Pictorial History of Gynecology and Obstetrics*, Philadelphia: F.A. Davis.

Wiesner, M.E. (1993) 'The midwives of south Germany and the public/private dichotomy' in H. Marland (ed.) *The Art of Midwifery: Early Modern Midwives in Europe*, London: Routledge, pp.77–94.

Wiesner, M.E. (2000) *Women and Gender in Early Modern Europe*, Cambridge: Cambridge University Press.

Wilson, A. (1995) *The Making of Man-Midwifery: Childbirth in England 1660–1770*, London: University College Press.

Source Book readings

B. Duden, *The Woman beneath the Skin: A Doctor's Patients in Eighteenth-Century Germany*, translated by T. Dunlap, Cambridge and London: Harvard University Press, 1991, pp.130–5 (Reading 8.1).

A. McLaren, 'The pleasures of procreation: traditional and biomedical theories of conception' in W.F. Bynum and R. Porter (eds) *William Hunter and the Eighteenth-Century Medical World*, Cambridge: Cambridge University Press, 1985, pp.332–40 (Reading 8.2).

L. Bourgeois, *Récit Veritable de la Naissance de Messeigneurs et Dames les Enfans de France. Fidelle Relation de l'Accouchement, Maladie et Ouverture du Corps de Feu Madame. Suivie de l'Ouverture du Corps de Feu Madame. Remonstrance a Madame Bourcier, touchant son Apologie*, ed. by F. Rouget, Geneva: Droz, 2000, pp.99–108, 111–20; translation by E. Rabone (Reading 8.3).

D. Evenden, 'Mothers and their midwives in seventeenth-century London' in H. Marland (ed.) *The Art of Midwifery: Early Modern Midwives in Europe*, London: Routledge, 1993, pp.9–19 (Reading 8.4).

A. Wilson, *The Making of Man-Midwifery: Childbirth in England 1660–1770*, London: UCL Press, 1995, pp.185–92 (Reading 8.5).

9

The Care and Cure of Mental Illness

Peter Elmer

Objectives

When you have completed this chapter, you should be able to:

- examine ways in which ideas relating to the care and cure of the mentally ill evolved and changed in the period from the Renaissance to the Enlightenment;

- demonstrate how medical understanding of the mad and definitions of madness were shaped by the wider concerns of early modern culture and society.

9.1   Introduction

In this chapter, I discuss two aspects of a very large and complex body of historical material relating to the experience and treatment of mental illness in early modern Europe. In the first half, I focus on the way in which contemporaries – patients and practitioners, lay people and medical experts – understood and defined what it meant to be mentally ill in the period from the Renaissance to the Enlightenment. A large body of evidence survives to illustrate the various ways in which the men and women of this period experienced madness. Books, diaries, official documents and the case notes of practitioners all provide fascinating insights into how madness was conceptualized and treated, and I look at some examples of these to illustrate the broad and eclectic nature of the response to mental illness in this period. In the second half of the chapter, I focus on the way in which those who were deemed to be suffering from some form of mental affliction were treated and cared for by their families and communities. In particular, I look at changing attitudes in society to the mad, and the emergence of more formal, institutional solutions to the care and cure of the insane as epitomized by the creation of special hospitals or asylums in the late seventeenth and eighteenth centuries.

In addressing these two broad themes, one is faced by fundamental, and often controversial, issues relating to what it means to discuss mental illness in a period so radically different from our own. Problems of definition lie at the heart of such concerns; you will need to keep them to the forefront of your thinking as we proceed. For the historian, who seeks to understand and explain how the people of the past experienced and understood mental suffering, two contrasting, though not entirely exclusive, approaches have traditionally guided work in this field. On the one hand, there is the temptation to reduce all past manifestations of mental anguish and insanity to disease categories familiar to the modern psychiatric profession. On the other, we are encouraged to accept as 'real' the definitions of mental illness widely subscribed to by the people of the past, even if we do not share those convictions today.

These two approaches represent radically different ways of understanding the impact of disease on past societies. In particular, by taking the first approach, we are led to *judge* the past, and to *mistrust* the definitions and categories of mental illness favoured by contemporaries. From our current vantage point, we are tempted to offer the benefits of retro-diagnosis, and so set the historical record straight – a case well illustrated in our period by those historians of witchcraft who have detected delusory and psychotic behaviour in the actions of accused witches and their persecutors. If, however, one adopts the alternative approach of accepting at face value the definitions of mental illness preferred by those who actually experienced the behaviour of the mad, we are unlikely to want to make such judgements or retrospective diagnoses. On this view, madness is widely perceived as culturally and historically specific, the product of particular societies at given moments in their evolution.

At its most extreme, some observers in the west have been led to conclude that madness or mental dysfunction does not in fact exist, and that it is wholly the product of the modern, western political system. According to this school of thought – popularized by writers like Thomas Szasz and historians such as Michel Foucault – madness came to be utilized by the ruling classes of industrial Europe as an instrument of repression and social control, epitomized for Foucault by what he termed the 'great incarceration' of the eighteenth century in France and the genesis of the modern asylum movement. This was in contrast with the period that went before, which Foucault envisaged as a 'golden age' for the insane, when the mad were treated with respect and even accredited with acts of divine inspiration.

Foucault himself saw the war on the mentally ill as part of a larger process of governmental centralization and control that occurred simultaneously with the first stirrings of the industrial revolution. This was no coincidence. According to Foucault, the desire to redefine and incarcerate the deviant clearly possessed an important economic, as well as a political, motive. The need to create a more compliant workforce that was willing to accept the new routines of an automated, industrial society, compelled governments, in his view, to impose new restraints on the mentally ill, as well as on others demonstrating deviant behaviour. Prisons, workhouses and asylums were all geared to this end, as the urge to define what was normal and morally acceptable increasingly became a feature of industrial society (Foucault, 1965; Szasz, 1972).

Today, it is probably fair to say that much of Foucault's legacy has been either debunked or radically challenged by historians of madness working in the field. Among other criticisms levelled at him, the most damning of all, at least from the perspective of the historian, concerns the extent to which it has proved virtually impossible to find concrete evidence in the sources for Foucault's larger claims. Not only have early modernists rejected his view of their period as a 'golden age' for the mad, but others have found little evidence for a 'great incarceration' in the eighteenth century (for example, Midelfort, 1999; Porter, 1987, pp.6–9). On the positive side, most historians writing on this subject nonetheless continue to pay a debt of obligation to Foucault for raising the whole issue of the extent to which concepts of madness and sanity were, or might have been, culturally and historically fashioned – an approach that has now become the dominant idiom for the study of insanity in the past (see, for example, Scull, 1993, p.5).

Throughout this chapter, I use a variety of terms to describe the wider phenomenon of 'madness', including the somewhat anachronistic phrase, 'mental illness'. In doing so, I should like to stress from the outset that I am not subscribing to an **essentialist** view of madness that perceives it as a universal given of western history – something that has remained constant in our past. The term 'mental illness' is invoked rather as a convenient phrase to cover the various categories used by contemporaries, both 'specialists' and lay people, in describing the range of symptoms and mental states exhibited by those suffering from some form of mental disturbance. As a recent historian of early modern madness has noted, the term 'mental illness' is itself a historical construct, the product of the late Enlightenment, when for the first time it became possible to talk of the mind as susceptible to physical degeneration and sickness. Prior to the mid-eighteenth century, it was virtually impossible to conceive of the mind as sick or diseased because of the inviolable nature of the immortal human soul and the fact that this was virtually synonymous with the mind in the thinking of early modern Europeans (Suzuki, 1995, p.418).

9.2   Richard Napier and his patients: a case study

In 1981, the American historian Michael MacDonald published a groundbreaking study concerned with the incidence of mental illness in the medical practice of an English country physician, Richard Napier (1559–1634) (Figure 9.1). Based on the case notes of over 2,000 'obscure rustics', it provides a unique insight into the way in which mental affliction was understood in its time, not just by the so-called experts such as Napier, but most importantly from the perspective of those who either experienced madness itself or saw others in its throes. In what follows, I rely extensively on this seminal research, which remains unchallenged as a source for the subject. In many respects, the approach of the university-educated Napier to the diagnosis and cure of the mentally ill was typical of that of a learned practitioner in the healing arts, even if his status as a cleric caused bitter professional rivalries.

Avowedly of the belief that 'the criteria for identifying mental afflictions vary between cultures and historical periods' (MacDonald, 1981, p.1), MacDonald's work is informed throughout by the need to explain how contemporary definitions of madness were firmly rooted in the social, material and cultural world of the seventeenth century. In some respects, these are familiar to the modern observer: MacDonald, for example, emphasizes the role of the family in both the genesis and the care of the mentally ill. In other respects, contemporary definitions are profoundly unfamiliar, as seen, for example, in MacDonald's discussion of the role of religion and religious belief in determining the mental state of an individual. In this section, I shall look at numerous examples of the way in which such factors impinged on definitions of madness as well as on the subsequent care and treatment of the mentally ill. I shall begin, however, by exploring Napier's practice and clientele in order to determine, if possible, the broad social profile of mental affliction in Napier's neighbourhood in the first three decades of the seventeenth century.

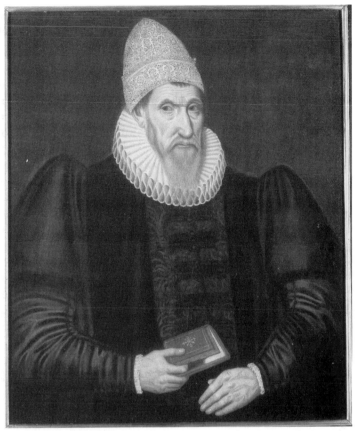

Figure 9.1   Portrait of the Reverend Richard Napier, who served as rector of Great Linford in Buckinghamshire from 1590 until his death in 1634. Throughout this period, he administered medicine and medical advice to thousands of patients in the neighbouring area, despite the fact that he had no formal training (that is, a doctor's degree) in medicine. His casebooks survive in the Bodleian Library, Oxford. Ashmolean Museum, Oxford

Locating the mad in early modern England

Exercise

Read extract (i) of 'Madness in early modern England: the casebooks of Richard Napier' (Source Book 1, Reading 9.1), and under the headings 'gender', 'age', 'marital status' and 'social status', note down the chief characteristics of Napier's anguished or mad clients. How does MacDonald relate these to the specific social and cultural contexts of early modern England?

Discussion

In the case of *gender*, MacDonald detects a notable imbalance in the mental health of Napier's patients, with more women than men reporting and being diagnosed as having mental illness and related complaints. MacDonald relates some of these complaints to the nature of women's role in early modern society. In particular, he points to the fact that one in five of the mentally afflicted women who visited Napier also complained of gynaecological and obstetrical problems. Given the very real dangers and complications surrounding childbirth in the seventeenth century, it is perhaps not surprising that many women exhibited mental anguish and despair. In addition, MacDonald suggests that the socially constrained role that women typically performed in what was a patriarchal society was a further factor in accounting for the high rates of mental illness found among women in Napier's clientele.

With respect to *age*, MacDonald detects a number of interesting anomalies. A disproportionate preponderance of young adults in their twenties is balanced by a reciprocal under-reporting of cases of mental illness among the very young and the very old. Cultural factors once again suggest an explanation for these statistics. In the case of infants and children, who were numerically very prominent in early modern communities, he suggests that their absence from Napier's practice was in all probability a reflection of the general tendency in this period to regard children as incapable of rational thought and action. If this was the case, then it was impossible to envisage how they might be susceptible to mental disorders, since such afflictions, by their very nature, demanded a capacity to think and act according to the dictates of reason.

In the case of young adults, who comprised such a large percentage of Napier's mentally ill patients (more than double the number one might expect from their proportion of the total population), again, cultural and social factors loom large in explaining such a discrepancy. The anxieties generated by courting, marriage, childrearing and the desire to create an independent economic household all produced a gamut of problems (for example, marital difficulties, infant death and economic frustration) that might easily foster mental strife and conflict. Less convincing is MacDonald's explanation for the general paucity of the aged among Napier's caseload. Proverbially given to gloom and despondency, one might expect them to have figured far more prominently in MacDonald's sample. However, one practical factor, overlooked here, is the difficulty caused by the need for Napier's patients to travel to him for consultation. Travelling in early modern England was never easy or comfortable. For the aged it must have acted as a very real deterrent, especially in light of the fact that Napier never visited his patients but relied on them to come to him.

In terms of *marital status*, MacDonald claims that his figures bear direct comparison with modern rates of reported mental illness among married and single men and women. Early modern marriage was largely a 'paradise for husbands and a purgatory for wives'. Married women outnumbered married men in Napier's sample, with single and widowed men constituting a significant minority.

With respect to *social status*, MacDonald's research demonstrates that Napier's 'mad and troubled clients' represented 'a faithful cross section of the social composition of the top two-thirds or so of rural society', with only the very poorest excluded from his practice. MacDonald himself speculates that Napier's fees (12d (60p) for a consultation – the equivalent of one day's wages for a labourer) may have deterred those at the very bottom of early modern society from availing themselves of his services. But even excluding this significant minority, one is nonetheless impressed by the broad social composition of Napier's medical practice.

Contrary perhaps to both popular belief and the theoretical assumptions of Foucault, MacDonald's analysis of the practice of Richard Napier suggests that rural, pre-industrial societies were just as likely to produce mental illness as their modern, industrial and post-industrial successors. Equally, when mental illness struck, it affected all sectors of early modern society, regardless of economic, social and geographic background, though some people, as we have seen, were seemingly more susceptible than others to mental anguish and breakdown. In seeking to explain the contours of mental stress and anxiety depicted in his analysis of Napier's caseload, MacDonald places particular emphasis on the role of the family and community in the genesis of mental illness in early modern England. Emotional disturbance and stress were more often than not related to conflict and crisis within the nuclear family, with women the major sufferers. Troubled courtships, marital problems, bereavement and unrequited love affected men and women equally, but it was women who bore the brunt of such disappointments. Mothers, in particular, seem to have succumbed to grief following the loss of a child. They were also more likely to express infanticidal urges as well as to experience anxiety as a result of barrenness. Women's dominance of the domestic sphere – a by-product of the patriarchal nature of early modern society – was undoubtedly a further factor in accounting for the high rates of mental stress and anxiety found among Napier's female clients.

An additional factor here – well worth bearing in mind when seeking to locate the social and cultural roots of madness in early modern Europe – is the lack of privacy that characterized social relations of all kinds in this period. Life, as MacDonald notes, was often 'oppressively public' in the seventeenth century. In the absence of organized policing, early modern communities regularly relied on the prying eyes of neighbours to report misdemeanours and other violations of the moral and legal code. Both formally, through the secular and ecclesiastical courts, and informally through local customs and rites, neighbours played a central role in upholding common moral, sexual and social standards of behaviour. On occasion, such behaviour led to highly tense and disturbing situations that might induce mental imbalance or even madness. The incidence of witchcraft in Napier's casebooks provides a case in point. More than 500 of Napier's patients reported that they were bewitched. Of these, over half were considered by Napier also to suffer from some form of mental illness. In the vast majority of cases, the root cause of the bewitchment was understood by the patient to have followed from the sufferer's refusal to grant alms to a poor neighbour. Historians of witchcraft have long argued that such an infringement of the social code induced a guilt-inspired accusation of witchcraft, which frequently left the innocent party prey to all manner of physical and psychological torments (Macfarlane, 1970; Thomas, 1971).

The large number of patients in Napier's casebooks who claimed that they were the victims of witches, and Napier's response to their predicament, suggests that early modern medical practitioners possessed an etiology of madness that was very different from our own. Whereas we today might happily declare anyone who claimed to be bewitched or possessed as suffering from some form of psychotic disturbance, Napier and his contemporaries applied a different set of criteria by which to judge the sufferer. While not excluding the possibility that those who claimed to suffer witch-related illnesses may have suffered from some form of mental disturbance or delusion, most early modern physicians were only too willing to speculate on a wide range of possible explanations – physical, mental, demonic or a combination of all three – before passing judgement on individual cases. In so doing, they were reflecting a general diversity of approach in medical practice, shared among the laity, with regard to the diagnosis and cure of mental illness in early modern Europe.

Defining the insane in early modern England

Citing contemporary pamphlets and the views of Napier's patients, MacDonald concludes that there was no single, authoritative voice in determining who was mad in seventeenth-century England. In the absence of a psychiatric profession, popular lay opinion was crucial in defining the varieties of mental illness – a point borne out by MacDonald's study in which he attempts to codify the different categories of mental anguish and insanity according to the terms used by those in despair. Once again, the benefit of this approach is that it prioritizes the extent to which the symptoms of mental disorder, expressed in the distinctive language of the mad, are 'culturally relative and are viewed as violations of particular social norms' (MacDonald, 1981, pp.114–15). By adopting this method, we avoid the temptation of employing anachronistic comparisons. It does, however, create problems in attempting to generalize about the incidence and nature of madness across time. On the basis of a vast range of symptoms described in almost 2,500 consultations undertaken by Napier, MacDonald identifies four distinct varieties of mental illness in early modern England, all of which can be found in contemporary literature, legal records and medical treatises before 1640:

> The most severe kinds of insanity were identified with two patterns of behaviour, one of which resembled criminality, the other sickness. Both of these stereotypes were characterized by terrible energy and mental incoherence, and both of them were called by a variety of names, including, respectively, *madness*, *lunacy* or *distraction* and *mania*, *distraction* or *light-headedness*. The less violent types of mental disorder were also loosely organized into two patterns of thought, mood, and action. These disorders were typified by physical torpor and by emotional disturbances, faulty perceptions, or delusions. One of these stereotypes was the most fashionable malady of the age, melancholy; the other was a much less prestigious affliction, usually referred to by such unflattering terms as mopishness, lethargy, or (in later works) insensibility.
>
> (MacDonald, 1981, p.120)

Within the category of mad, lunatic or distracted, Napier identified two main groups: those whose insanity was manifest in their violent or menacing behaviour, and those whose madness disposed them to incoherent raving and wild utterances. In both cases, an ability to establish lunacy was important since under the law, lunatics, like children and idiots, were not responsible for their actions. The need to establish criminal responsibility was particularly acute in the case of lunatics, since it was widely believed that one of the chief characteristics of mad behaviour was its proximity to criminality. Mad crime, however, might be distinguished from the actions of regular criminals by the unnatural and unreasonable way in which the criminally insane sought to threaten or destroy those people and things that ought to have been most cherished by them. Typically, then, the deeds of the mad involved acts against their own families and breaches of the most fundamental communal norms. An inability to recognize one's family or to take any pleasure from the role of parent or spouse was commonly seen, therefore, as indicative of a mad frame of mind. Infanticide was a case in point. Any woman who killed her baby or child was, more often than not, automatically assumed to be mad (MacDonald, 1981, p.128).

In a related fashion, acts of wanton destruction were also regularly invoked as evidence of insanity. As today, but even more so in early modern Europe, possessions 'articulated one's place in the social hierarchy'. The destruction of luxury objects, such as windows, for example, was thus widely perceived as an indicator of madness. Of all material possessions, however, the most inviolate within the context of this period were clothes. Nakedness itself was widely seen as akin to bestiality and antithetical to civilized values. Consequently, destruction of one's clothing represented a symbolic gesture of rejection of the moral and social values of contemporary society (MacDonald, 1981, p.131).

In the cases of madness so far cited, it is evident that early modern definitions of mental instability were firmly linked to the wider social and cultural values of the period. Behaviour which we today might not consider as evidence of lunacy – a disregard for one's physical appearance, for example – was widely construed as such in the sixteenth and seventeenth centuries. In the same way, much that we might currently consider as evidence of mental derangement was not necessarily perceived as such by our early modern forebears. Prior to the middle of the seventeenth century, for example, men and women who claimed to have received messages from God, or to have communed with angels and spirits, would not necessarily have been regarded as mentally unbalanced or in need of medical care. Indeed, Napier himself recorded frequent 'conversations' with angels and good demons, whom he often consulted in the course of his regular medical practice. Early modern 'specialists' – theologians, physicians and lawyers – possessed a range of possible explanations for such behaviour, of which insanity or delusion was only one. Only after 1660, and the emergence of a radical religious tradition that threatened to subvert the political and social order, were such acts of religious 'enthusiasm' widely considered as manifestations of mental illness. In this way, groups such as the **Quakers** and the **Methodists** were routinely stigmatized as breeding grounds of irrationality and insanity – a judgement that was facilitated in the case of the early Quakers because of the predilection of some of their members to 'go naked for a sign', that is, to express their spiritual rebirth through the symbolism of bodily nakedness (Godlee, 1985; Spierenburg, 1991, pp.174–5).

Another example cited by MacDonald further highlights the way in which madness in early modern Europe can be seen as the product of the prevailing cultural norms of the age. Suicide, which today is widely perceived as the product of mental instability, was rarely seen in the sixteenth and seventeenth centuries as prima facie evidence of insanity. From both a legal and a theological perspective, suicide was a case of wanton and self-willed destruction. It implied collusion with that great tempter, the devil, and as such was widely vilified in both pulpit and press. Thus, despite the fact it was accepted that men and women might take their own lives while temporarily out of their wits or mad, the fact of suicide itself was never alone considered sufficient proof of mental illness. The distinction was a crucial one in early modern society since the penalties for suicide, a serious felony, were draconian. The insanity defence was widely recognized in most early modern legal codes, and was frequently resorted to in the case of relatives eager to prove that in a given instance suicide was the result of temporary mental impairment. Failure to secure such a verdict, however, entailed dire consequences for the family of the deceased. In the most extreme cases, rights of inheritance were annulled and the estate of the suicide forfeited to the crown.

In opposition to the frantically mad or 'lunatic' were those whom Napier characterized as 'distracted' or 'light-headed'. The distinctive feature of this group was their proneness to 'verbal pandemonium'; their erratic behaviour was often compared to the symptoms of those who suffered from delirium caused by physical illness. Typically, such people spoke nonsense and were unaware of what they had said. Their message, however, was not totally incomprehensible to onlookers since, more often than not, it was couched in the conventional and symbolic language of the age that was characterized in the main by a deep-seated belief in the religious conflict between good and evil. Most of the ramblings and utterances of Napier's patients betray this essential fact. Many talked incessantly about the devil, or communicated conversations that they claimed to have had with him or with his evil minions. Others described what sounds like an internal war of words between the forces of good and evil, which frequently left the patient exhausted and broken. The common denominator in most of these consultations was a deeply held fear or panic surrounding the state of one's soul and impending judgement followed by divine retribution. Applying modern criteria, we might be tempted to ascribe such symptoms as classically those pertaining to schizophrenia or multiple personality disorder. The value of such an approach is, however, open to question, not least because of the way in which it threatens to deny the validity of the mad person's moral and spiritual concerns by reducing them to universal or essentialist categories of mental illness. Whether or not such people were mad – Napier himself adopted a number of different stances – is ultimately perhaps irrelevant. What is important from the point of view of the historian of madness is the way in which Napier's judgement in such cases was informed and constrained by the prevailing religious and cultural standards of the age.

Categories of mental illness in early modern Europe: the case of melancholy

Perhaps one of the most important findings in MacDonald's work is the extent to which he finds that those whom Napier termed chronically mad or insane, and who required close care and attention, constituted only a very small minority of his mentally disturbed clientele. Far more common were those who suffered from a range of lesser maladies, which MacDonald has categorized as 'afflictions of mood and perception'. If we are to believe the claims of contemporaries, by the end of the sixteenth century Europe was in the throes of a veritable epidemic of mental anguish, grief and madness. Whether this constitutes real evidence for the growth of insanity in early modern culture is debatable. It strongly suggests, however, that, as MacDonald has argued in respect of the English, Europeans were becoming 'more aware of mental suffering' at this time than ever before (MacDonald, 1981, p.149). But what shapes did these common, though lesser, forms of mental strife take? Here, clearly, contemporaries were in uncharted territory, as they sought to provide labels and descriptions for the various forms of mental suffering that they encountered on a daily basis. Some of the terms were familiar and probably long lived; others were of more recent provenance. In most cases, these conditions were thought to be the product of excessive, immoderate or inappropriate passion or emotional response – typically an over-reaction to a day-to-day problem. Among Napier's patients, such conditions prompted a variety of symptoms, the most common being sleeplessness, fear and anxiety, light-headedness, thoughts of suicide and religious anxiety. A large proportion of those so affected, however, were diagnosed with two conditions that were not ascribed to excess of emotion. Napier referred to these as melancholy and mopishness. Both provide valuable evidence for the way in which early modern attitudes to the mentally ill were informed by a variety of topical concerns, not all of which were purely medical in nature.

Exercise

Read extract (ii) of 'Madness in early modern England: the casebooks of Richard Napier' (Source Book 1, Reading 9.1) and 'Melancholy: a physician's view' (Source Book 1, Reading 9.2).

1   How did Napier's view of melancholy, as described by MacDonald, differ from that of Barrough?

2   What evidence does MacDonald's analysis of Napier's melancholic and mopish clients provide for disease as a social and cultural construct?

Discussion

1   Barrough's definition of melancholy is broad and all-inclusive. In seeking to lump together all the known symptoms of madness under one category, or disease, 'melancholy', he clearly seeks to redefine madness itself. Napier on the other hand, who was confronted on a daily basis with a bewildering variety of symptoms and complaints, is more discriminating, applying the label 'melancholy'

only in certain specific instances – that is, to patients who exhibited the symptoms of deluded fear and excessive and unwonted sorrow.

2   Despite the fact that Napier's melancholic and mopish patients presented very similar symptoms, they were distinguished on the grounds of social status. The melancholic were largely drawn from the upper ranks of society who were literate and thus more likely to be sensitive to the labels attached to their maladies. Mopishness, on the other hand, was confined to the lower social classes, who were largely ignorant of their condition. 'This socially pejorative aura' was also reflected in the different explanations that Napier provided for the origin of the two conditions. Whereas melancholy was inflicted on its sufferers (with the implication that they could not help but 'catch' it), the mopish are described as naturally idle and given to indolence. They, in other words, bring the disease on themselves. In contemporary medical parlance, the mopish were inferior in every way since their condition was primarily seen as a disturbance of the sensitive faculty. The melancholic, on the other hand, were the victims of a malady that impaired one of the most vital functions of the human body, man's capacity to reason. This was a hierarchical distinction that mirrored the social gap between those who suffered from these two complaints in the seventeenth century.

By stressing the physical origins of the disease (Barrough, for example, is typical in ascribing the mental disturbances associated with melancholy to traditional notions of causation based on humoral theory), a rational explanation was provided for what was otherwise inexplicable behaviour. Like certain afflictions today that have been labelled by some as 'middle-class' diseases, melancholia was clearly a fashionable complaint that owed much to social and cultural expectations.

The growing popularity of melancholy as a diagnostic label for the mad was in all likelihood related to the popularization of the concept in medical circles from the late sixteenth century onward. It is probably no coincidence that there was a discernible rise in the number of patients described as melancholic among Napier's clientele after 1621 following the publication of the bestseller *The Anatomy of Melancholy* (Figure 9.2) by Robert Burton (1577–1640).

Erik Midelfort has found a similar trend in Germany. In a detailed study of admissions and dismissals from a new foundation, the Juliusspital (1576) in Würzburg, between 1580 and 1630, he detected not only a gradual rise in the number of patients suffering from some form of mental affliction, but a distinct growth in patients described as melancholic (Midelfort, 1999, pp.376–8). Intriguingly, he also found evidence to suggest that over time ordinary people, as well as the educated elite, who suffered some form of mental illness were increasingly likely to be described as subject to melancholy. Like MacDonald, Midelfort has argued that the popularization of melancholy owed most to the growing discussion of the condition in professional medical circles, and its widespread appearance in print. Again, it was probably no coincidence that the hospital at Würzburg had close links with the medical faculty of the city's university (Midelfort, 1999, pp.376–8).

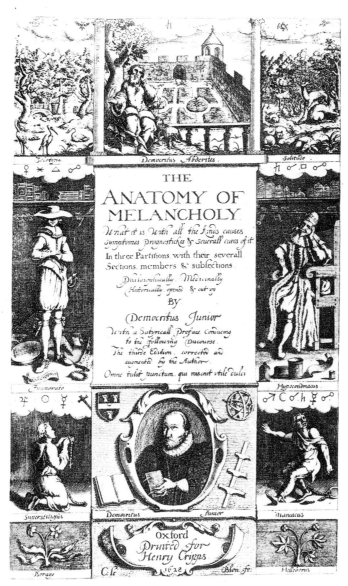

Figure 9.2   This engraved frontispiece first appeared in the third edition of *The Anatomy of Melancholy* in 1628. The work rapidly became the standard text on the diagnosis and treatment of the 'fashionable' disease of melancholy. The illustrated frontispiece depicts the multifaceted nature of melancholy as understood by learned men like Burton. The numbered items (just visible) are described in the accompanying doggerel verse that appeared in the 1632 edition: 1. 'Old *Democritus* under a tree ... Over his head appeares the skye, And *Saturne* Lord of Melancholy'; 2. 'Toth' left a Landskip of *Jealousye*; 3. 'The next of *Solitarinesse*'; 4. 'Inth' under Columne there doth stand, *Inamorato* with folded hande'; 5. *Hypocondriacus* leanes on his arme, Winde in his side doth him much harme ... About him pottes and glasses lye, Newly brought from's Apothecary; 6. 'Beneath them kneeling on his knee, A *Superstitious* man you see'; 7. But see the *Madman* rage downe right, With furious lookes, a ghastly sight. Naked in chaines bound doth he lye, And roares amaine he knowes not why?'; 8. And 9. '*Borage* and *Hellebor* fill two sceanes, Soveraigne plants to purge the veines, Of melancholy ...'; 10. 'Now last of all to fill a place, Presented is the *Authors* face'. Wellcome Library, London

The diagnosis and treatment of the insane in early modern Europe

It is evident from Napier's case notes that early modern medical practitioners utilized a variety of techniques in treating the mentally ill that reflected the eclectic nature of contemporary explanations for the origins of madness. Mental disorders might be caused by natural or supernatural means, or indeed by a combination of the two. In the case of those said to be suffering from bewitchment, for example, mental torment might proceed directly from the intervention of the devil and his minions (with God's permission) or indirectly through the devil's manipulation of a pre-existing physical condition, such as melancholy. Regardless of the origins of psychological disturbance, practitioners like Napier adopted a varied approach to the diagnosis and cure of such afflictions. Napier himself favoured astrological medicine combined with the traditional remedies prescribed by Galenic practitioners. Others – especially local folk healers – preferred the use of charms, amulets and exorcisms. The competitive nature of the early modern medical marketplace was particularly evident in the case of those who sought cures for madness. Napier, it should be remembered, was a clergyman by profession, whose medical practice was theoretically subservient to the higher goal of saving souls. He was not alone, however, as a minister in arguing for an active role for the clergy in medical matters, particularly in those borderline cases such as mental illness where the boundary between mind, body and soul was unclear and contested.

In many respects, such thinking was firmly embedded in early modern medical psychology, which was itself a synthesis of ancient classical science and medieval Christian thinking. According to this view, the human soul was divided into three distinct, but interconnected, parts: the vegetal, animal and rational souls. The vegetal soul oversaw nutrition, growth and generation. The animal or sensitive soul controlled the powers of perception and motivation. The rational soul was the seat of reason, understanding and will. This tripartite division of the soul thus incorporated the chief characteristics of all living things (vegetal, animal and angelic or spiritual) and enabled contemporaries to talk of man as unique in the divine creation – a microcosm of the whole. Mental illness was thus understood to proceed from impairment of one of the two higher faculties, the animal or rational souls. Extremes of madness and outright lunacy, which as we have seen were relatively rare, were the product of a disturbance in the highest faculty of the rational soul. More commonly, however, mental turmoil and affliction resulted from the defective working of the animal or sensitive soul – that faculty which contained the five external senses (smell, hearing, taste, sight and touch) and three internal senses (common sense, memory and imagination).

Of all these, it was the power of the imagination that most concerned early modern 'psychologists'. It played a crucial role in rousing the passions and stirring men and women to action. Under normal circumstances, it was kept in check by the superior authority of reason, thus ensuring that men and women controlled the bestial side of their natures. Reason – located in the rational soul – acted as a break on the imagination and passions. It alone contained the power of judgement, comprehension and reflection, as well as the power of will, which gave it command of the senses 'so that the potent drama of imagination conforms to judgment's script and thus to control human passion and behavior' (MacDonald, 1981, p.180). But when reason, for whatever cause, no longer exerted such control and allowed the imagination to run riot, then madness soon followed. As Robert Burton declared:

> That melancholy men and sick men conceive to many phantastical visions, apparitions ... and have such absurd suppositions, as that they are kings, lords, cocks, bears, apes, owls; that they are heavy, light, transparent, great and little, senseless and dead ... can be imputed to naught else but a corrupt, false and violent imagination.
>
> (quoted in MacDonald, 1981, p.180)

It was also widely believed that the imagination was capable of transforming the passions, counterfeiting images of reality and inducing extraordinary emotions until the point where they became pathological. Moreover, it was the imagination, according to MacDonald, that was 'the amplifying power that transformed the griefs and fears of many of Napier's patients into destructive passions that sickened their minds and bodies' (MacDonald, 1981, p.181). Because of the widely held view in early modern Europe that soul, mind and body were linked and mutually interactive, it was generally believed that a disordered imagination might inflict harm on both body and soul. Fear, sadness, despair and sorrow were all perceived as potentially fatal. Among Napier's clients, for example, a wide range of physical ailments, including consumption, rheumatism, lameness and fevers, were blamed on emotional distress. The puritan physician Stephen Bradwell was not alone in arguing that those who were most fearful of the plague were also most likely to contract the disease (MacDonald, 1981, pp.181–2).

Stephen Bradwell is discussed in Chapter 6.

Contemporary physicians explained such incidents by recourse to a humoral view of the body that envisaged mental turmoil as transmitted to the heart, where the inflamed passions caused a rise in bodily temperature with a concomitant disturbance in the balance of the humours. It is probably fair to say, however, that understanding of the precise physiological mechanisms connecting mind and body was only poorly developed in this period. For the vast majority of people, a more accessible explanation for the operation of the mind on the body, and vice versa, was the belief in correspondences and action by sympathy, based as it was on the premise that events in certain planes of existence affected those on other levels:

> The concepts of sympathy and correspondence permitted people to organize popular ideas about the fragility of body and mind into a coherent system by providing them with an explanation of how events on apparently separate levels of existence – physical, social, and moral – could cause sickness and insanity.
>
> (MacDonald, 1981, p.183)

Man was thought to be subject to such influences because of his unique place in the creation. It was precisely for this reason that astrological medicine gained such a purchase on both the popular and the educated mind, encouraging the view that alterations in the natural world might impact on the individual bodies and souls of men and women.

The classification of psychological types (melancholy, sanguine, choleric and phlegmatic) in the early modern era also provided an explanation as to why individuals were susceptible to certain physical and mental illnesses, and provided an important guide to therapy. It was commonly understood that men and women were predisposed to suffer from specific ailments that resulted from a dangerous excess of their own particular humoral type. For humanist-trained physicians and those who chose to emulate their methods, a whole range of physical remedies was available, most notably purging and bleeding. Napier himself commonly resorted to such methods. Like so many contemporary healers, however, Napier was a thorough eclectic when it came to prescribing the specific drugs or compounds that might be used alongside conventional therapies. Many of the concoctions he recommended to his mentally disturbed clients contained inorganic substances or drugs imported from the New World and Asia. Among the former, he frequently advocated the new mineral-based compounds favoured by the Paracelsians, which he produced in his own laboratory.

In addition to traditional humour-based therapies, classically trained physicians offered advice to the mentally ill in relation to their wider environment and social setting. This was achieved by focusing on the so-called six 'non-naturals' – diet, retention and evacuation, air, exercise, sleeping and waking, and the passions. Typically, therapists like Napier might admonish their clients to avoid excessive drinking and laziness, or promote the curative properties of listening to music or enjoying good company. Regular church-going was widely believed to promote sanity. Even flogging might, on occasions, be authorized in order to tame the wild passions.

I shall conclude this section by looking at Napier's response to a specific complaint that from our perspective looks suspiciously like a form of madness, but that to the minds of Napier and his contemporaries, rich and poor, educated and ignorant, provoked a very ambiguous response: bewitchment or possession.

Exercise

Look at Table 9.1. What general points might one infer about the nature of Napier's patients who were either obsessed with, or possessed by, demons?

Discussion

The first point to note is the relative rarity of such patients as a percentage of Napier's caseload (just 164 consultations, or 148 cases, in a sample of almost 2,500 patients). Second, it is apparent that the majority of his possessed clients displayed fairly mundane and unspectacular symptoms ('troubled in mind' and 'religious anxiety'). And third, there is the existence of a distinct minority, about a quarter of the total sample, who claimed to have witnessed the presence of supernatural beings or spirits ('hallucinations').

MacDonald's analysis of these figures, and the individual consultations that constitute the sample, suggest once again just how important cultural factors were in defining mental illness in this period. Today, we commonly assert that those who

Table 9.1 Napier's patients who either feared demons or claimed to be possessed. Figures are expressed as a percentage of consultations in which these symptoms appeared

	All mentally disturbed (N = 2,483)	Demoniacs (N = 164)
Mad, lunatic, distracted	10.3	4.8
Light-headed	15.0	9.8
Melancholy	19.9	11.0
Troubled in mind	32.0	41.5
Suicidal	6.4	17.1
Tempted	5.3	18.3
Evil thoughts	3.6	8.5
Religious anxiety	11.8	28.0
Hallucinations	5.1	26.8
Mopish	15.2	11.6

claim to experience hallucinations are suffering from some form of delusional or psychotic disturbance. Napier and his contemporaries, however, were able to choose from a much broader set of potential explanations, which included supernatural as well as physical causes. As MacDonald comments, '[i]n the early seventeenth century perceptions of the invisible world were taken very seriously [and] [e]ncounters with spirits and angels [though] rare ... were not by themselves signs of abnormality' (MacDonald, 1981, p.200). Though Napier was quite capable, on occasions, of dismissing the stories told by his possessed clients as 'strange fancies' or 'conceits', he was equally likely to accept at face value other accounts of supernatural activity or the appearance of the devil. In line with other contemporary physicians, he employed a vast array of diagnostic techniques, including magic and astrology, in order to determine whether men and women were truly afflicted. In certain cases, he readily proffered natural explanations for seemingly supernatural complaints, as for example in the case of hysterical women afflicted by the **suffocation of the mother**, a disease in which the womb was believed to move around and press on the other organs of the body. In others, he was more than happy to collude with those of his patients who saw local witches as the root cause of their mental and physical affliction. Just how he managed to discriminate between individual cases is not always clear. But one point is inescapable. In making his judgement, Napier was not influenced by medical factors alone: '[t]he patient's personality, the credibility of his accusations, and the public response to the case all influenced his decision' (MacDonald, 1981, p.212).

There was, then, no simple, agreed, response among early modern healers and patients to the phenomenon of mental illness in this period. Though Napier's practice in the East Midlands of England may have been singular in certain respects, it does seem to have been fairly typical in many others, most notably in the broad eclecticism that he brought to bear on the diagnosis and cure of the mentally sick. Since the publication of MacDonald's pioneering work, other studies have sought to broaden our picture of the state of mental health, and its treatment, in early modern Europe. By and large, most have confirmed the broad features outlined by MacDonald. Nonetheless, some of his findings have been questioned, most notably his assertion that early modern women were more subject than men to mental illness. Historical data from Germany, Spain, the Low Countries and Scotland, spanning the period from 1500 to 1800, suggests that there was no such gender bias in the numbers of those admitted to early modern asylums, and that in this respect at least, Napier's clientele may have represented the exception rather than the rule (Fernández-Doctor, 1993, p.377; Houston, 2000, pp.110–11, 123–5; Midelfort, 1999, pp.364–5; Spierenburg, 1991, p.187). On the other hand, virtually all these studies, and many others, have reaffirmed MacDonald's view that early modern understanding of mad behaviour was gendered (see, for example, Houston, 2002, pp.319–20).

On the whole, however, Napier was representative of his age – never more so than in terms of his deep religiosity which so often helped to shape and determine his understanding of madness. As a result of the close interaction between soul and body, madness was never considered the sole prerogative of the physician, nor was psychiatry likely to evolve as a specialist branch of medicine in early modern Europe. By the end of the seventeenth century, however, such restraints were beginning to erode as growing secularization – most often associated with the values of the Enlightenment – began to subvert the magical and theological underpinnings of Napier's universe.

The medical consequences of the spread of Enlightenment values was profound. They also had an impact on approaches to mental health, most notably in the extent to which the eighteenth century witnessed the gradual emergence of a specialized field of medicine and practitioners devoted to madness and diseases of the mind. The new 'models of the body', discussed in Chapter 7, many of which incorporated the rational materialism of the Enlightenment, were eagerly taken up by 'mad doctors', who now found a learned rationale for their specialism. In particular, notions of the body that prioritized the role of the nerves began to provide a new, more comprehensive medical explanation for ailments that had previously been contested by those 'physicians of the soul', the clergy.

Hysteria provides a case in point. As we have seen in the case of Napier's clientele, there were several competing explanations for hysteria in the early seventeenth century. Some claimed that it was the result of diabolical possession; others that it proceeded from purely physical causes, located in the 'wanderings' of the uterus (the so-called 'suffocation of the mother'). In both cases, the condition was seen as largely confined to women. Beginning with Thomas Willis in 1667, hysteria, alongside other 'convulsive distempers', came increasingly to be understood as a complaint that proceeded from damage to the nervous system. A century later, in 1769, the celebrated Scottish physician William Cullen reclassified hysteria under a new category of ailments which he termed 'neuroses', that is 'generalized diseases caused by a malfunction of the nervous system which involved changes in sensibility and motion' (Risse, 1988, p.15). Under the influence of these ideas, the language of modern psychiatry and a new profession, devoted to explaining the physical origins of mental illness, began to take embryonic form (Risse, 1988; Suzuki, 1995). At the same time, a disease that had hitherto been seen as the exclusive property of women – hysteria – was no longer seen as gender-specific.

I shall conclude this chapter by looking at the impact of these and other changes on the care and cure of the mentally ill in eighteenth-century Europe, focusing in particular on the creation of designated spaces, or asylums, which catered specifically for the needs of the insane.

9.3 Caring for the mad in eighteenth-century Europe: a 'psychiatric dark age'?

Despite the introduction of new theoretical explanations for the causes of mental illness in eighteenth-century Europe, historians of madness have traditionally depicted the eighteenth century as a 'psychiatric dark age' and 'a disaster for the insane' (MacDonald, 1981, p.230; Porter, 1987, pp.4–5). Echoing Foucault, they point to the growing containment and management of the mad in this period, while stressing the lack of innovative thinking with regard to their care and treatment. Seemingly untouched by the benign influence of enlightened rationalism, the prevailing image of the insane in this period remains Hogarth's much reprinted engraving of the treatment afforded to Tom Rakewell in Bedlam, where he lies half-naked and manacled, surrounded by various scenes of mayhem and lunacy (Figure 9.3).

Therapeutic innovation, by most accounts, did not take place until the early years of the nineteenth century when a new, more positive and humane approach to the treatment of the mentally ill emerged in the movement for asylum reform associated with the Quakers at York. Why have historians, until recently, projected such a negative image of the care and cure of the insane in Enlightenment Europe? And is the stereotype justified? In this section I shall look more closely, first, at how and why this view of the eighteenth century has proved so enduring, and then at some of the arguments of those who are slowly beginning to challenge such an approach.

The origins of the asylum movement in early modern Europe

One of the most distinctive features of the eighteenth century in terms of the fate of those deemed mentally ill or defective was the extent to which such people were increasingly subjected to the discipline of mad-houses operated by men and women who claimed a specialist expertise in the care and cure of the insane. Prior to 1700, it was the norm for those suffering from some form of mental affliction to be cared for in the homes of their next of kin or close family (this continued to be the case throughout the eighteenth century, despite the growth in the number of private and public asylums). Alternatively, in Catholic countries, the afflicted might resort to healing shrines such as that at Altötting in Bavaria where miraculous cures of the mad were widely reported (Figure 9.4).

Occasionally, the mad or their dependants were able to gain access to institutional care, though this was usually temporary and selective. In the Protestant territories

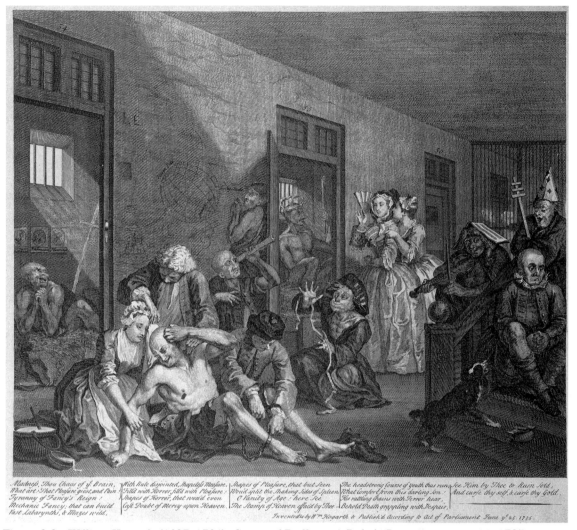

Figure 9.3   William Hogarth (1697–1764), *Scene of Bedlam, A Rake's Progress*, scene viii, 1735, engraving. A stereotypical depiction of the chaos and misery associated with Bethlem Hospital in London, in which Hogarth presents the rise and fall of the libertine Tom Rakewell. Among the lunatics shown here are a mad scientist, an astronomer, a king, a papist and a religious enthusiast, the latter depicted in his own cell where he mistakes the light from his window for a divine revelation. The two young women are clearly visitors amused by the spectacle but oblivious to the plight of the subject, Tom, who is being attended by a physician and a guard. Wellcome Library, London

of Germany, for example, monasteries were often converted into hospitals, to which the mad poor, along with those suffering from other ailments, were admitted. At Haina, in Hesse (Figure 9.5), the mad patients were segregated from the rest of the community and were housed in individual cells, where they were cared for by special overseers. Similar initiatives can be found in Catholic Germany. At Würzburg, for example, the Juliusspital (Figure 9.6), catered for a

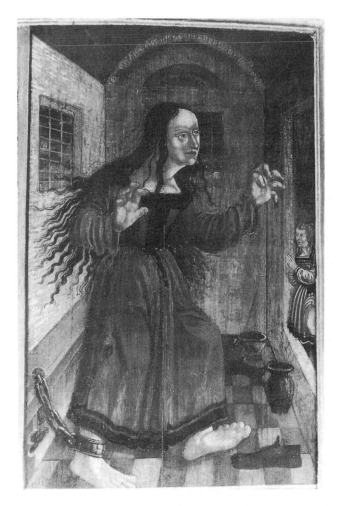

Figure 9.4 Anonymous, *The Mad Woman, Margreth*, 1520, panel from the Gnadentalfel, Heilige Kapelle, Altötting. Margreth was the daughter of Hanns Eyseleis from Mündraching who, having been unwell for about four years, was taken to the shrine at Altötting, a centre of Marian devotion 50 miles (80 kilometres) east of Munich, where she was cured of her madness. The painting depicts a wild and dishevelled young woman chained to the wall for her own safety. By permission of Hans Strauss, Altötting

large range of patients, including those designated as mad. Its rules were very similar to those at Haina, though Midelfort has detected some interesting differences in approach between the two institutions (Midelfort, 1999, Chapter 7).

Exercise

Read 'The hospitalisation of the insane in early modern Germany: Protestant Haina and Catholic Würzburg' (Source Book 1, Reading 9.3). How do these accounts of two early modern German hospitals contradict traditional historical descriptions of the provision of institutional care for the mad in this period?

Discussion

Most significant perhaps is what Midelfort refers to as the climate of 'therapeutic optimism' which characterized the regime at Würzburg and, to a lesser extent, at Haina. At the former, the short average length of stay for mental patients helps to dispel the myth of the early modern asylum or hospital as a place of incarceration,

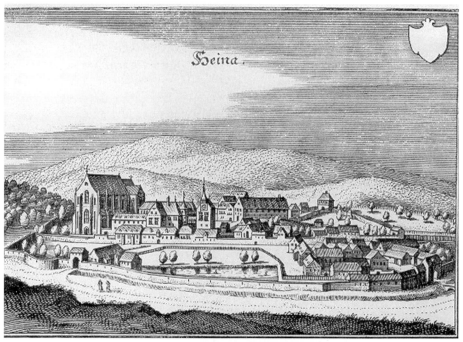

Figure 9.5   Matthäus Merian, the Protestant hospital at Haina in Hesse, first half of seventeenth century, copperplate. The hospital was established by Philipp, landgrave of Hesse, after the Reformation on the site of an old monastery. It was based on the twin principles of Christian charity and piety and offered spiritual as well as material succour to the sick, poor and mentally ill. Archiv des Landeswohlfahrtsverbandes Hessen, Fotosammlung

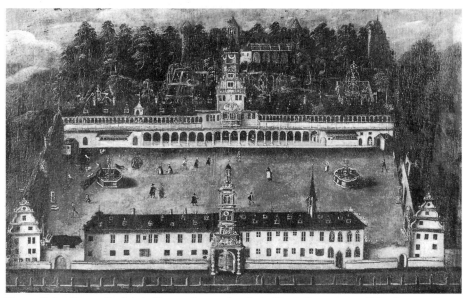

Figure 9.6   Georg Rudolph Hennenberg, the Catholic Juliusspital at Würzburg, oil on canvas. The hospital, constructed in the 1570s, was the brainchild of the prince-bishop of Würzburg, Julius Echter (1545–1617), an enthusiastic supporter of the Counter-Reformation in Germany. Reproduced from Midelfort (1999), p.336 by courtesy of Stiftung Juliusspital, Würzburg

as does the general level of care and concern exhibited by the rules governing the institution. Though one needs to be wary of accepting the degree to which such care was carried out in practice, the overall impression gained from close study of the two institutions is that they were popular with patients and neighbouring communities – increasingly so as the years progressed – and that they aspired to cure rather than contain.

Midelfort's emphasis on the care shown to the mentally sick in sixteenth- and seventeenth-century Germany marks an important departure in our understanding of the purpose of the early asylum movement. Where early modern institutions for the mentally ill were previously viewed as little more than holding institutions designed to remove the socially and morally dysfunctional elements from open society, historians of madness are now beginning to question such assumptions and to challenge prevailing myths about their repressive nature. Within a British context, the most famous – indeed the only one of its kind before the middle of the seventeenth century – was the London hospital, Bethlem. What can we learn about changing attitudes to the mad in England from a study of seventeenth- and eighteenth-century Bethlem?

Bedlam: fact or fiction?

In 1985, the archivist of Bethlem Royal Hospital, Patricia Allderidge, questioned for the first time the prevailing image of Bethlem in the seventeenth and eighteenth centuries as a house of horrors, where little attention was paid to either the care or the cure of the inmates (Allderidge, 1985). At the heart of her critique is a plea for historians and others to go back to original sources before forming judgements about the nature of the regime at the hospital, rather than repeating ad nauseam discredited sources or the well-worn clichés perpetuated by dramatists and popular writers. A particular target of Allderidge was the frequently repeated assertion that the mad were treated as objects of amusement for the sadistic pleasure of the London masses. She suggests that the doors of Bethlem were thrown open to the public only on rare occasions, and then as a way of raising much needed money to supplement the income of the cash-strapped institution. Following the lead of Allderidge, scholars like Jonathan Andrews and Andrew Scull have now begun to paint a picture of Bethlem that threatens to challenge our whole image of what it meant to be incarcerated in an asylum in the period before 1800. Bethlem was the only public institution in England before the middle of the eighteenth century to specialize in the care and treatment of the insane. Refounded in the sixteenth century by Henry VIII, Bethlem was very much a 'state institution', its principal patrons and benefactors being the crown and the corporation of the city of London. Whether or not it operated in the Foucauldian sense as a repressive arm of the state, designed to suppress all forms of religious, political and social dissent, is open to question. Though Andrews has found some evidence to support the notion that a few individuals were incarcerated in Bethlem prior to 1800 for 'political' reasons, these were very few in number and represented only a small percentage of the total population of the hospital (Andrews, 1995). It is also worth remembering that the hospital itself, even after it was rebuilt in the 1670s and removed to

Moorfields (Figure 9.7), never accommodated more than a few hundred patients at a time.

If Bethlem provides little evidence to support Foucault's thesis of a state-sponsored institution whose principle aim was to discipline the unruly in eighteenth-century England, what might it tell us about changing attitudes to the mad in both public and medical circles? Andrews and Scull have attempted to paint a rather different picture of the conditions experienced by mad patients at the hospital in the heyday of its notoriety – that is, around the middle decades of the eighteenth century. With respect to public visiting, for example, and the unseemly nature of charging spectators to view the inmates at Bethlem, it has been argued not only that the incidence of such an open door policy has been exaggerated, but that the imposition of restrictions on visiting, implemented in 1770, may in the last resort have proved to the disadvantage of the incarcerated. Deprived of contact with the outside world, many patients may well have suffered unduly from this new form of enforced isolation and segregation (Andrews and Scull, 2001, pp.27–8).

Bethlem's reputation among historians and others has also suffered through comparison with those newer institutions founded in the eighteenth century that

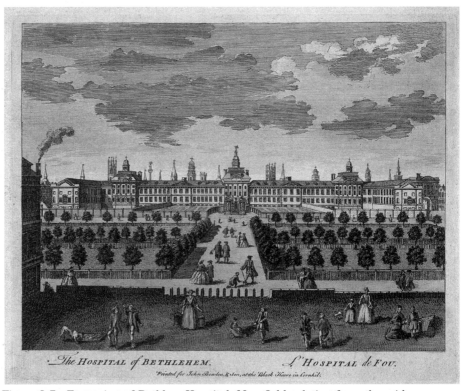

The HOSPITAL of BETHLEHEM.   L'HOSPITAL de FOU.

Printed for John Bowles & Son, at the Black Horse in Cornhill.

Figure 9.7 Engraving of Bethlem Hospital, Moorfields, dating from the mid-eighteenth century. It shows the new hospital, built (*c.*1675–6) to the design of Robert Hooke, with two recent additions, the incurable wards for male and female patients, situated at each end of the original façade. Wellcome Library, London

were designed to treat and care for the insane. Most important in this respect was the establishment of St Luke's in London in 1751 (Figure 9.8). Built close to Bethlem, it set out from the start to challenge the older hospital in every way. Even its architecture – plain and unadorned – represented a subtle criticism of Bethlem, the ornamented façade of which was considered by some as 'very improper for a hospital for madmen' (Andrews and Scull, 2001, p.45).

Likewise, the governors of St Luke's distanced themselves from previous associations between charitable hospitals and unnecessary grandeur by encouraging discreet, subscriptions-based funding and anonymous donations. Here, there was not to be found the vainglorious celebration of benefactors mounted on large tablets on the walls of the hospital – a radical departure from the usual practice at Bethlem and other London hospitals such as St Bartholomew's (Andrews and Scull, 2001, pp.45–6).

The reputation of Bethlem, and its physicians, has also suffered by contrast with the man who was appointed as first physician to St Luke's, the appropriately named William Battie (1703–76) (Figure 9.9). It was probably Battie, an ex-governor of Bethlem, who was responsible for instituting from the outset a ban on visiting at St Luke's – a position that formed part of a self-consciously new approach to the care and cure of those confined to asylums. In contrast, Bethlem's physician for much of the mid-eighteenth century, the famous mad-doctor, John Monro (1715–91), has

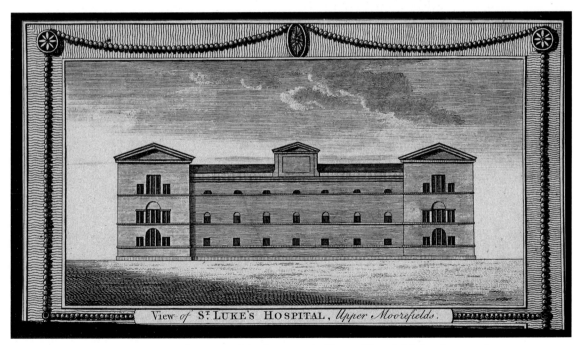

Figure 9.8 Engraving of St Luke's Hospital for Lunatics in Upper Moorfields by the pseudonymous Walter Harrison, 1775. It depicts the hospital's first building, designed by the architect George Dance the elder (1695–1768). Its austere façade is in stark contrast to neighbouring Bethlem and was partly designed as an overt criticism of the grandeur and ornamentation employed in the construction of the latter. Wellcome Library, London

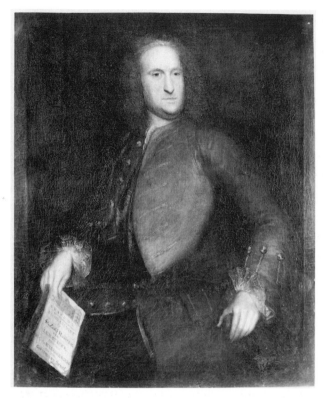

Figure 9.9   Portrait of Dr William Battie, physician at St Luke's Hospital, by Thomas Hudson (1701–79). This was painted about 1752 and depicts Battie clutching a copy of *Reasons for the Establishing and Further Encouragement of St Luke's Hospital for Lunaticks*, 1751, a blueprint for a new asylum for the insane inspired by Battie's desire to rectify the faults that he saw as prevalent at Bethlem. Reproduced by permission from the Witt Library, Courtauld Institute of Art, London

been widely depicted in the literature of madness as a medical traditionalist averse to any form of innovation. This was evident both in the way he continued to prescribe traditional Galenic remedies (purges, vomits, bleedings, etc.) and in his thinly veiled therapeutic pessimism. According to Monro:

> Madness is a distemper of such a nature, that very little of real use can be said concerning it; the immediate causes will for ever disappoint our search, and the cure of that disorder depends on management as much as medicine.

(quoted in Andrews and Scull, 2001, p.56)

Exercise

Read 'New approaches to curing the mad?: William Battie's *A Treatise on Madness* (1758)' (Source Book 1, Reading 9.4). On the balance of the evidence presented here, to what extent would it be fair to label Battie a 'progressive' in matters relating to the diagnosis, care and cure of the mad?

Discussion

The evidence would appear to be ambiguous. On the one hand, Battie adopted a 'modern' approach to madness, both in terms of demanding a clearer definition of the malady and in applying up-to-date medical theories to account for the causes of mental affliction. Hopefully, you will have noted Battie's debt to the nervous model of the body discussed in Chapter 7. In addition, Battie criticized others, whom he stigmatized as 'Empiricks', for failing to share their specialist knowledge in this field, and throughout he emphasized the need to create an environment characterized by high-quality care, cleanliness and recreation. There is little doubt that these barbed comments were part of an ongoing controversy focused on undermining the reputation of Bethlem and its principal physician, John Monro.

On the debit side, however, Battie's therapeutic optimism is tempered by a number of factors. 'Original madness', that is, mental illness resulting from an inherent fault in the nervous system, was deemed incurable. All other forms of the disease ('consequential madness') are considered susceptible to cure, but even here the measures that Battie advocated are hardly novel and differ little from those administered two centuries earlier. The 'lancet and the cupping glass' still ruled at St Luke's, as elsewhere, including Monro's Bethlem. Moreover, the benefits of Battie's more 'modern' regime, and his disparagement of those asylums that sought to treat the mad as 'criminals or nusances to [the] society', are open to question given the emphasis he placed on the confinement and isolation of patients, even to the extent of excluding friends and family from visiting the sick.

On balance, the gap between Battie and those he sought to criticize for their failure to care for and cure the mentally ill was probably much narrower than we might otherwise suspect from the verdict of earlier generations of historians of madness.

9.4 Conclusion

This brief excursion into the medical regime that operated at Bethlem in the eighteenth century suggests a number of ways in which attitudes to the mad in this period may have been unfairly judged by historians and others. It should also be remembered that in England, as in much of the rest of Europe, incarceration in public and private asylums was very much the exception rather than the rule. Throughout the eighteenth century, with the possible exception of France, the vast majority of those deemed to be suffering from some form of mental illness continued to be cared for within the confines of home and family. In other respects, too, continuity with the immediate past is evident. Despite the plethora of new ideas relating to the origins of madness – in particular those associated with the development of nervous theory – the various methods of care and cure remained much the same as in Napier's day. Vomiting, bleeding and other forms of evacuation remained the most popular treatment for the mentally ill and were as much part of the therapeutic programme at St Luke's as they were at Bethlem. One of the few discernible differences between the regimes operated by Battie and Monro was the greater optimism of the former with regard to the curability of most mental afflictions. There is no evidence to suggest, however, that Battie's approach to his St Luke's patients was any more successful than that of Monro at Bethlem.

But if there were few changes in the way in which the mad were treated in society at large, and in institutions in particular, between 1600 and 1800, that is not to say that all aspects of contemporary understanding of mental illness stayed the same. Important inroads were made into legal and medical definitions of madness, as philosophical and scientific rationalism took centre-stage. During the course of the eighteenth century, suicide was no longer treated as a form of spiritual apostasy, a self-conscious rejection of God, but instead was widely interpreted as a product of mental instability. In a similar vein, those who claimed to be possessed by demons were now far more likely to be treated as mentally ill rather than indulged as the victims of supernatural forces. With these and other developments in mind, historians now incline to speak of two distinct phases in the history of early modern madness – pre- and post-medicalization – characterized by the emergence after about 1750 of a new group of specialists devoted to exploring the physical or somatic origins of psychological disorders. Under the pressure of such changes, old diseases such as melancholia metamorphosed into new mental states such as 'depression' (first coined in its modern medical sense by Samuel Johnson in the 1750s) (Rousseau, 2000, p.72). Given the prominence of the medical marketplace in this period, it was also inevitable that unlicensed and irregular practitioners would increasingly find ways to market new and exotic remedies for the mad. The fad for 'electrical medicine', for example, offered new methods of treatment presaging electro-convulsive therapy in the twentieth century. Other medical entrepreneurs pioneered mechanical chairs and swings as an early form of shock therapy.

The medical marketplace is discussed in Chapter 13.

The extent to which such innovation constituted a major turning point in the care and treatment of the insane is, however, open to question. Generally speaking, historians of madness have been inclined to view the period around 1800 as marking a more significant watershed. Its landmarks, according to Roy Porter, included the 'madness' of George III, the opening of York Retreat – a Quaker asylum that introduced a new form of 'moral therapy' for mental patients – and the first stirrings of legal and parliamentary intervention into the establishment and running of asylums (Porter, 1987, p.3). It was these changes, or so the conventional story runs, that facilitated the growth of a new psychiatric profession in the nineteenth century, one that established its own specialized body of knowledge and practice in a way unimaginable before. Here, perhaps, one might find more sustained evidence for Foucault's 'great incarceration'.

References

Allderidge, P. (1985) 'Bedlam: fact or fantasy?' in W.F. Bynum, R. Porter and M. Shepherd (eds) *The Anatomy of Madness: Essays in the History of Psychiatry*, vol.2, London: Tavistock, pp.17–33.

Andrews, J. (1995) 'The politics of committal to early Bethlem' in R. Porter (ed.) *Medicine in the Enlightenment*, Amsterdam: Rodopi, pp.64–112.

Andrews, J. and Scull, A. (2001) *Undertaker of the Mind: John Monro and Mad-Doctoring in Eighteenth-Century England*, Berkeley: University of California Press.

Fernández-Doctor, A. (1993) 'Psychiatric care in Zaragoza in the eighteenth century', *History of Psychiatry*, vol.4, pp.373–93.

Foucault, M. (1965) *Madness and Civilization: A History of Insanity in the Age of Reason*, translated by R. Howard, New York: Random House.

Godlee, F. (1985) 'Aspects of non-conformity: Quakers and the lunatic fringe' in W.F. Bynum, R. Porter and M. Shepherd (eds) *The Anatomy of Madness: Essays in the History of Psychiatry*, vol.2, London: Tavistock, pp.73–85.

Houston, R.A. (2000) *Madness and Society in Eighteenth-Century Scotland*, Oxford: Clarendon Press.

Houston, R.A. (2002) 'Madness and gender in the long eighteenth century', *Social History*, vol.27, pp.309–26.

MacDonald, M. (1981) *Mystical Bedlam: Madness, Anxiety, and Healing in Seventeenth-Century England*, Cambridge: Cambridge University Press.

Macfarlane, A. (1970) *Witchcraft in Tudor and Stuart England*, London: Routledge & Kegan Paul.

Midelfort, H.C.E. (1999) *A History of Madness in Sixteenth-Century Germany*, Stanford, CA: Stanford University Press.

Porter, R. (1987) *Mind-Forg'd Manacles: A History of Madness in England from the Restoration to the Regency*, Cambridge, MA: Harvard University Press.

Risse, G.B. (1988) 'Hysteria at the Edinburgh Infirmary: the construction and treatment of a disease, 1770–1800', *Medical History*, vol.32, pp.1–22.

Rousseau, G. (2000) 'Depression's forgotten genealogy: notes towards a history of depression', *History of Psychiatry*, vol.11, pp.71–106.

Scull, A. (1993) *The Most Solitary of Afflictions: Madness and Society in Britain 1700–1900*, New Haven and London: Yale University Press.

Spierenburg, P. (1991) *The Broken Spell: A Cultural and Anthropological History of Preindustrial Europe*, Basingstoke: Macmillan.

Suzuki, A. (1995) 'Dualism and the transformation of psychiatric language in the seventeenth and eighteenth centuries', *History of Science*, vol.33, pp.417–47.

Szasz, T.S. (1972) *The Myth of Mental Illness*, London: Granada.

Thomas, K. (1971) *Religion and the Decline of Magic*, London: Weidenfeld & Nicolson.

Source Book readings

M. MacDonald, *Mystical Bedlam: Madness, Anxiety and Healing in Seventeenth-Century England*, Cambridge: Cambridge University Press, 1981, pp.33–54, 160–4 (Reading 9.1).

P. Barrough, *The Methode of Phisicke, Conteyning the Causes, Signes, and Cures of Inward Diseases in Mans Body from the Head to the Foote*, London: Thomas Vautroullier, 1583, pp.35–6 (Reading 9.2).

H.C.E. Midelfort, *A History of Madness in Sixteenth-Century Germany*, Stanford: Stanford University Press, 1999, pp.356–65, 369–84 (Reading 9.3).

W. Battie, *A Treatise on Madness*, London: J. Whiston & B. White, 1758, pp.1–3, 43–4, 61–2, 68–72, 74–5, 93 (Reading 9.4).

10

War, Medicine and the Military Revolution

Ole Peter Grell

Objectives

When you have completed this chapter, you should be able to:

- explain how and why surgery and medicine may have developed as a consequence of the changing nature of warfare;

- describe how and why military hygiene and epidemic disease became major concerns for military doctors and surgeons in the eighteenth century;

- demonstrate how and why the military hospital came into existence and developed.

10.1 Introduction

Since the days of Hippocrates, war has been considered an excellent training ground for medical men, especially surgeons. The range and quantity of wounds and injuries they were likely to encounter during times of war surpassed anything they were likely to come across in civilian life. This invaluable training was something about which, during the early modern period, surgeons did not hesitate to boast when they returned to civilian life. It was evidently a highly marketable experience.

As Roy Porter writes in *The Greatest Benefit to Mankind*:

> War is often good for medicine. It gives the medical profession ample opportunities to develop its skills and hone its practices. It can also create a postwar mood eager to beat swords into scalpels.
>
> (Porter, 1999, p.652)

This statement precedes Porter's account of the significance of antibiotics and the National Health Service in the medical developments that followed the Second World War. If true for the twentieth century, does this assertion hold true for the developments in medicine that followed what historians have described as the military revolution of the sixteenth and seventeenth centuries? Did the new approaches to surgery, health care and medicine that developed during this period originate primarily among doctors and surgeons who had experienced military service? Likewise, did the military hospitals serve as templates for the somewhat later changes and improvements to civilian hospitals towards the end of the eighteenth century? Is it purely coincidental that nearly all of the French and English physicians and surgeons associated with the reforms of surgery and clinical medicine from the sixteenth to the eighteenth centuries had experienced service with the army or the navy? These are some of the questions I shall attempt to answer in this chapter.

10.2 Changes to warfare in the early modern period

War has always been an integral part of human life. Before 1494, however, warfare in Europe had been characterized by brief and irregular campaigns, such as the Wars of the Roses in England (1455–85) and the Hundred Years War between France and England (1337–1453). By comparison, the sixteenth and seventeenth centuries proved unusually belligerent, with less than ten years of complete peace during the whole period, and no more than a couple of years of peace in the first half of the seventeenth century.

Among the most significant changes was the growth in the size of armies. Between 1500 and 1800 they grew dramatically, at least ten- or twelve-fold. In the 1490s, a large army would have consisted of fewer than 20,000 men; by the 1550s, it would have been twice that, while towards the end of the Thirty Years War (1618–48) the leading European states fielded armies of close to 150,000 men. By the end of the eighteenth century, armies had become even larger, especially those of France.

Reasons for this increase in the incidence and scale of warfare lie in the breakdown of the traditional social structure of late medieval society. The stable feudal system that had served the European aristocracy so well had come under considerable stress towards the end of the fifteenth century, as had the associated political structure, as a result of pressures generated by population growth. This weakening of feudal society provided territorial rulers or princes with the chance to strengthen their personal power and expand their lands, often on the basis of dynastic and therefore 'legitimate' claims of inheritance.

A consequence of the increased incidence of war between much larger forces was that armies acquired greater permanence during the early modern period. Military campaigns became lengthier, and were no longer restricted to the spring and summer seasons. The increased need to be able to wage war at any time encouraged states to retain large troops of professional soldiers in peacetime. These served as a core to which further and less experienced troops could be added at short notice. By the beginning of the seventeenth century, a number of small and medium-sized states were maintaining larger forces than before, whether at peace or at war.

One of the consequences of the growth in the size of armies was heightened anxiety on the part of princes and commanders alike about military discipline. Wanton destruction and pillaging, and uncontrolled suicidal actions could devastate the theatre of war and prevent further military action. This period therefore witnessed the issue of an increasing number of more detailed military codes.

The growing armies of the sixteenth and early seventeenth centuries consisted predominantly of volunteers from the poorer regions of Europe or those deprived and cast adrift by the effects of war engulfing their regions. However, no armies in early modern Europe consisted exclusively of combatants. Most soldiers were accompanied by prostitutes, mistresses, wives and children, servants, camp-hawkers and sutlers. Camp followers in the Spanish army of Flanders in the sixteenth century appear to have constituted more than half its number, and up to 28 per cent of these were female (Parker, 1990, p.288).

Early modern armies had to be supplied by boats and barges along coastlines or navigable rivers; only exceptionally, when troops moved along a known route such as the '**Spanish Road**', could suitable victuals be prepared and stocked beforehand. The provisioning requirements were staggering: it has been calculated that the daily needs of an army of 30,000 men would have been 20 tons (20 tonnes) of bread, 20,000 gallons (91,000 litres) of beer and 30,000 pounds (14,000 kilograms) of meat. These figures do not include the requirements of some 20,000 horses needed by the cavalry, the officers, the baggage wagons and the growing number of artillery guns. These animals would have needed 90 tons (90 tonnes) of fodder or 400 acres (162 hectares) of grazing daily.

During the eighteenth century, both armies and navies continued to grow, and most national governments were faced with the need to find new ways of recruiting soldiers and seamen. The importance of the military entrepreneur – the private individual who raised, trained and paid for troops on behalf of governments and had been such a dominant figure in the Thirty Years War (1618–48) – declined as his role was taken over by the state. The expanding bureaucratic machinery of increasingly powerful states made it possible to raise the larger armies and navies of the eighteenth century through voluntary enlistment and/or impressment.

Technological innovations served dramatically to change the nature and scale of warfare in this period. By the sixteenth century, heavily armoured knights on horseback had been replaced by infantry pikemen fighting together in tightly knit units or squares. It was, however, the growing number of firearms that proved of greatest significance. As early as the 1520s, it had become generally accepted that handguns could wreak havoc on the massed pikemen who had controlled the battlefield for the previous forty years. As a result, by 1570, the Spanish army had one handgun for every three pikemen, while thirty years later, it had as many handguns as pikes; by 1590, the Dutch army, then the most modern in Europe, had two handguns for every pike. The growing number of handguns and cannons changed the nature of warfare dramatically, causing injuries to combatants that were both more numerous and more atrocious.

In the sixteenth century, the most common type of firearm was the arquebus. It was fired by pulling a trigger that lowered a piece of smouldering cord into the gunpowder in the priming pan, a mechanism known as the matchlock. Unfortunately, the rate of misfire may have been as high as 50 per cent; if the gunpowder in the priming pan exploded, causing a 'flash in the pan', it could permanently blind the soldier and inflict horrendous burns, particularly to his face. Still, the matchlocked arquebus was a relatively cheap and effective tool of destruction, with reasonable accuracy when fired inside 60 yards (55 metres), compared with other weapons available at the time.

From the middle of the sixteenth century, the longer and heavier musket, which needed a metal fork for support, gradually replaced the arquebus. It was a far more powerful weapon. It fired a 2-ounce (57-gram) ball that could kill a man in shot-proof armour a hundred paces away or bring down a horse at the same distance, and when loaded with scattershot it was horribly effective at close range. By the eighteenth century, firearms had become even more accurate and deadly, and were being mass-produced according to national standards in most countries.

Artillery pieces were also developing. They had come into their own in the late fifteenth century as siege-guns. Their great size and weight made them extremely cumbersome to move, and therefore unsuitable as field-guns, but lack of mobility did not matter in a siege.

However, from the 1630s, artillery became increasingly mobile, not least because of the introduction of lighter field-guns by the Swedish King Gustavus Adolphus in the Thirty Years War. This development reached a new peak in the eighteenth century with the introduction of mass-produced, flexible and lighter field artillery with longer firing ranges (Cunningham and Grell, 2000, pp.92–124).

10.3 New wounds and old diseases

With the increased use of gunpowder, injuries to combatants posed new problems for the growing number of army surgeons who sought to treat them. Gunpowder presented surgeons with three new types of battlefield injury, namely **compound fractures**, burns and gunshot wounds. Before the use of firearms, compound fractures had been relatively unusual, not least because hand-wielded weapons could not generate sufficient impact to break bones in several places. When a bone was broken, it normally broke in one place, making it relatively easy to set. Hippocrates had considered compound fractures to be generally fatal and recommended amputation of the injured limb as the only treatment. Most early modern firearms fired lead balls, which were heavy and soft, and travelled at low speed, causing terrible injuries. When they struck a bone, the victim usually suffered a compound fracture. Even when this did not occur, the lead balls caused horrible wounds.

Furthermore, the new weaponry also resulted in new military tactics that dispersed infantry in much thinner and wider formations, which made it much more difficult to locate and assist the wounded. Consequently, many either died or were seriously weakened before they could receive medical assistance.

On the whole, the nature of injuries sustained by naval personnel did not differ materially from those suffered by soldiers on land. However, the wooden construction of ships and the limited space available aboard them did often serve to aggravate injuries. For example, heavy cannon balls, often fired at close distance, could shred wooden decks, masts and railings, creating a high volume of large splinters travelling at speed. Likewise, the not infrequent explosions of poorly cast cannons on the narrow decks close to where gunpowder had to be stored presented the sailor with added dangers. Medical treatment by ships' surgeons was provided in small, dark and badly ventilated rooms below deck, known as 'cockpits', which were too low-ceilinged for the surgeons and their helpers to stand erect.

As well as these new types of wound, armies and navies had to contend with a number of 'old' diseases, many of which proved more devastating to the much larger armies and navies of the era. Military campaigns were regularly affected or even halted by the outbreak of serious epidemics such as plague, camp fever, typhus, smallpox and dysentery. It was only from around the middle of the eighteenth century that military doctors and surgeons sought to tackle these problems. Once they had begun, however, they did not restrict their investigations to questions of hygiene, but also took a considerable interest in the dietary aspects of military life. In the case of the navy this resulted in the discovery of a remedy for scurvy, the greatest killer of naval personnel in the eighteenth century.

In order to illustrate how doctors and surgeons tackled these issues I focus in this chapter on four prominent surgeons and doctors who acquired fame for their efforts in these areas. The first, Ambroise Paré (Figure 10.1), served the French armies of the sixteenth century. Two served the English navy in the seventeenth and eighteenth centuries, namely the Plymouth surgeon James Yonge (1647–1721) and Dr James Lind (1716–94) (Figure 10.2), 'the father of nautical medicine' as his pupil Dr Thomas Trotter labelled him. The fourth, Sir John Pringle (1707–82) (Figure 10.3), served the English army in the eighteenth century.

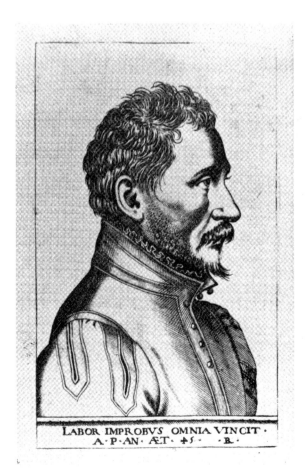

LABOR IMPROBVS OMNIA VINCIT ·
A · P · AN · ÆT · 45 · · R ·

Figure 10.1 Portrait of Ambroise Paré, aged 45, attributed to Jean Le Royer, 1561, engraving. Wellcome Library, London

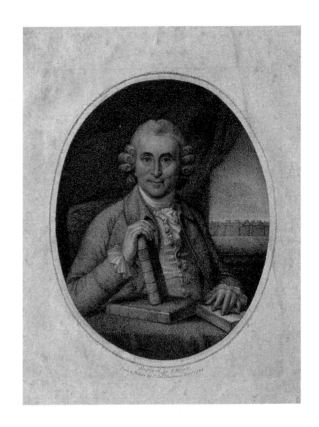

Figure 10.2   Portrait of James Lind by Wright, after Chalmers, engraving. Wellcome Library, London

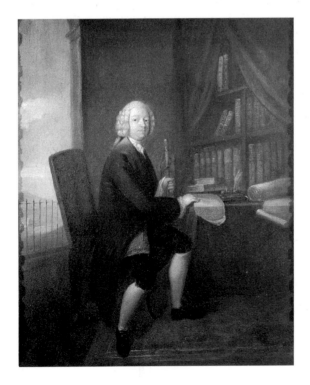

Figure 10.3   Portrait of Sir John Pringle, oil on canvas, 42 × 34.5 cm. Wellcome Library, London

The French surgeon Ambroise Paré, who served in more than forty military campaigns and wrote a number of bestselling medical/surgical treatises, became the leading exponent of new approaches to surgery that eventually led to significant improvements in a variety of areas. The most important of his books, *Method of Treating Gunshot Wounds*, first published in 1545, publicized his new techniques for treating gunshot wounds and performing battlefield amputations. In addition, Paré discussed mines and burning or explosive missiles which blew up many soldiers and caused others 'to burne in their harnesse, no waters being sufficiently powerfull to restraine and quench the raging and wasting violence of such fire cruelly spreading over the body and bowells' (quoted in Keynes, 1968, pp.132–3).

10.4 Surgical treatment of gunshot wounds

Major changes in the treatment of gunshot wounds were introduced in the sixteenth century by prominent army surgeons. In addition to Paré, whose publications had a significant impact throughout Europe, there were the English surgeon Thomas Gale (1507–87), Felix Wurtz of Zurich (1518–75?) and Bartholomeo Maggi of Bologna (1477–1552). Until this time, surgeons believed that gunshot wounds were poisoned by the gunpowder that was carried into the body by the bullet, as can be seen in the influential *The Book of Wound Dressing* (1497) written by the Alsatian army surgeon Hieronymus Brunschwig (1450–1533). His suggested treatment was to draw a silken cord through the wound to remove the poisonous powder. In 1514, the Spaniard Giovanni da Vigo (1450?–1525), personal physician to Pope Julius, published his *Practica Copiosa in Arte Chirurgica* [Rich Handbook in the Art of Surgery] in which he recommended cauterizing the wound with boiling oil, if necessary followed by the sealing of any severed arteries with a red-hot iron. This publication went through no less than forty editions during the sixteenth and seventeenth centuries, and supplanted the former treatment. The myth of the poisonous gunshot wound probably had a lot to do with the fact that the most efficient firearm of the day, the musket, which fired lead balls that flattened on impact, often carried parts of the soldier's clothing into the wound. Even without the further complication of fractured bones, such wounds were difficult to treat. Belief in the poisonous gunshot wound led to the practice of attempting to remove the bullet with fingers, probes and extractors, all of which enlarged the wound and significantly increased the risk of infection. Matters were not improved by the doctrine of **suppuration** practised by physicians as well as surgeons, which had originally come about as a result of a mistranslation of Hippocrates and Galen. As a result of this misunderstanding surgeons tended to stuff wounds with all sorts of material in order to produce the effect considered necessary for healing.

Exercise

Read extract (i) of 'Medicine, surgery and warfare in sixteenth-century Europe: Ambroise Paré' (Source Book 1, Reading 10.1) and describe how Paré made his discoveries.

During his first campaign, in 1536, Paré stumbled on a new treatment for gunshot wounds that convinced him such wounds were not poisonous and that cauterizing them with boiling oil caused more harm than good. After the assault by French forces on the castle of Villane, Paré and his fellow surgeons treated a large number of soldiers who had suffered gunshot wounds. At the start, the young and inexperienced Paré treated his patients in the same way as the more senior surgeons, according to the instructions of Vigo, despite the realization that it caused great pain to the victims. He ran out of oil, however, and so to the wounds of the remaining injured he proceeded to apply a dressing of egg yolk, oil of roses and turpentine. The next morning he found that those treated with this liniment had fared much better than those who had had their wounds cauterized: they not only had slept well but also had no fever, and their wounds were not inflamed. From then on he advocated the use of soothing liniments and bandages instead of boiling oil, emphasizing the need to remove dead tissue and foreign matter to prevent infection. Clearly, it was necessity that led Paré down the avenue of experimentation – forced by circumstance, he had to abandon traditional medical theories and deal with his patients on a case-by-case basis using the medical supplies available and often under extremely difficult conditions.

Paré also realized from his experiences in the field that gunpowder was not poisonous. As he explained to Jacques Dubois, the royal professor of medicine in Paris, his own early acceptance of the poisonous nature of gunpowder was reversed by his observation of soldiers drinking gunpowder mixed with wine before going into battle in an attempt to avoid poisoning should they be injured by gunshot. He saw that they suffered no negative side effects. Nor, for that matter, did the bullets fired become 'caustick', as was also commonly believed. Paré had conducted a simple experiment: firing a gun against a stone and picking up the bullet immediately after, he found that it did not burn his hands.

Read extract (ii) of 'Medicine, surgery and warfare in sixteenth-century Europe: Ambroise Paré' (Source Book 1, Reading 10.1). How did Paré develop new techniques for locating bullets in gunshot wounds?

Paré was asked to attend de Brissac, who had been injured in the shoulder by a musket shot, only after the three or four army surgeons had failed to locate the bullet. Instead of trying to find the bullet while the patient was lying down, as attempted by his colleagues, Paré insisted on him getting out of bed and taking up a position similar to the one he had held when shot, 'taking a javelin betweene his hands as [he] held the Pike in the skirmish', thus making it possible to determine the angle at which the bullet had entered the body. Paré was thus able to locate the bullet. It was through trial and experimentation such as this that Paré developed his approach to surgery and to medical treatment generally.

Later changes in the treatment of wounds

Paré's rejection of boiling oil and hot irons remained the only major improvement to the treatment of gunshot wounds until the end of the eighteenth century and the publication in 1794 of *Treatise of the Blood, Inflammation, and Gun Shot Wounds* by the Scottish physician and surgeon John Hunter (1728–93). Hunter had acquired his expertise while serving as a surgeon with the British army during the Seven Years War (1756–63), where he gained valuable first-hand experience in France at the battle of Belle Isle. Based on this experience he argued for a minimal method in treating gunshot wounds, rejecting the practice of enlarging the wounds and the traditional Galenic practice of bloodletting patients.

Use of oils, ointments and dressings of various sorts continued, however. Some of these practices, more by accident than design, contained substances that had an antiseptic effect; others relied on what can best be described as the miraculous, such as the 'weapon salve' or the so-called 'sympathetic powder', a Paracelsian remedy that was applied to the weapon rather than the wound. The popularity of such dressings was, of course, closely linked to the extremely high infection rate of gunshot wounds. Despite the fact that military surgeons and physicians were willing to try nearly anything, the positive results obtained by using dry bandages moistened with water ensured that their use gradually gained ground during the eighteenth century.

During the seventeenth and eighteenth centuries in particular, army and navy surgeons were also helped by the development of surgical tools. Increasingly, such instruments were made by highly skilled silversmiths and cutlers. The variety and specialization of such instruments can be seen in early modern books about surgical instruments, with illustrations of instruments drawn to scale and demonstrating their specific application. New types of surgical instrument proliferated during the eighteenth century. By the end of that century, their number and diversity had become so great that catalogues of surgical instruments were regularly published.

10.5 Wounds to the head and the disappearance of the helmet

The end of the seventeenth century saw the total dominance of firearms within the theatre of war. A consequence of the growth of firearms was the gradual disappearance of body armour and helmets. The abandonment of this protective gear for more than three hundred years is somewhat surprising given that the helmet in particular would have offered excellent protection against exploding cannon balls, grenades and pieces of shrapnel.

The increase of wounds to the head became a focus of the surgical literature of the period. The English military surgeon Richard Wiseman (1622–76), who had been on active service as a soldier, dedicated a considerable part of his writings to the treatment of wounds to the skull. As had already been recognized by military surgeons of the sixteenth century such as Paré, medical assistance in these difficult cases did not stand much of a chance when the **dura**, or outer membrane, of the brain had been penetrated. In 1542, while treating a soldier who had received 'a stroke with an Halbard upon the head penetrating even to the left ventricle of the brain', Paré realized immediately that the soldier would die despite the fact that he had been able to walk to his own lodgings after having his wound 'dressed' (Keynes, 1968, p.29).

James Yonge, appointed surgeon in charge of the first naval hospital in Plymouth at the age of 23, had greater success when treating a 4-year-old boy who had suffered a serious head injury. As was common at the time, Yonge supplemented his income from the navy with a considerable private practice, and he had been summoned by the boy's father. The boy had been hit on the head by a falling gate which had caused two fractures of the skull, 'one opposite to the other on each **bregma**'. Yonge removed a large piece of the skull on the left side of the head, which had penetrated the brain and caused a part of it, the size of a hazelnut, to come out. Despite the seriousness of the injury, Yonge succeeded in curing the boy within ten to twelve weeks. A couple of years later his claims to success in this case were questioned by a certain Dr Dunstan, who claimed that wounds of the brain were incurable. Yonge challenged him to a public debate in a local coffee house, but Dr Dunstan did not attend. Instead, Yonge went on to present his case in print, to which he added supporting evidence from a host of medical authors, in his *Wounds of the Brain Proved Curable*, published in 1682 (Poynter, 1963, pp.163, 186).

10.6 Treatment of burns

The increased use of gunpowder, as mentioned above, presented army and navy surgeons with a growing number of serious burn cases. Early modern cannons were not only unreliable but likely to explode, killing and burning the gunners, while insufficient cleaning of barrels caused a high incidence of flashburns among the crews. Musketeers, stressed in the midst of battle, often poured too much powder into the flashpans of their weapons, causing minor explosions that resulted in severe facial burns. The horror of such injuries was immediately evident to Paré at the start of his career as a military surgeon. In 1537, during the Turin campaign, he encountered by chance three stunned soldiers with terribly burned and disfigured faces, and their clothes still on fire from gunpowder. When their veteran companion discovered from Paré that he could do nothing to help them, he unceremoniously, and to Paré's horror, cut their throats, declaring that he hoped someone would do the same for him should he find himself in a similar situation. The event evidently made a deep impression on Paré, who was elated when later during the same campaign he was able to introduce a new and improved treatment for burns.

Read extract (iii) of 'Medicine, surgery and warfare in sixteenth-century Europe: Ambroise Paré' (Source Book 1, Reading 10.1).

1   How did Paré develop his new treatment for burns?

2   Why do you think surgeons such as Paré were willing to act in this way?

1   In this case Paré appears to have indulged in a couple of human experiments. A kitchen boy in the service of the marshal of Montejan had accidentally fallen into a cauldron of boiling oil. On his way to treat him, Paré had stopped at the nearest apothecary to pick up 'refrigerating medicines commonly used in this case'. An old countrywoman, overhearing his request, told him to use a dressing of crushed onions and salt, which, according to her, would reduce the blistering and scarring. Paré took the opportunity to experiment on 'this greasy scullion', and covered part of the boy's burns with the onion paste and part with the traditional remedies. The next day he discovered that the area treated with the paste was free of blisters while the rest of the burned area was full of them. Shortly afterwards he was able to repeat the experiment on a German soldier serving the marshal of Montejan who had burned his face and hands badly when his container of gunpowder had caught fire. He applied the onion paste to one half of the soldier's face and the medicines traditionally relied on by surgeons to the other half. Once more the onion paste produced wonderful results, while the rest of the affected area was covered in blisters and excoriation.

2   Paré's willingness to take advice from lay people and to use popular medicine is important here. He did not consider himself to be bound by the rules of traditional, Galenic medicine. Instead, he was prepared to experiment and to revise his approach on the basis of empirical discoveries. The need to produce results often led army surgeons to regard as obsolete the traditional medicine in which they had been trained.

Such is the value of the onion dressing that it is reported to have remained in use for burns among Russian army surgeons as late as the Second World War.

10.7 Amputations

The practice of ligature prior to amputation, which had been lost since Celsus in the first century, was reintroduced by surgeons such as Paré and William Clowes, who served the Earl of Leicester's expeditionary corps in the Netherlands in the 1580s. This was due in part to the success of the Renaissance and humanist enterprise of retrieving classical medical texts, and reduced the risk of patients bleeding to death. Thus, Clowes claimed to be able to remove legs yet cause his patients to lose less than 4 ounces of blood in the process. Other improvements included covering the stump of the amputated limb with flaps of skin and muscle, as already advocated in Hans von Gersdorff's *Feldbuch der Wundartzney* [Handbook for the Treatment of Wounds] (1517), which helped prevent infection, while the risk of gangrene was reduced by amputating well above the wound. Owing to its labour intensiveness – the surgeon needed at least a couple of assistants – the practice of ligature gained ground only slowly. In fact, military surgeons who were acquainted with the ligature technique, such as Paré's biographer and pupil Jacques Guillemeau (1550?–1613), gave up using it because of difficulties in applying it under the far from ideal conditions in which surgeons had to work during military campaigns. Instead they reverted to stopping the bleeding from the amputated limb by using cautery and boiling oil.

Furthermore, the ligature as applied by Paré and Clowes worked only on amputations below the knee, in which the **femoral artery** need not be tied off. Amputations above the knee could not be successfully undertaken until the beginning of the eighteenth century, when the screw tourniquet was introduced by the French surgeon Jean-Louis Petit (1674–1750) (Figure 10.4). This invention made it possible temporarily to halt the flow of blood in thigh and leg amputations by compression of the femoral artery in the groin. In effect, the screw tourniquet served to reintroduce ligature in surgical amputations.

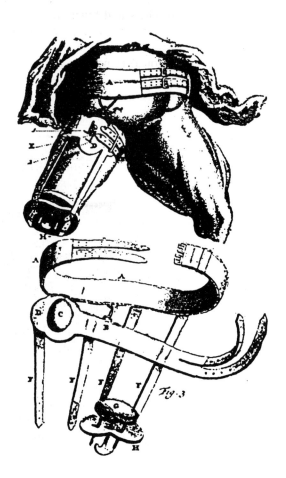

Figure 10.4   Jean-Louis Petit's screw tourniquet, engraving. Reproduced from Gabriel and Metz (1992), p.104, Figure 4.1. Copyright © 1992 Greenwood Publishing. Reprinted by permission of Greenwood Publishing, Inc., Westport, CT

Even if surgeons such as Paré and Clowes were exceptional in the sixteenth century, and allowing for the fact that their improved techniques and treatments filtered through only gradually, soldiers must have stood a reasonable chance of surviving amputations, as can be seen from the many pictures of the period which depict limbless ex-soldiers begging on the streets.

Obviously, the injured soldier's survival depended to a considerable extent on the quality and availability of medical care. While princes and great noblemen were attended by their personal physicians and surgeons, only a limited number of barber-surgeons were available to the rank and file from the sixteenth to the eighteenth centuries. However, the number and quality of barber-surgeons continued to improve throughout the early modern period. The Danish King Christian IV (1588–1648), for example, encouraged surgeons to settle throughout his kingdom. Here, despite reservations on the part of local guilds, he developed a network of such people stretching from Copenhagen to all the major provincial towns of his realm. This was achieved as much to supply his army and navy with qualified medical personnel as to give the provincial population reasonable access to medical care. Thus, in early 1611 a number of provincial towns were instructed by the king to provide him with a quota of surgeons by Easter. Again in 1645, when a naval force was being equipped, he informed local administrators that a number of cities and towns were to be prepared at short notice to send surgeons to the capital 'with well-supplied chests'. These chests contained everything the surgeons would need for a military campaign, from surgical instruments and bandages to medical remedies. Typically, they would contain some thirty instruments and a wide variety of drugs, and could weigh well over 300 pounds (136 kilograms) (Figures 10.5 and 10.6).

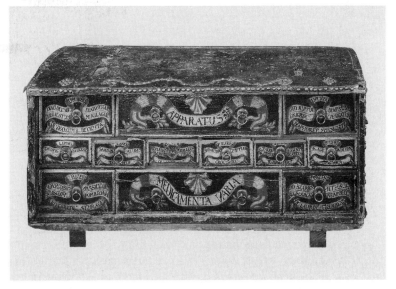

Figure 10.5   Army surgeon's chest from Zurich from the second half of the seventeenth century. Note the different drawers for surgical tools ('Apparatus') and medical remedies. Museum of Medical Health, University of Zurich

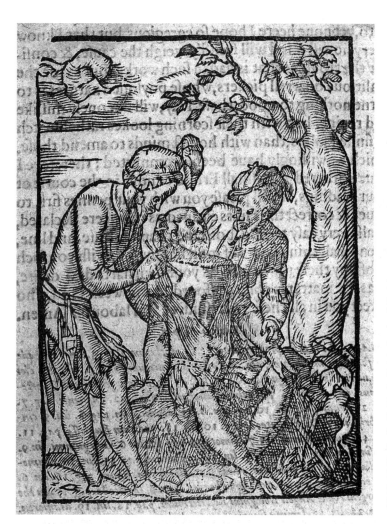

Figure 10.6 William Clowes, *Surgery in the Fields*, woodcut. The primitive working conditions with which army surgeons had to contend when in the field are portrayed in this woodcut, emphasizing Clowes's own observation that surgeons above all needed a good eye, a strong arm and a stout heart. The image shows a surgeon probing for a bullet in the shoulder of a soldier injured by a gunshot wound while the patient is being restrained by a colleague or the surgeon's assistant. Wellcome Library, London

Military service did not always appeal to the best surgeons and frequently those chosen for military service sought to supply substitutes, who were often considerably less skilful. Clowes undoubtedly came close to the truth when he complained about the many deaths caused by incompetent surgeons. Low pay, as well as the obvious dangers, served to discourage potential candidates. This was acknowledged by the English Privy Council in the 1580s when, in response to suggestions from officers of the English expeditionary corps in the Netherlands, it doubled surgeons' salaries – from 1s (5p) to 2s (10p) a day – thus enabling them to employ several assistants and simultaneously doubling their number. On average, surgeons were better paid than many officers. According to figures quoted by the military writer John Cruso, quartermaster-generals in the armies of the United Provinces were paid 6s 8d (33p) per day, while the chief surgeon received 4s (20p) and surgeons 2s 6d (12.5p) a day – the same amount as quartermasters (Cruso, *Militarie Instructions*, 1632, p.24).

Exercise

Read extract (iv) of 'Medicine, surgery and warfare in sixteenth-century Europe: Ambroise Paré' (Source Book 1, Reading 10.1).

1   According to Paré, why were amputations necessary, and on which part of the limb should they be performed?

2   How were amputations to be performed?

Discussion

1   Like other surgeons, Paré recommended amputation in cases where limbs showed signs of gangrene, so as to avert the spread of mortification through the whole body. Amputations should be effected as soon as signs of gangrene were detected. He emphasized repeatedly that the surgeon should make his cut in the 'sound flesh' in order to avoid all risk of leaving behind any gangrenous flesh, which would have rendered the operation pointless, and in support of this view he cited Celsus. He pointed out, however, that there were other considerations to take into account, such as future mobility. In the case of gangrene involving the foot, for example, he argued for amputation of the leg as far as five fingers' breadth beneath the knee. This would allow the patient better use of the remainder of his leg and he would also be able to use a wooden leg rather than relying entirely on crutches.

2   Prior to the amputation, the strength of the patient must be the first consideration, and he should be given a nourishing and easily digestible meal. The surgeon should pull the muscles of the leg towards the sound part, tying them with a straight ligature just above the place where he planned to perform his incision. Eventually, the extra skin and muscle would cover the end of the cut bone and facilitate healing of the amputated limb.

Paré recommended that the surgeon begin his amputation with a large dismembering knife, but then switch to a crooked incision knife for the tough muscles lying between the bones and use a small saw only when the bones had been totally bared. He also underlined the importance of smoothing the end of the bone to improve the healing process. He recommended that the cut be allowed to bleed for a short time, depending on the strength of the individual patient, as a way of preventing inflammation of the wound. The veins and arteries should then be bound up, preferably with the use of the specialized instrument known as the 'Crowes beake'. This should be done speedily. Only then should the ligature be removed and the wound closed up with four cross-stitches, taking care that the bones were covered with flesh and muscles.

Paré also recommended that a number of lotions or ointments be applied to the wound after amputation. While some of these strike the modern reader as weird and wonderful, others incorporated **aqua vitae**, which must have had some antiseptic effect. Similarly, the bandages, which he recommended should be dipped in oxycrate, a mixture primarily of vinegar and saffron, would have been antiseptic to some degree. Finally, Paré attacked the prevalent practice of using hot irons and oil to stop bleeding after the amputation. In his view, some patients were killed by the shock, or developed fever or complications as a consequence. Cauterization of the wound, Paré believed, caused serious damage to the healthy part of the newly amputated limb, as well as hampering the healing process. It often resulted in permanent ulcers on the end of the limb, making the use of artificial legs and arms impossible.

Paré did not restrict his innovations to the surgical aspects of amputation, but took a significant interest in the construction of artificial limbs. This can be seen from a number of illustrated editions of his works, which contain detailed instructions for the construction of wooden legs 'for poore men' (Figure 10.7) and far more complex artificial limbs made in iron, often of an intricate mechanical nature (Figures 10.8a and 10.8b). He also offered detailed instruction on how to deal with fractures and how best to set dislocated bones (Figures 10.9 and 10.10). Amazingly, he even found time to engage in something akin to plastic surgery, for example in his development of special brackets for sewing together deep facial cuts (Figure 10.11).

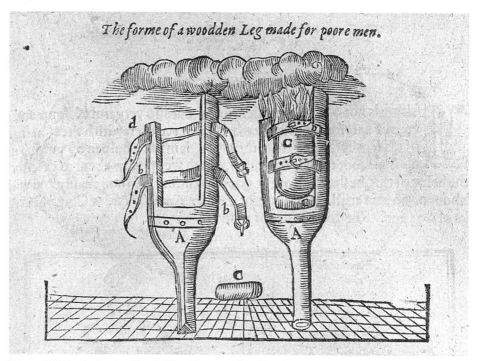

Figure 10.7 Ambroise Paré, *The Forme of a Wooden Leg Made for Poore Men*, engraving. Wellcome Library, London

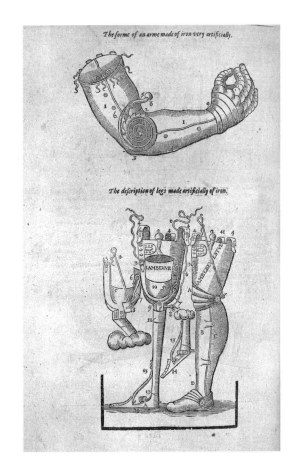

Figures 10.8a and 10.8b   Ambroise Paré, *Artificial Arm and a Leg Made of Iron*, engravings. Wellcome Library, London

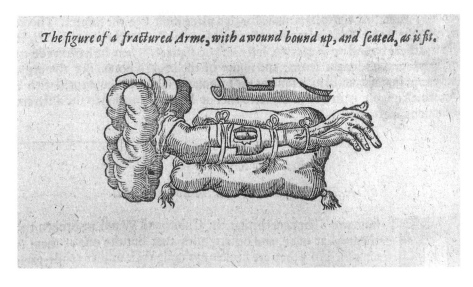

Figure 10.9 Ambroise Paré, *The Figure of a Fractured Arme*, engraving. Wellcome Library, London

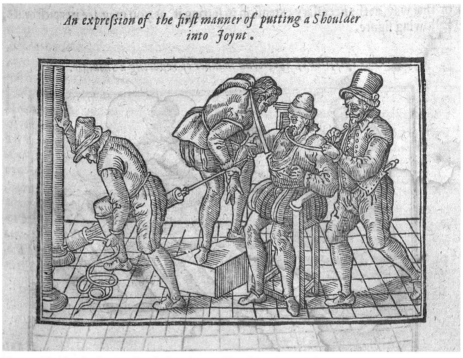

Figure 10.10 Ambroise Paré, *Putting a Shoulder into Joint*, engraving. Wellcome Library, London

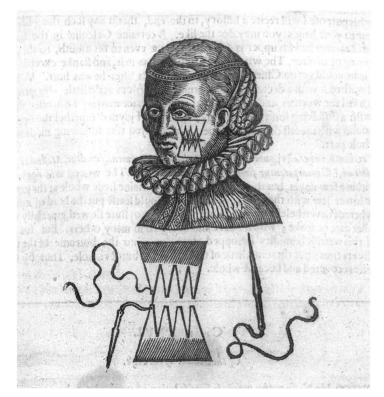

Figure 10.11 Ambroise Paré, *How to Sew a Facial Wound*, engraving. Wellcome Library, London

10.8 Foot rot and shell shock

Early modern soldiers were far more likely to die from diseases such as dysentery, typhoid, smallpox, malaria, or plague than from wounds sustained in battle. Another danger to both their health and their fitness for battle was 'foot rot', which besieging troops encountered on a considerable scale. In the twentieth century this became known as 'trench foot' when it materialized as a serious problem for troops serving in the trenches of the First World War. The clergyman George Storey recorded during the confrontation between the troops of William and Mary and James II in Ireland in 1689 that toes and whole feet sometimes fell off while the surgeons were dressing them. Clearly, peripheral blood circulation had been so badly affected that gangrene had developed well before the soldiers could be attended by a surgeon.

The stress induced by constant violent explosions, which in the twentieth century came to be known as 'shell shock', was also known to early modern army physicians and surgeons. In the Spanish army of Flanders fighting the Dutch in the seventeenth century, some soldiers were known to suffer from *el mal de corazón* (heart pain). This clearly referred to some kind of stress or psychological disorder, expressed physically as a heart condition, which made the soldier unfit for service. More often than not it was induced by sustained exposure to battle or sieges.

Increased use of artillery from the sixteenth century onwards guaranteed that shell shock came to be seen as a new medical problem by army surgeons such as Paré.

Exercise

Read extract (v) of 'Medicine, surgery and warfare in sixteenth-century Europe: Ambroise Paré' (Source Book 1, Reading 10.1). How did Paré explain the failure of many of his patients to recover during the siege of the castle of Hedin?

Discussion

Paré obviously had a large number of injured patients to attend to. His 'field hospital' in the great tower of the castle was unable to provide most of them with proper beds and bedding. The diet he could offer them was clearly dreadful, consisting mainly of old, salt beef which was hardly edible. Likewise the bandages were often dirty and they had to be dried next to the fire, which made them hard as parchment. Conditions were evidently difficult, but the constant firing of cannons caused the patients to suffer further psychological and physical damage. The sound constantly reverberating through the building caused physical pain to many of the wounded, whose groans and cries prevented others from resting. The stress, or shell shock, caused wounds to open up again and to bleed even more than they had initially, eventually resulting in many deaths.

10.9 Scurvy

Scurvy quickly became the greatest killer within the growing naval forces of the late seventeenth and early eighteenth centuries. The disease had, of course, been known for centuries, but the increasingly long journeys undertaken by navies and merchant fleets, involving ever larger ships, meant that its effects became far more widespread and serious. On long voyages a ship could lose between a quarter and a third of its crew to the disease, not to mention those who were temporarily incapacitated. The condition became a topic of particular interest to a young English naval surgeon, James Lind, who had joined the navy as a surgeon's mate in 1739, aged only 22. Lind was undoubtedly inspired by the high mortality rate from scurvy suffered by the naval personnel involved in Lord Anson's voyage around the world during which more than half of the 2,000 men died. While serving as a surgeon on the sixty-gun ship *Salisbury* in the English Channel in 1747, Lind carried out a dietary experiment on those sailors who fell ill with scurvy. The results of his research were published in his *Treatise of the Scurvy* published in 1753. Lind's book proved a success – three editions were published during his lifetime, and it was quickly translated. However, his proposals for prevention of the disease were not adopted by the Admiralty until 1795 when, owing primarily to the efforts of Lind's pupils Gilbert Blane and Thomas Trotter, the naval authorities ordered that lemon juice should be distributed to crews who had been on salted provisions for six weeks. It is noteworthy that it took the merchant navy a further fifty years to make similar provisions.

A more immediate effect of Lind's treatise on scurvy was his appointment in 1758, five years after publication, as senior physician to the recently opened naval hospital, Royal Haslar at Portsmouth, where he remained until 1783. His appointment may well have been influenced, too, by the opportune dedication of his book to Lord Anson.

Exercise

Read 'The cause, diagnosis and treatment of scurvy: James Lind's *A Treatise of the Scurvy* (1753)' (Source Book I, Reading 10.2).

1   According to Lind, what were the main causes of scurvy?

2   How did he diagnose the disease?

3   What preventive measures did he suggest?

4   How did he achieve his results?

Discussion

1   From his observations Lind concluded that there were three main causes of the disease. He considered the principal cause to be the diet of sailors at sea. Not only must the condition of the provisions – 'putrid beef, rancid pork, mouldy biscuits and flour' – have had a detrimental effect, but the food was extremely

hard to digest, whether fresh, such as the pound of biscuit each sailor received per day, or salted, such as the beef, pork and butter.

Second was the influence of weather and environment. Lind considered cold and wet weather, as opposed to fine and sunny weather, to be conducive to the spread of the disease. This explained why the incidence of scurvy was much higher on some cruises than others. Linked to this was the quality of the air and the wet environment. Lind saw moister conditions as the explanation for the higher incidence of scurvy at sea than on land. While at sea sailors had to breathe this moister air day and night while frequently sleeping in wet 'bed clothes'. According to Lind, this situation was further aggravated by the lack of ventilation below deck, which caused the moist air to stagnate to an intolerable degree.

Third, relying on traditional humoral pathology, Lind was convinced that certain people were more likely than others to contract scurvy. The more susceptible group included those who were already weakened through earlier illness, those who suffered from melancholy, and those who were of a lazy and inactive disposition. Lind added the further observation that those who had recovered from a serious case of the disease were more likely to catch it again, as he had observed in some of those who had been on Lord Anson's voyage.

2   Lind described the symptoms of scurvy in the order they most commonly appeared. He considered the disease to have three distinct stages. The first indication was the development of a pale, yellow and bloated complexion accompanied by a disinclination to undertake any physical activity. This aversion to movement was quickly followed by a stiffness of the knees in particular. Then the patient's gums would start to bleed, followed by bleeding from other parts of the body, while black spots and ulcers would develop, particularly on the legs.

In the second stage of the disease, patients often lost the use of their limbs, which became severely swollen. The time they spent immobile increased, and they were prone to fainting when making the slightest attempt to move. Often when moved or exposed to fresh air they would suddenly die.

If patients reached the third stage of the disease, ulcers that had previously healed would develop again, while the swellings on their legs would shoot out 'bloody fungus'. Some would develop putrid fevers, others would discharge 'rotten blood' with their stool and urine, and through the nose, and others would develop jaundice or dropsy. Not surprisingly this caused a deep melancholy in the patients. Before death some would find it difficult to breathe, while others would start to breathe rapidly before suddenly dying.

3   In order to find out how best to prevent scurvy, Lind embarked on an experiment in May 1747 while serving as a surgeon on the *Salisbury*. By 20 May, he had twelve patients who showed the same signs of the disease. He proceeded to establish a separate sickroom for these patients in the 'fore-hold' of the ship and gave them the same food. In addition to this food, he ordered every two patients to consume a different substance every day. Two were to drink a measure of cider, another two a couple of spoonfuls of vinegar, while two each ate two oranges and one lemon. There were those who consumed a measure of **elixir vitriol** every day, or half a pint of sea water each, and there were two

who were purged three or four times a day by means of an electuary recommended by a hospital surgeon. After six days, the two who had been eating lemons and oranges were fit enough to report for duty. Lind had no doubt that the result of all his experiments showed that oranges and lemons were the most effective remedy against scurvy.

4   Despite relying on traditional humoral pathology Lind's interest in the environment and in diet helped him in his search for measures against scurvy. He achieved his results through experiment and observation. It was empiricism and *not* traditional, learned medicine with its emphasis on natural philosophy which proved successful.

As Lind himself put it:

> It is indeed not probable that a remedy for the scurvy will ever be discovered from a preconceived hypothesis, or by speculative men in the closet, who never saw the disease, or who have seen, at most, only a few cases of it.

(quoted in Lloyd, 1965, p.24)

10.10 Hygiene

Already during the sixteenth century the increasing number of outbreaks of epidemic disease within their expanding armies was forcing military commanders to pay greater attention to matters of hygiene. Thus, the disciplinary code of the Earl of Leicester for his expeditionary corps in the Netherlands stipulated that soldiers were to use latrines to relieve themselves, while animals were to be slaughtered only at appointed places outside camps and garrisons. All carrion and entrails were to be buried, and all personnel were warned not to 'defile the waters adioyning, but in the lower part of the stream some good distance from the Camp, upon payne of imprisonment'. At the same time it was also recognized that to camp near bogs and moors exposed the troops to unnecessary risk of disease 'by the stenches and infectious vapours thereof'. By the eighteenth century, for a growing number of medical men stench came to equal disease (Cunningham and Grell, 2000, p.135).

However, by this period, the role of the state and national governments in military medical care and military hygiene had grown considerably. By 1750, all major armies had begun to create institutionalized systems of medical care, including military hospitals and army medical schools. Another aspect of the state's concern for the medical care of its soldiers is evident in its attempts to prevent disease and maintain the health of soldiers. In 1726, the French army had begun regular medical examinations of new recruits. Despite voluntary enlistment, European armies still recruited mainly from among the poorer sections of the population whose general health was far from good. However, medical examinations of recruits did not become common within most European armies until the end of the century.

Further improvements to military hygiene were achieved by the creation of permanent military camps with barracks, ensuring that all troops were quartered to certain minimum standards, rather than being billeted in private houses and inns. The general health of soldiers also improved with the introduction in the eighteenth century of the standard military ration, which meant that soldiers ate better and more regularly. Further improvements followed the introduction of government-issued uniforms, even if the quality was not always of the best.

However, epidemic disease continued to be the greatest problem for armies throughout the eighteenth century, despite attempts at preventive medical care by army surgeons and physicians. Thus, more than 80 per cent of all deaths in the British army in the eighteenth century were caused by disease. Furthermore the diseases, plague apart, remained the same as in the sixteenth century, for example smallpox, fevers, dysentery, and jail or hospital fever, which was a disease similar to typhus (Gabriel and Metz, 1992, vol.2, pp.101–22).

By the mid-eighteenth century, military hygiene and the associated epidemic diseases had become a focus of interest for Sir John Pringle. He served the British army first as physician from 1742, then as physician-general from 1745, until he retired from military life in 1748 to pursue a highly lucrative private practice in London. Based on his experiences on active service, Pringle published in 1752 what has been described as the most important work on military hygiene in the eighteenth century, *Observations on the Diseases of the Army*. Here he identified jail and hospital fever as the same disease and suggested treatment for it, while pointing out the need for proper ventilation in military hospitals.

Exercise

Read 'Military medicine in the eighteenth century: John Pringle's *Observations on the Diseases of the Army* (1764)' (Source Book 1, Reading 10.3), an extract from a later edition of this work.

1 Why did Pringle decide to write his book? And what were the foundations for his deductions?

2 In what ways can Pringle's text be seen as a product of the Enlightenment?

Discussion

1 Pringle felt that he was filling a most important gap in contemporary knowledge for the simple reason that none of the 'ancient physicians' nor any of the moderns who had any direct experience of military life had written on military diseases. According to Pringle, he would have been unable to write this book, built as it is on empiricism, without the practical experience of active service. Pringle began by noting down his observations while serving with the army. His main aim was to collect materials that would make it possible for him to trace the causes of the most prominent military diseases. By doing so, he hoped to be able to suggest ways of preventing or minimizing the effect of such diseases on future military campaigns.

2   Pringle stated that he had taken his notes about the most evident causes of disease among British troops in order that they could be prevented or at least reduced in future military campaigns. He was convinced that his efforts contributed to 'Natural Knowledge', which he considered to be 'daily improving'. These are all clear expressions of Enlightenment optimism. Overall, Pringle expressed a typical Enlightenment concern for hygiene and public health, in his case specifically for the health of army personnel.

10.11 Military hospitals

Military hospitals were slow to be established in the early modern period. The first appears to have been set up in 1567 in the city of Mechelen by the Spanish duke of Alva on his arrival in the Netherlands. Initially, the hospital survived for only a year, probably because of lack of funds. It is noteworthy, however, that among the complaints of Spanish mutineers between 1574 and 1576 the lack of proper medical care for the troops, including a hospital, featured prominently. In 1585, the military hospital in Mechelen reopened with a staff of around 50 and with 330 beds. It appears to have treated not only combat injuries but also diseases such as malaria and the pox, and psychological disorders such as shell shock. The Spanish government appears to have paid most of the expenses connected with the hospital, but the veteran Spanish and Italian troops for whose benefit it had been established contributed one *real* of their monthly salary. Gradually, more military hospitals came into existence during the early seventeenth century. Thus in 1638, the Swedish government created a military hospital in the former monastery of Vadstena, though the nature of this institution seems to have resembled the nursing home for crippled and maimed soldiers established by the Spanish government at the garrison of Our Lady of Hal (Cunningham and Grell, 2000, p.136). Other states eventually followed suit. In France, the Hôtel des Invalides was established in 1670, and in Britain military hospitals were set up at Dublin in 1681 and Chelsea in 1684. By the seventeenth century, leading statesmen such as Cardinal Richelieu had become very supportive of military hospitals, not least for reasons of state. Thus Richelieu stated: '2000 men leaving hospital cured, and in some sense broken in to the profession, are far more valuable than even 6000 new recruits' (Jones, 1989, p.210).

Exercise

Read 'Military and naval medicine in eighteenth-century France' (Source Book 1, Reading 10.4). What was the role and significance, according to Brockliss and Jones, of the military hospital in France in the eighteenth century?

Discussion

Even if the establishment of the Hôtel des Invalides had its roots in the French crown's ambition to confine maimed and demobilized army personnel, it nevertheless went a long way to demonstrate the importance of medical care for military personnel in the eyes of the French absolutist state. The new hospital was designed with lofty, airy and hygienic wards. Considerable effort was expended in the provision of an efficient system of water supply and waste disposal. There were separate wards for those with venereal diseases and for the mad. By the early eighteenth century, the Invalides had become the leading teaching hospital in France, especially in surgery and anatomy. It was the cornerstone in a network of French military hospitals founded during the eighteenth century, and it has come to be seen as a pioneer of the medicalized hospital in France. Not surprisingly, the new military hospitals employed a high proportion of surgeons and many of them, like the Invalides, quickly developed into teaching hospitals. The teaching was clinically orientated and, contrary to the situation in most contemporary civilian hospitals, there was no shortage of corpses for dissections and anatomy. As discussed above, salaries for medical personnel in both the army and the navy improved dramatically in the eighteenth century, as did the social status of military physicians and surgeons. According to Brockliss and Jones, military hospitals can be seen to have inspired the new civilian, medicalized hospitals, where cure rather than care takes priority, which came into existence in the same period.

When the English philanthropist John Howard visited the Great Hospital in Vienna in 1778 he was clearly impressed by the medical care provided in the military section of the hospital, where the 551 patients were attended by no less than 30 surgeons, of whom 14 were resident at any given time, reporting to a superintendent surgeon (Howard, 1789, p.68). In Britain it was the new naval hospitals, such as the Royal Haslar Hospital under the guidance of James Lind, which led the way in setting standards for medicalized hospitals. Howard visited the Royal Haslar and later included features of it in his plans for an ideal hospital.

The practice of establishing field hospitals followed a similar pattern. In the seventeenth century, something akin to field hospitals were often set up during major sieges or campaigns. They were generally recognized and protected by the warring parties, as can be seen from events surrounding the siege of Maastricht in 1632. Here, when the articles of surrender were concluded between the Spanish forces, who had defended the town, and the Prince of Orange, an article was included which stated that all injured and sick soldiers and officers could remain until fully recovered, either privately with their hosts or in their respective hospitals.

It was not until the eighteenth century, however, that real field hospitals were created. During the War of Austrian Succession (1740–8), the British army developed a system of small mobile hospitals in tents close to the battlefield. Each could offer initial treatment to around 200 until they could be transported further back to general hospitals some 12 to 40 miles (19 to 64 kilometres) to the rear. The development of this system, in which Sir John Pringle was instrumental, significantly improved the chances of survival of the wounded. It was later agreed with the opposing French forces that hospitals on both sides should be mutually protected as sanctuaries for the sick.

10.12 Conclusion

The growing incidence of warfare combined with the increased use of more destructive weapons in the early modern period caused greater and more horrific injuries to military personnel than ever before. This led to the discovery of better treatment of gunshot wounds and amputation techniques by the growing number of surgeons who were employed in early modern armies and navies. Often reacting to the circumstances in which they found themselves, as we have seen in the case of Ambroise Paré, surgeons were willing to consider innovative and unorthodox approaches and remedies in order to save their patients. Many, like William Clowes, were positively inclined towards Paracelsianism. Paracelsus, it should be noted, had started his medical career as an army surgeon and among his most famous works was his book on surgery, *Grosse Wundartzney* [Big Book of Surgery], which was first published in 1536. Paracelsus' advice to the surgeon to protect the wound by keeping it clean and open and not sealing it off obviously inspired Clowes and other surgeons.

During the eighteenth century, a number of army and navy surgeons began to take greater note of the environment and of hygiene in general as factors involved in reducing the risk of epidemic disease, which remained by far the largest killer of military personnel. On the basis of observation and experimentation doctors such as Sir John Pringle and James Lind found new ways to avoid or at least minimize the risk of the much feared jail or hospital fever. For a variety of practical and bureaucratic reasons, however, a considerable length of time often elapsed before these discoveries resulted in real improvements.

Greater state involvement in medical care for military personnel led to the creation of increasingly medicalized military hospitals towards the end of the seventeenth century. In many ways these hospitals set a pattern for the new medicalized civilian hospitals which were established in the eighteenth century.

References

Cruso, J. (1632) *Military Instructions for the Cavall'rie*, Cambridge: printer to Cambridge University.

Cunningham, A. and Grell, O.P. (2000) *The Four Horsemen of the Apocalypse. Religion, War, Famine and Death in Reformation Europe*, Cambridge: Cambridge University Press.

Gabriel, R.A. and Metz, K.S. (1992) *A History of Military Medicine*, 2 vols, New York: Greenwood.

Howard, J. (1789) *An Account of the Principal Lazarettos in Europe: Together with Further Observations on Some Foreign Prisons and Hospitals*, Warrington.

Jones, C. (1989) *The Charitable Imperative: Hospitals and Nursing in Ancien Régime and Revolutionary France*, London: Routledge.

Keynes, G. (ed.) (1968) *The Apologie and Treatise of Ambroise Paré*, New York: Dover.

Lloyd, C. (ed.) (1965) *The Health of Seamen: Selections from the Works of Dr James Lind, Sir Gilbert Blane and Dr Thomas Trotter*, Greenwich: Navy Records Society.

Parker, G. (1990) *The Army of Flanders and the Spanish Road 1567–1659*, Cambridge: Cambridge University Press.

Porter, R. (1999) *The Greatest Benefit to Mankind: A Medical History of Humanity from Antiquity to the Present*, London: Fontana.

Poynter, F.N.L. (ed.) (1963) *The Journal of James Yonge (1647–1721) Plymouth Surgeon*, London: Longman.

Source Book readings

A. Paré, *The Apologie and Treatise of Ambroise Paré containing the Voyages Made into Divers Places with many of His Writings upon Surgery*, ed. by G. Keynes, New York: Dover, 1968, pp.137–8, 28, 140, 147–52, 50–1 (Reading 10.1).

C. Lloyd (ed.), *The Health of Seamen: Selections from the Works of Dr James Lind, Sir Gilbert Blane and Dr Thomas Trotter*, London: Navy Records Society, 1965, pp.12–21 (Reading 10.2).

J. Pringle, *Observations on the Diseases of the Army*, London: A. Millar, D. Wilson & T. Payne, [1752] 1764, pp.iii–xiv (Reading 10.3).

L. Brockliss and C. Jones, *The Medical World of Early Modern France*, Oxford: Clarendon Press, 1997, pp.689–700 (Reading 10.4).

$$11$$

Environment, Health and Population

Mark Jenner

Objectives

When you have completed this chapter, you should be able to:

* understand the connection between health and environment in early modern Europe;

* appreciate the role of broader political and cultural factors in shaping early modern attitudes to environmental health;

* analyse the growing role of the state in formulating policies with regard to health and the environment in early modern Europe.

11.1 Introduction

In September 1524, the Dutch humanist Desiderius Erasmus sent a letter to John Fisher, bishop of Rochester, who was not well. 'I suspect', he wrote:

> that a large part of your ill health is caused by the place where you live ... Your being near the sea and the mud which is repeatedly laid bare at low tides means an unhealthy climate, and your library has walls of glass all round, the chinks of which let through an air which is tenuous and, as the physicians call it, filtered, which is very dangerous for those who are sparely built and not robust ... Personally, if I spent three hours together in such a place, I should fall sick. You would be much better suited by a room with a wooden floor and wooden panelling ... some sort of miasma issues from the bricks and mortar.
>
> (Erasmus, 1992, p.368)

The modern media sometimes talk of 'sick-building syndrome', suggesting that a particular space causes sickness among those forced to live or work in it. Erasmus similarly attributed his friend's afflictions to his habitation and workplace. This chapter explores various aspects of the connection between health and environment in Europe between 1500 and 1800. It is a topic which can be explored in numerous ways. Historical demographers, for example, continue to debate the relative significance of health interventions and environmental changes in accounting for the decline of mortality in the later eighteenth century (see, for example, Razzell, 1993; Riley, 1986; Wrigley, 1983). In this chapter, I concentrate on the social, cultural and intellectual aspects of health and environment. In particular, I focus on medical and lay perceptions of what constituted a healthy or an unhealthy environment, and I foreground the political and ideological context of interventions designed to reduce mortality. In the early part of the chapter I have deliberately left these questions to one side, however, because I wish to concentrate on two other aspects of the history of health and environment. First, I feel it is important to ask how we 'know' peoples and places, and to think about how the way we discuss and categorize the world shapes our perceptions of the environment. These perceptions have clearly changed over time. Second, I consider that it is important not to assume that it is 'natural' for governments to intervene in matters of public health in any particular way. Such interventions and policies are profoundly ideological, and are based upon conscious or unconscious decisions about the remit of the state with reference to the population or the environment. Early modern Europeans possessed a different understanding of the natural world, and its impact on the body, from that with which we are familiar today. They also worked with different notions of the responsibility of the state from those that generally apply within modern western European democracies with a degree of public healthcare provision. In this chapter, I explore these differences in order to build a more complete picture of the complex and changing relationship between health and environment in the period from 1500 to 1800.

11.2 Airs, waters, places

If you return to the quotation from Erasmus, you will see that he was principally concerned about how Fisher's setting was affecting his body. In particular, he draws attention to the dangers presented to the bishop's health by miasma, or malign qualities in the air. These were sometimes thought – as in this case – to emanate from the fabric of particular buildings. More commonly, they were believed to affect much wider areas and to be caused by, among other things, earthquakes or unfavourable conjunctions of the stars or planets. Miasma could also result from a range of other environmental factors. The putrefaction of organic matter, for instance, was widely held to create an evil air, or miasma, which in turn provided a suitable medium for the propagation of plague and pestilence. A chronicler of the Dutch town of Amersfoort, for example, recorded in 1629 that it had been occupied by troops who led a:

> bad, reckless and irregular life, [so] the ... city was totally infected by the quantity of dead horses, cattle, sheep, pigs and other animals, which ... were found everywhere in the streets, roads and canals. And although it was ordered to ... bury all those dead animals ... this did not prevent, that a great number of citizens was attacked by the plague.
>
> (quoted in Van Andel, 1913, pp.438–9)

Plagues and other epidemics often led to a redoubling of efforts to cleanse and improve city streets and airs in order to remove sources of corruption. The medical boards of seventeenth-century Italy did not simply set out quarantine rules and policies of household isolation; in addition, they energetically surveyed insanitary conditions and commanded the removal of waste at times of epidemics. In 1622, for instance, the Health Magistracy of the Grand Duchy of Tuscany issued an order for a general cleansing of streets, sewers and houses 'in order to ward off all disorders in such dangerous times' and to minimize the possible 'damage [to] health by foul vapours' (Cipolla, 1992, p.10). Similar instructions were issued in towns and cities throughout much of early modern Europe.

Although these orders were much easier to proclaim than to enforce, they nonetheless betrayed a strong sensitivity to bad smells, and a determination to eradicate corruption of the air. Plague orders and advice books for the plague routinely recommended a range of measures designed to correct the air and combat stench with powerful fumigants. Typical was the French physician, François Vallériole (1504–80), who recommended the use of rosemary, juniper and laurel in homes as a preventive measure in warding off the 'evill vapours' of the plague. He added that it 'is not amisse likewise at every corner of the street ... to make ... Bonefires to consume the malignant vapours of the ayre' (Lodge, 1963, vol.4, p.23). Evidence of this kind suggests that we need to revise the common assumption that pre-modern people had no conception of the importance of private and public hygiene. They may have lacked the economic resources and technological knowledge which sustain modern systems of sanitation and public health, but they clearly linked disease with 'dirty' environments. Injunctions to clean streets and correct the air represented an intensification of the previous norms, rather than the panic-stricken introduction of innovation in ideas and practices relating to public health. Indeed, they were often articulated with reference to wider notions of good government and social order, as you have seen in Chapter 6.

If you return once again, however, to Erasmus's letter, you will see that it is the site of Fisher's episcopal palace near the muddy banks of the river Medway in Kent, not any failure of sanitation, that the author holds responsible for its unhealthy climate. Erasmus was clearly drawing more general connections between place and disease. In fact, there was a long tradition of medical writing related to the impact of environment upon health. Many of the works associated with the Greek doctor Hippocrates, most notably his *Airs, Waters, Places* and *Epidemics*, had drawn attention to the various ways in which the seasons, climate, geology and other natural factors affected health; he subsequently stressed the need for the physician to be aware of such connections. In these works, Hippocrates explained how the body's humours were influenced by the weather – the coldness and wetness of winter, for example, increased the amount of phlegm in the human constitution. The Hippocratic corpus discussed many other factors that we might term environmental. The prevailing winds and the nature of the water supply, for instance, were both seen as substantially determining what kinds of illness might affect the inhabitants of a particular place. Some locations were especially dangerous to health. Marshes were linked with fevers and debilitating conditions, while the inhabitants of cities exposed to hot winds were thought to suffer from poor digestion and low fertility (Hippocrates, 1923, vol.1, pp.85, 75).

Such arguments were well known in early modern medical circles. *Airs, Waters, Places* and *Epidemics* had been translated into Latin in the Middle Ages, and Latin and Greek editions of the whole Hippocratic corpus were published in the sixteenth and seventeenth centuries (Lonie, 1985; Nutton, 1989). Moreover, an analogous understanding of cosmology and climate was integral to the wider culture of the period, and permeated popular notions of health. It is evident, for example, in the cheap almanacs and pamphlets that proliferated in this period and which recommended, among other things, the right time to let blood and to undergo other forms of medical treatment (Figure 11.1).

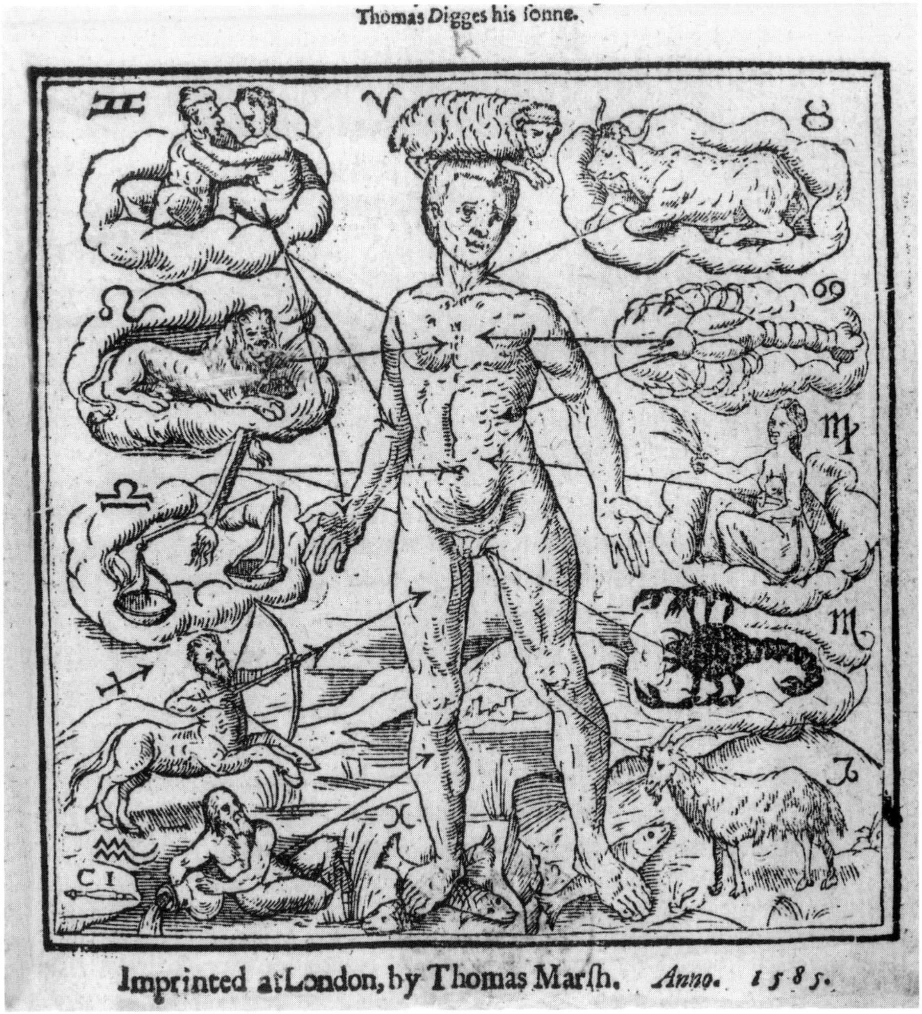

Thomas *Digges* his fonne.

Imprinted at London, by Thomas Marfh. *Anno.* 1585.

Figure 11.1   Figure from Leonard Digges, *A Prognostication Everlasting*, corrected and augmented by Thomas Digges, 1585 edition, fol. 19. Most almanacs contained a similar figure of a man and the signs of the zodiac. The picture indicates which sign is associated with particular parts of the body. Thus the image of the ram perched rather improbably on top of this man's head indicates the association of Aries, the Ram, with the head and the face, while Sagittarius is associated with the thighs. © The British Library

Geological and geographical thinking also prompted many health-related recommendations. In providing advice on how and where to build a house, the English diplomat, Sir Henry Wotton, directed that its site should not be 'subiect to any foggy noysomnesse, from *Fenns* or *Marshes*', nor to any '*Mineral* exhalations' from the soil (Wotton, 1968, p.3). Much early modern topographical writing was preoccupied with issues of salubrity. Descriptions of places were often informed by notions of temperament – the idea that the physical and psychological nature of a particular group of people was shaped by the soil, water and, above all, the air they breathed. As the Oxford scholar and cleric, Robert Burton, explained in 1621:

as the air is, so are the inhabitants, dull, heavy, witty, subtle, neat, cleanly, clownish, sick, and sound. In Périgord in France the air is subtile ... but hilly and barren: the men sound, nimble and lusty; but in some parts of Guienne, full of moors and marshes, the people dull, heavy, and subject to many infirmities.

(Burton, 1968, vol.2, p.61)

Environmental themes informed another important strand of medical thinking – the regulation of the six non-naturals through regimen. While in theory individual physicians were best placed to advise about the regimen most suited to the individual's humoral balance, from the mid-sixteenth century a printed health advice literature developed which set out recommended regimens structured around the non-naturals. Much of this advice was essentially dietetic, but it also included much discussion of the importance of air quality in the maintenance of health. Moreover, such advice was not concerned exclusively with the dangers posed by pestilential and fatal diseases. At the end of the sixteenth century, the French physician, André du Laurens (1558–1609), discussed the preservation of eyesight with reference to the quality of the air.

Exercise

Read 'Air and good health in Renaissance medicine' (Source Book 1, Reading 11.1).

1 Why did Laurens pay such attention to air in his discussion of diet?

2 What kinds of air did he suggest one should avoid in order to preserve sight, and why?

Discussion

1 The first point to note is that Laurens used the term diet in a much wider sense than most modern usages. He described it as 'the manner of living' rather than eating and drinking. He focused on the air as it was essential for life, was continually ingested, and had a rapid impact upon the body. Moreover, he invoked the authority of Hippocrates for this position, indicating that the nature or constitution of the air determined the health or otherwise of the humours.

2 Laurens emphasized temperance and the avoidance of climatic extremes, of temperature as well as humidity. He particularly highlighted the dangers of marshy, wet and low-lying areas. He echoed the advice of Hippocrates that northerly and southerly winds were potentially dangerous – the former stinging the eyes because of its sharpness, the latter because it bred gross spirits and a heaviness of the head, which impaired all aspects of the function of the senses, including sight. He also stressed the lethal nature of metallic fumes, advising those with sensitive eyes to avoid such pursuits as alchemy. He concluded by warning of the danger of excessively bright lights which were encouraged by light airs.

So far you have seen how some places were perceived as naturally unhealthy or how they might become so through pollution. By contrast, other parts of the natural world were considered beneficial to human health and were thought to assist physical recovery. Wells, springs and other waters provide one such example, for drinking from, or bathing in, particular waters was widely believed to relieve or cure a range of ailments. From the thirteenth century onwards, the reputation of the healing properties of hot baths, such as those at Pozzuoli in Naples, was widely celebrated in poetry and prose, by both laymen and physicians (Palmer, 1990; Park, 1999). Although it is possible that people had been visiting such places since pre-Christian times, by 1500 many healing springs had become firmly associated with the cult of various saints. Thus, for example, the revealingly named Holywell in north Wales was associated with the cult of St Winifred, and a spring at Ventas con Peña Aguilera, near Toledo in Spain, which was recommended for eye complaints, was dedicated to St Lucy (Christian, 1981, p.84). Despite, or perhaps because of, their popularity these healing places often lay outside the jurisdiction of the medical, secular and ecclesiastical authorities. Their therapeutic powers found no place in university medicine, and the saints venerated at these sites were not always approved or even recognized by the church. However, between 1500 and 1800 there were repeated attempts, only partially successful, to bring healing waters and spas under closer medical and religious supervision.

Early in the sixteenth century, a number of Catholic reformers expressed disquiet at what they saw as the superstitious practices that had grown up around wells and shrines. In the 1520s, for example, Erasmus satirized the notion that the wells at the pilgrimage site of Our Lady of Walsingham in East Anglia had 'suddenly shot up from the ground at the command of the Most Holy Virgin', and the belief that they were not only 'wonderfully cold' and 'good for headache and stomach troubles', but also sacred to her (Erasmus, 1997, pp.631–2). In the later sixteenth and seventeenth centuries, this unease developed into active hostility as Roman Catholic missions, led by preaching orders such as the Jesuits, attempted to bring 'true Christianity' to what they saw as the dark and superstitious corners of Europe. In the early seventeenth century, for instance, Father Michel le Nobletz denounced the way that Breton villagers made offerings of bread and butter to local fountains every New Year's Day (Delumeau, 1977, pp.161–2). In the place of such popular cults, missions promoted sanctioned therapies such as Xavier water, mass produced by priests dipping the relics of St Francis Xavier (1506–52) in water. Alternatively, they brought such shrines firmly under church control by building chapels near the source of the waters (Forster, 2001, pp.72–5; Johnson, 1996, pp.195–8).

Protestant reformers, hostile to the veneration of both objects and saints, initially regarded holy waters with great suspicion and on occasions tried to close them down. In 1538, for example, a royal official enforcing the early stages of the English Reformation locked up the shrine of St Anne at Buxton, in Derbyshire, and carried away all the crutches left behind by people who had been cured there. Likewise in Lutheran Denmark in 1570, King Frederik II (1559–88) ordered one of his officials to prevent people resorting in a superstitious manner to a healing spring in the parish of Vesternæs (Johansen, 1997, pp.61–2; Walsham, 1999, pp.232–3). Some of the most sustained campaigns to outlaw such practices were initiated in Calvinist Scotland, where the records of **kirk sessions** contain numerous prosecutions of people for such practices.

Read 'Visiting wells and springs in Protestant Scotland' (Source Book 1, Reading 11.2).

1 How does Todd account for the significance of visiting wells in Scottish popular culture?

2 What aspects of these practices did Protestant clergymen find offensive and why did they seek to repress them?

1 Todd argues that visiting wells and springs was an ancient custom in early modern Scotland and that it was thoroughly integrated into the forms and routines of popular culture. The custom was markedly calendrical, being associated with specific times of the year, especially May Day. Well-visiting was, moreover, a social activity and was generally done in groups. It specifically formed a part of women's sociability. Behaviour at wells and springs was also highly ritualized, and incorporated aspects of exchange, most notably when objects such as pins or pieces of cloth were left behind after water was taken.

2 The Protestant clergy prosecuted well-visiting for a number of reasons. First, because they saw it as encouraging immorality and superstition. Recreational activities at the wells included music and dancing, which were routinely castigated by the kirk as immoral. Second, these practices competed with attendance at the kirk services on the sabbath, and thus undermined devotion to spiritual duties. And third, and most important, the practices at the waters were widely thought to be idolatrous or magical. In particular, the elders of the kirk sessions were worried that women were ascribing powers to the waters which more properly belonged either to God or the devil. As the case of Isabell Haldane shows, such beliefs could often lead to charges of magic or diabolic witchcraft being levelled against those who lauded the therapeutic powers of the waters.

As well as attracting the attention of the clergy, wells, baths and springs increasingly attracted the interest of the medical authorities, who investigated, publicized, and sought to control their use. During the sixteenth century, the papal physician Andrea Bacci (1524–1600) and the German polymath Conrad Gesner (1516–65) began the task of collecting information about the range of waters across Europe, noting in particular their properties and the afflictions they were said to cure. Such catalogues of waters effectively constituted a natural history of spas. This was, however, just one aspect of a much grander intellectual project that aimed to collect and catalogue all kinds of natural phenomena. Both Gesner and Bacci, for example, also investigated the medical properties of precious stones (Findlen, 1994; Palmer, 1990).

The supposed healing properties of waters presented both doctors and ecclesiastics with various problems of interpretation and authority. How did the waters work? Were reported cures the result of the intercession of a particular saint, or were they due entirely to the natural properties of the water? Even Protestants rarely dismissed all waters as having no efficacy. Rather, they argued that in those cases where efficacy was proved it came about as a result of the God-given natural quality inherent in the source. Catholics who claimed that cures were effected by the intercession of saints were accused by their Protestant opponents of perpetrating fraud on the common people. For their part, Catholic priests and doctors continued to defend holy healing while at the same time recognizing the natural properties and effects of the waters on the body. Not surprisingly, there was little unanimity as to why certain waters were effective in relieving specific complaints such as gout or helping women conceive.

Such questions were fiercely debated in the sixteenth and seventeenth centuries. Some authorities, such as the English physician John Jones (*fl.*1562–79), discussed the curative power of water within the framework of Galenism and the non-naturals. However, there was comparatively little on baths and water cures in the classical medical corpus, and the use of such cures was fundamentally empirical – that is, based on trial and error. From the Middle Ages, medical writings on mineral waters were rooted in that branch of medical learning known as *practica,* which concerned itself with the treatment of particular diseases, rather than with general medical knowledge, and was thus less reverential towards classical authorities (Park, 1999). We should not be surprised therefore to find that some of the first major challenges to Galenic orthodoxy came from Paracelsian practitioners who operated in this field. The Paracelsians were especially sympathetic to the use of mineral waters because so many contained those metals and minerals, such as iron and sulphur, which they championed in their own medical practice. In France, for instance, many of the sixteenth-century partisans of water cures were Paracelsian in theoretical orientation, though mineral waters were incorporated in the medical mainstream by the middle of the seventeenth century.

Discussion surrounding the origins of the therapeutic properties of the waters raised another question: how should these waters be used? Physicians were as one in emphasizing that water cures should be taken only under proper medical supervision. In books and pamphlets, they sought to 'medicalize' the waters, stressing that because they were so powerful they should be taken only in a carefully controlled course of treatment. Tunbridge Wells water could be as dangerous as 'a Sword in a *Mad-Mans* hand', warned one English physician in 1687. A decade later, a French medic told the cautionary tale of a foreign visitor who had gulped down a dozen glasses of the spa water at Forges, in northern France, and was subsequently struck down with dreadful pain that required urgent medical attention (Brockliss, 1990, pp.43–4; Harley, 1990, p.50). It is hard to tell how many people heeded these warnings. In a culture where physicians possessed little coercive power and only limited prestige, many people incorporated medicinal baths and the consumption of mineral waters into their regimes of self-medication. The French philosopher Michel de Montaigne (1533–95) was typical of this trend. When he visited the baths at Lucca in Tuscany he cheerfully

Paracelsianism is discussed in Chapters 4 and 5.

ignored every medical recommendation about how best to use them. When, two centuries later, the Welsh gentleman Lewis Morris went to take the waters at Llandrindod he took along a microscope which he used to investigate the mineral salts in the various springs. Only then did he decide which to drink (Owen, 1949, pp.484–5; Palmer, 1990, p.17).

Medical authors regularly bewailed the number of people who were ignoring their advice and going in for self-help water cures. Such complaints were not, however, purely altruistic. During the course of the seventeenth and eighteenth centuries, many spas and mineral waters were becoming thoroughly commercialized. The supplies of some sources were bottled and sold all over Europe. The more successful spa towns were growing into major resorts where large numbers of the leisured classes passed weeks and months seeking better health, and where the local inhabitants gained work providing a range of services to these visitors. Such developments presented new opportunities and challenges to medical practitioners.

The growth and commercial success of English spas was particularly notable. New sources such as those at Tunbridge Wells were developed in the seventeenth century, and by the 1690s a regular summer coach service had been established to carry wealthy Londoners and courtiers to take the waters there. But none matched the success of eighteenth-century Bath. Long renowned for the curative properties of its hot springs, the town became a centre of fashionable society in which taking the waters was accompanied by concerts, dances and the rounds of polite society. The wealth generated by the growth of Bath as a major centre of medical recuperation and leisurely pursuits is still evident today in the grand, classical-style public buildings that were erected to house the baths and the pumps (Figure 11.2).

No continental resort could rival Bath. The town of Spa itself, located in the eighteenth century in the Austrian Netherlands (modern-day Belgium; see plate 9), was by comparison a modest market town with few striking architectural features (Figure 11.3). A number of French spas did turn into significant therapeutic centres. Aix-les-Bains and Vichy, for example, attracted aristocrats and wealthy townspeople in search of a cure. Neither, however, achieved Bath's blend of medicine and high fashion, and by the mid-eighteenth century the population of Aix-les-Bains was only 1,300 (Mackaman, 1998, Chapter 1). If society did not travel to Spa or Vichy, Spa and Vichy could nonetheless come to them by the bottle and, indeed, by the gallon. 'I have good *Spaw-Water*', the London merchant, John Houghton, announced regularly in the advertisement columns of his newspaper in the 1690s. Sixteen types of bottled mineral water good for everything from chest complaints to anal fistulas were on sale in Paris in 1760. This market continued to grow and diversify; twenty-five varieties were available by 1777. Mineral waters had become big business (Brockliss and Jones, 1997, p.639; Franklin, 1891, pp.181–7).

The development of more commercial medicines, whether in a free market or under state control, is discussed in Chapter 13.

This process, in turn, encouraged the development of more commercial forms of medicine. In Britain, there was a relatively free market in cures, ranging from patent medicines to mineral waters. Elsewhere in Europe, greater state and corporate control was exercised over medicine. This did not, however, inhibit the commercial exploitation of these therapies in mainland Europe. Here, as in Britain,

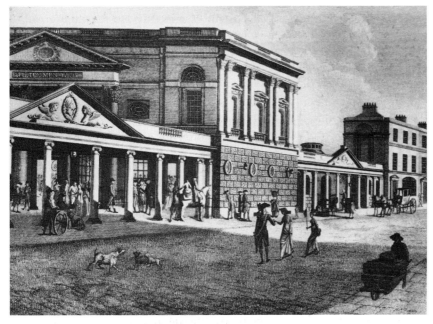

Figure 11.2 This engraving of 1801 shows the grandeur of the New Private Baths and the Pump Room, completed in 1788 and 1796 respectively. The very fact that these buildings were considered worthy of portrayal, and that the image was put on sale as something that would provide visual pleasure, indicates how they had escaped from their purely therapeutic meaning and had been assimilated into polite culture. Victoria Art Gallery, Bath, and North East Somerset Council

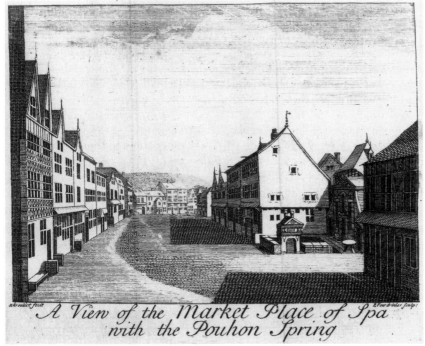

A View of the Market Place of Spa with the Pouhon Spring

Figure 11.3 This engraving was the frontispiece to Henry Eyre's *An Account of the Mineral Waters of Spa*, 1733. It represents the marketplace of the small market town in the Austrian Netherlands (modern Belgium) and the site of the Pouhon spring – one of the main sources of the town's mineral waters and the one from which Eyre drew his supplies. The image hammers home Eyre's emphasis that his supplies were the 'real thing', taken at source, but the contrast with Figure 11.2 reveals how much less the town is being presented as a site of fashionable sociability (no people are shown and the architecture is not highly fashionable).© The British Library

much effort was invested in promoting the sale of mineral waters. Supplies had to be marketed, and customers required reassurance in respect of the therapeutic qualities and authenticity of the waters they purchased (see, for example, the activities of the English merchant, Henry Eyre in 'An account of the mineral waters of Spa (1733)', Source Book 1, Reading 11.3).

Exercise

Read 'The commercialisation of spa waters in eighteenth-century France' (Source Book 1, Reading 11.4). In this passage, Brockliss and Jones identify a number of different social and economic routes by which mineral waters were marketed in France. How novel were these developments?

Discussion

Brockliss and Jones suggest that in some cases the 'traditional' ecclesiastical promoters of water cures were elbowed aside by more secular and commercial forces – the Cordeliers were undermined by manufacturers who counterfeited their supplies. However, the authors generally emphasize the extent to which many established groups were involved in the commercialization of mineral waters. Many sections of the state – the ministry of war, for example – sponsored the development of resorts. Court contacts, family and patronage ties are all identified as being important in the establishment of mineral water businesses by individuals such as Bordeu. The authors thus imply that the traditional forms of social connection were harnessed for the pursuit of profit as readily as the improvements in transport infrastructure, advertising and policing.

If anything, commercialization intensified medical debates about the nature and efficacy of mineral waters. After all, if a physician recommended Malvern water, he implied that it was better than the waters of rival spas, such as those at Buxton or Bath. Throughout the seventeenth and eighteenth centuries there were fierce pamphlet wars between advocates of different spas, with partisans denouncing other sources as useless or positively dangerous while trumpeting the virtues of their own. There was no easy solution to such disputes. Participants invoked different forms of analysis in order to establish their case, and there was no consensus as to how to determine the composition of waters. The simplest ways involved descriptions of taste, smell and visual appearance. Other tests were equally ancient – oak galls, for instance, which change colour in iron-rich water, were extensively employed. Various people, including the Italian physician Gabriele Fallopia and the English natural philosopher Robert Boyle, tried to systematize the analysis of waters, cataloguing the colours produced by the presence of particular chemicals. From the late seventeenth century onward, chemistry was increasingly deployed to investigate sources and even to manufacture artificial mineral waters. Samples were evaporated and residues analysed. During the eighteenth century, improved chemical techniques enabled analysts to isolate and identify gases dissolved in waters. All this work remained highly controversial. In the 1770s, a Swedish professor of chemistry, Torbern Bergman (1735–84), published a widely acclaimed set of essays outlining the experiments that he had conducted on a large selection of mineral waters (these included the use of evaporation techniques, the measurement of specific gravity, and the use of reagents). He concluded that an accurate analysis of these waters would enable a natural philosopher to synthesize the water for himself. Although his methods were subsequently subjected to telling intellectual and methodological critiques, the tables he produced (see, for example, Figure 11.4) seemed to set out accurate and convincing descriptions and catalogues of mineral waters in much the same way that Enlightenment natural historians such as Karl Linnaeus (1707–78) were cataloguing the species of animals and plants (Hamlin, 1990, pp.24–30).

TABLE of CONTENTS of the cold medicated Waters, in Grains.

	Seydfchutz.	Seltzer.	Spa.	Pyrmont.
Aerated lime	$4\frac{1}{2}$	17	$8\frac{1}{2}$	20
Vitriolated lime	$24\frac{1}{2}$	—	—	$38\frac{1}{2}$
Aerated magnefia	$12\frac{1}{2}$	$29\frac{1}{2}$	20	45
Vitriolated magnefia	$859\frac{1}{2}$	—	—	25
Salited magnefia	$21\frac{1}{4}$			
Aerated mineral alkali	—	24	$8\frac{1}{2}$	
Salited mineral alkali	—	$109\frac{1}{2}$	1	7
Aerated iron	—	—	$3\frac{1}{4}$	$3\frac{1}{4}$
Sum total	$922\frac{1}{4}$	180	$41\frac{1}{2}$	$138\frac{1}{4}$
Greateft quantity of aerial acid, in cubic inches	4	60	45	90
Pure air	2	1		
Specific gravity	1,0060	1,0027	1,0010	1,0024

Figure 11.4   This table of contents setting out the amounts of various substances in four mineral waters – Seydschutz, Seltzer, Spa and Pyrmont – exemplifies the way in which chemists sought authoritatively to fix and determine numerically and in tabular form the physical properties of mineral waters. Reproduced from Bergman (1784), vol.1, p.225. British Library. © The British Library

11.3 Analysing places, analysing populations

In considering airs, waters and places, and by seeking to determine the composition of mineral waters, early modern medical practitioners and natural philosophers were making the analysis of the natural world part of their search for new and more effective therapies. In the second half of the seventeenth century, the English physician Thomas Sydenham (1624–89) extended this approach to the very notion of disease. A pious Protestant, Sydenham was strongly committed to reforming medical practice so that it was based upon empirical grounds. Following the English philosopher Francis Bacon (1561–1626), he emphasized the importance of observation and the accumulation of data in scientific practice. He was also convinced of the divinely sanctioned regularity and order of the natural world. His strong conviction that 'Nature, in the production of disease, is uniform and consistent' led him to maintain that diseases were knowable entities, which, like plants, could be catalogued according to their peculiar properties (Sydenham, 1848–50, vol.1, p.15).

This proposition represented a direct challenge to the standard approach of learned physicians. As Andrew Cunningham has observed, when the latter treated a patient with a fever (or, for that matter, any other disease) 'they treated ... *the fevers of individual patients*. It was not the fever which was their starting-point, but the pre-disposition of their *patient* to suffer from it, and the particular capacity of their *patient* to withstand and overcome it' (Cunningham, 1989, pp.176–7; emphases in original). The physician thus sought to remedy or alleviate the general indisposition, or the disease, of the individual, by attending to the patient's manner of life and physical characteristics. Sydenham, by contrast, aimed to redirect medical attention to the disease, which he presented as having a distinct ontological status, or being. Now the emphasis was on understanding the disease rather than the patient. Identifying diseases thus required particular skills in observation, description and discrimination.

Sydenham argued that an individual disease could be isolated and known by charting its history, that is, by recording the sequence of symptoms displayed by patients over the course of their affliction and by using large numbers of such descriptions to construct a general account of specific diseases. The symptoms were not themselves the disease, but rather the signs which indicated the natural processes employed by the body to combat a malady. The task of the physician was to work with nature in this process of recovery. In particular, Sydenham devoted much attention to the study of those epidemic diseases, especially fevers, which affected the population of London between 1661 and 1676. He thus analysed an entire population over many years and concluded that the capital suffered from different epidemic diseases in different years.

Exercise

Read 'New approaches to understanding disease: Thomas Sydenham (1624–89)' (Source Book 1, Reading 11.5).

1 How, according to Sydenham, should one construct the history of a disease?

2 What faults did Sydenham identify in existing approaches to the analysis and categorization of diseases?

Discussion

1 In this passage, Sydenham identified four things to keep in mind when constructing the history of a disease. First, one should discriminate between the different species of diseases in much the same way as the botanist distinguishes species of plants. Second, he recommended that general laws, theories and hypotheses should be set aside. Third, he counselled caution because it was often difficult to differentiate between what he termed 'peculiar and perpetual' symptoms and the 'accidental and adventitious'. Finally, he emphasized the need for careful observation of the effect of the seasons on the occurrence of diseases.

2   Sydenham was particularly critical of those whose views on disease were largely determined by philosophical speculation rather than acute observation. He wrote disparagingly of those who fitted the evidence to suit their preconceived theories and omitted that which inconveniently conflicted with their a priori assumptions. He also condemned the use of fine-sounding, but meaningless, phrases such as 'Morbifick Cause' in discussions of disease which he implied disguised the ignorance of physicians.

Sydenham was unable to offer confident explanations of his own for the cause of these epidemics; indeed, he felt that it would be arrogant and premature to do so. Consequently, his work was more important for its methodological recommendations than for any therapeutic breakthrough. In particular, he stressed the need for the physician to be aware of the seasons and to note those months in which epidemics became prevalent. He noted, moreover, that different years had different 'constitutions' and hypothesized that particular qualities of the air or weather in a given year might produce specific epidemic diseases. Invoking Hippocrates as an authority, Sydenham encouraged other physicians to focus on the role of climate and the environment in order to understand the patterns of disease. Despite this 'macro' approach, however, we should note that Sydenham's observations were traditional in that they were qualitative and descriptive in their language. As we shall see, many of his contemporaries and successors shared his preoccupation with the analysis of the medical experiences of whole populations while adopting a more quantitative approach.

It is, of course, difficult to think quantitatively, if you do not have numerical data with which to make calculations. The new, more number-based approach made use of two new sources of information about population and mortality which emerged after 1500. During the sixteenth century it became obligatory in most European countries to register baptisms, marriages and burials in every parish. An Act of Parliament made such registration compulsory in England in 1538; the Ordinance of Villers-Cotterêts did the same for France in the following year. In 1563, the Council of Trent ordered Roman Catholic priests to keep records of marriages and baptisms, and in 1614 Pope Paul V (1605–21) issued detailed instructions for the registration of baptisms, marriages and burials. Initially, this information was retained locally, and only limited use was made of it. In time, as we shall see, such registers provided valuable raw data for calculations about population trends.

Another, more immediately useful, source of information was bills of mortality. In their crudest form, these constituted the weekly totals of burials in a given community. However, these were supplemented by the numbers of baptisms and by lists which detailed the causes of death. Originally introduced as a way of detecting the onset and severity of plague epidemics, the information was sometimes published in weekly and annual summaries. Among the most widely diffused and printed were the bills of mortality for London (Figure 11.5). From 1627, when cause of death was added to the London bills, it was possible to see at a glance how many Londoners had died of the plague or the pox in a specific year. By

A general BILL for this prefent year, ending the 19. of *December*, 1665. according to *n° 14* the report made to the KINGS moft Excellent MAJESTY.

By the Company of Parifh Clerks of *London*, &c.

	Buried	Pla.		Buried	Pla.		Buried	Pla.		Buried	Pla.
St Albans Woodftreet	200	121	St Clements Eaftcheap	18	20	St Margaret Mofes	38	25	St Michael Cornhill	104	52
St Alhallowes Barking	514	330	St Dionis Back-church	78	27	St Margaret Newfifh	114	66	St Michael Crookedla.	179	133
St Alhallowes Breadfr.	35	16	St Dunftans Eaft	265	150	St Margaret Pattons	49	24	St Michael Queenbith.	203	112
St Alhallowes Great	455	426	St Edmunds Lumbard.	70	36	St Mary Abchurch	99	54	St Michael Querne	44	18
St Alhallowes Honila.	10	5	St Ethelborough.	195	106	St Mary Aldermanbury	181	109	St Michael Royal	152	116
'St Alhallowes Leffe	239	175	St Faiths	104	70	St Mary Aldermary	105	75	St Michael Woodftreet	122	62
St Alhall. Lumbardftr.	90	62	St Fofters	144	105	St Mary le Bow	64	36	St Mildred Breadftreet	59	26
St Alhallowes Staining	185	112	St Gabriel Fen-church	69	39	St Mary Bothaw.	55	30	St Mildred Poultrey	68	46
St Alhallowes the Wall	500	356	St George Botolphlane	41	27	St Mary Colechurch	17	6	St Nicholas Acons	46	28
St Alphage	271	115	St Gregories by Paul	376	232	St Mary Hill	94	64	St Nicholas Coleabby	125	91
St Andrew Hubbard	71	25	St Hellens	108	75	St Mary Mounthaw	56	37	St Nicholas Olaves	90	62
St Andrew Underfhaft	274	189	St James Dukes place	262	190	St Mary Summerfet	342	262	St Olaves Harefreet	237	160
St Andrew VVardrobe	476	308	St James Garlickhithe	189	118	St Mary Staynings	49	27	St Olaves Jewry	54	32
St Anne Alderfgate	282	197	St John Baptift	138	83	St Mary Woolchurch	65	33	St Olaves Silverftreet	250	132
St Anne Black-Friers	652	467	St John Evangelift	9		St Mary Woolnoth	75	38	St Pancras Soperlane	30	15
St Antholins Parifh	58	33	St John Zacharie	85	54	St Martins Iremonger	21	11	St Peters Cheape	61	35
St Auftins Parifh	43	40	St Katherine Coleman	299	213	St Martins Ludgate	196		St Peters Cornhill	128	76
St Barthol. Exchange	73	51	St Katherine Creechu.	135	231	St Martins Orgars	110	71	St Peters Pauls Wharf	114	86
St Bennet Fyrch	47	18	St Lawrence Jewry	94	48	St Martins Outwitch	60	34	St Peters Poor	79	47
St Benn. Grace-church	57	41	St Lawrence Pountney	214	140	St Martins Vintrey	417	349	St Stevens Colmanftr.	560	391
St Bennet Pauls Wharf	355	172	St Leonard Eaftcheap	42	27	St Matthew Fridayftr.	14	6	St Stevens Walbrooke	34	17
St Bennet Sherehog	11	1	St Leonard Fofterlane	335	255	St Maudlins Milkftreet	44	22	St Swithins	93	56
St Botolph Billingfgate	83	50	St Magnus Parifh	103	60	St Maudlins Oldfifhftr.	176	121	St Thomas Apoftle	163	110
Chrifts Church	653	467	St Margaret Lothbury	100	66	St Michael Baffifhaw	253		Trinity Parifh	115	79
St Chriftophers	60	47									

Buried in the 97 Parifhes within the Walls, ———— 15207 *Whereof, of the Plague,* ——— 9887

St Andrew Holborne	3958	3103	Bridewell Precinct	230	179	St Dunftans Weft	958	665	St Saviours Southwark	4235	3446
St Bartholomew Great	493	344	St Botolph Alderfga.	997	755	St George Southwark	1613	1260	St Sepulchres Parifh	4509	2746
St Bartholomew Leffe	193	139	St Botolph Algate	4926	4051	St Giles Cripplegate	8069	4838	St Thomas Southwark	475	371
St Bridget	2111	1427	St Botolph Bifhopfg.	3464	2500	St Olaves Southwark	4793	2785	Trinity Minories	168	123
									At the Pefthoufe	159	156

Buried in the 16 Parifhes without the walls, ———— 41351 *Whereof, of the Plague,* ——— 28888

St Giles in the Fields	4457	3216	St Katherines Tower	956	601	St Magdalen Bermon	1943	1362	St Mary Whitechappel	4766	3855
Hackney Parifh	232	132	Lambeth Parifh	798	537	St Mary Newington	1272	1004	Redriffe Parifh	304	210
St James Clarkenwell	1863	1377	St Leonard Shordicth	2669	1949	St Mary Iflington	696	593	Stepney Parifh	8598	6583

Buried in the 12 out Parifhes, in Middlefex and Surrey ——— 28554 *Whereof, of the Plague* ——— 21420

St Clement Danes	1969	1319	St Mary Savoy	303	198	
St Paul Covent Garden	408	261	St Margaret Weftminft.	4710	3742	
St Martins in the Field	4804	2883	*Whereof at the Pefthoufe*	156		

Buried in the 5 Parifhes in the City and Liberties of Weftminfter ——— 11194
Whereof, of the Plague ——— 8403

The Total of all the Chriftnings		9967
The Total of all the Burials this year		97306
Whereof, of the Plague		68596

The Difeafes and Cafualties this year.

Abortive and Stilborne	617	Executed	21	Palfie		30
Aged	1545	Flox and Small Pox	655	Plague		68596
Ague and Feaver	5257	Found dead in ftreets, fields, &c.	20	Planet		6
Appoplex and Suddenly	116	French Pox	86	Plurifie		15
Bedrid	10	Frighted	23	Purfeued		1
Blafted	5	Gout and Sciatica	27	Quinfie		35
Bleeding	16	Grief	46	Rickets		557
Bloody Flux, Scowring and Flux	185	Gripping in the Guts	1288	Rifing of the Lights		397
Burnt and Scalded	8	Hang'd and made away themfelves	7	Rupture		34
Calenture	3	Headmouldfhot and Mouldfallen	14	Scurvy		105
Cancer, Gangreene and Fiftula	56	Jaundies	110	Shingles and Swine Pox		2
Canker and Thrufh	111	Impofthume	227	Sores, Ulcers, broken and bruifed Limbs		82
Childbed	625	Kill'd by feveral accidents	46	Spleen		14
Chrifomes and Infants	1258	Kings Evil	86	Spotted Feaver and Purples		1929
Cold and Cough	68	Leprofie	2	Stopping of the ftomack		332
Chollick and Winde	134	Lethargy	14	Stone and Strangury		98
Confumption and Ptifick	4808	Livergrown	20	Surfet		1251
Convulfion and Mother	2036	Meagrom and Headach	12	Teeth and Worms		2614
Diftracted	5	Meafles	7	Vomiting		51
Dropfie and Timpany	1478	Murthered and Shot	9	Wenn		8
Drowned	50	Overlaid and Starved	45			

Chriftned {	Males	5114	Buried {	Males	48569
	Females	4853		Females	48737
	In all	9967		In all	97306

Of the Plague ——— 68596

Increafed in the Burials in the 130 Parifhes and at the Pefthoufe this year ——— 79009
Increafed of the Plague in the 130 Parifhes and at the Pefthoufe this year ——— 68590

Figure 11.5 This single sheet bill of mortality provides at a glance a range of information about the total numbers of deaths in London during the plague year of 1665. It summarizes totals by parish, but also gives the numbers of Londoners who died as a result of a wide range of afflictions. Such information was to provide the raw material for many subsequent calculations of the incidence of fatal diseases over time and according to place. University of London EEBO image http://wwwlib.umi.com/eebo/image/35765

the early eighteenth century, long runs of similar data were available for a number of other European cities, including Amsterdam, Dresden and Dublin.

Probably the earliest systematic analysis of the mortality figures contained in bills was John Graunt's *Natural and Political Observations ... made upon the Bills of Mortality ... with Reference to the Government, Religion, Trade, Growth, Ayre, Diseases, and the Several Changes of the said City* [1662] (1973). The title indicates the twin ambitions of what became known as 'political arithmetic'. In the first place, it sought to reconstruct or determine patterns in nature through an analysis of a sequence of events. And second, it was based on the fundamental assumption that matters of population were profoundly political, and amenable to manipulation and improvement. Graunt (1620–74) was a London merchant who applied arithmetical techniques derived from double-entry book-keeping to analyse the number of London's inhabitants over the preceding sixty years. By comparing the total numbers of burials and baptisms, he was able to show that more people had been buried than baptised in the capital in this period, and thus to prove that the recent growth in London's population was the result of immigration. Tabulating the totals derived from the bills and crudely correcting them for possible distortions, Graunt was able to address a range of other questions. He suggested, for instance, that patterns of mortality revealed that autumn was particularly unhealthy. He also constructed a rudimentary life table, in which he estimated how many in a sample of one hundred newborn Londoners would still be alive after ten, twenty or fifty years.

His work was further developed by his friend William Petty (1623–87), who saw in the analysis of such figures new ways of promoting the nation's wealth. In his *Political Arithmetic*, for instance, first published in 1690 (but written during the 1670s and 1680s), Petty set out to understand how a relatively small country such as the United Provinces (modern-day Netherlands) had come to be wealthier than its much larger neighbour, the kingdom of France. Petty was interested above all in the *productivity* of both land and people. An important strand of this concern was the number of hands that could be put to profitable work. Crucially, Petty and later political arithmeticians saw this as the business of the state. Governments could and should take action to promote populousness and productivity. Petty, for example, advocated reforms such as the foundation of public hospitals and the passage of laws designed to promote marriage. Both would increase the size of the labour force and thus make the nation wealthier. Such reforms, however, depended on the collection of accurate information by the state. According to Graunt, governments ought to know 'how many People there be of each Sex, Age, Religion, Trade, Rank or Degree', so that 'Trade and Government may be made more certain, and Regular' (Graunt, 1973, p.73). Similar ideas spread through Europe. During the 1680s, Sébastien Le Prestre de Vauban (1633–1707) suggested that his royal master, Louis XIV (1643–1715), should establish annual national censuses. It took some time, however, for such ambitious schemes to get off the ground. Some of the most impressive data collection was done in Scandinavia, and especially Sweden. From 1686, every minister was obliged to keep a register, which listed everyone in their parish by household, as well as recording all births, marriages and deaths. In 1748, another law was passed that required the clergy to draw up tables summarizing such data, which was then sent to Stockholm for analysis. As a result of this enterprise, national mortality tables were first published in 1766.

You may be thinking that this discussion takes us a long way from medicine. Crucially, though, these developments brought about a new technology and a new language whereby contemporaries were able to visualize and discuss the health of nations. Such arithmetical techniques rapidly became part of medical analysis in the eighteenth century. Bills of mortality and parish registers could now be read in order to determine whether or not nations were becoming healthier. Similarly, a new numerical language of statecraft became available. Manpower could now be represented and discussed in a variety of new ways, and enabled greater analysis and understanding of what the French philosopher Michel Foucault has termed 'biopower', or those human resources at the disposal of the state.

Exercise

Read 'Medical police and the state in eighteenth-century medicine' (Source Book 1, Reading 11.6). What reasons does Foucault suggest for the interest shown by eighteenth-century governments in issues of health and population?

Discussion

Foucault suggests two main reasons. First, he argues that the increase in population in this period presented governments with novel problems as to how they should ensure the successful integration and regulation of people. And second, he identifies state interest in the health of populations, and its successful 'policing', as evidence of a growing ideological shift in which the remit of state action extended to all aspects of the subject's life, including their economic and physical well-being.

The arithmetical and statistical methods discussed thus far were not, however, simply crude instruments of state-building. First, there was often a moral or religious dimension to this work. Many investigators, for example, had a strong sense that if one examined demographic change over time, then God-given natural regularities would emerge. Graunt clearly felt that the balance of population was part of the divine order. The Prussian cleric and political arithmetician Johann Peter Süssmilch (1707–77), gave his massive 1741 study of population the revealing title *Die Göttliche Ordnung* [The God-Given Order]. In a similar vein, the Sheffield physician Thomas Short (1690?–1772) published a book in 1767 which brought together close analysis of parish registers and bills of mortality in order not only to demonstrate how the nation might be made stronger and more populous, but also to hammer home the dire consequences of '*Vices, Intemperance, Irregularities, and Luxury*' (Short, 1973, p.i).

And second, eighteenth-century doctors promoted quantitative analyses of the relative healthiness of places because they wanted to develop the Hippocratic heritage of airs, waters and places into a more empirical and observation-based environmental medicine. Across Europe, a network of natural philosophers systematically measured rainfall and used barometers to chart day-to-day variations in atmospheric pressure. Some physicians sought to relate this topographical and meteorological data to patterns of disease. In the late 1750s and early 1760s, for instance, Jean Razoux (1723–98) compiled detailed monthly accounts of the diseases that afflicted patients in the Hôtel Dieu at Nîmes, which he summarized in tabular form alongside daily summaries of wind direction, temperature and atmospheric pressure for the same period. When he published his findings in 1767, he claimed to have established the connections between illness and climate (Rusnock, 2002, pp.129–35).

11.4 Changing populations? The case of inoculation

Political arithmeticians like William Petty did not simply want to count the state's population, but they wished to see it increase, because in their opinion national wealth was linked to populousness. Consequently, they advocated state policies to encourage marriage and large families and sought ways to make people healthier, or at the least, less likely to die prematurely. This could be achieved either by altering the bodies of the population in ways that made them more resistant to debilitating diseases or by creating a healthier environment.

In the eighteenth century, inoculation against smallpox offered the most dramatic solution to the problem of human susceptibility to fatal infections. As the plague receded (the last major epidemic in western Europe occurred in Marseille in 1720–2), smallpox became the most lethal epidemic disease afflicting Europeans. It was highly contagious, killing indiscriminately among both rich and poor. Moreover, those that recovered were often left with disfiguring pock marks. Its ravages were presented as particularly disastrous for women. However, it was widely recognized that if one recovered from the disease, immunity followed. Employers, for example, advertising in newspapers for servants often stated that they would hire only those who had previously contracted and survived smallpox. Inoculation exploited this aspect of the disease.

It is important to distinguish between inoculation and vaccination. Inoculation involved cutting or scratching a patient's arm and inserting matter taken from a smallpox pustule. This induced a relatively mild form of the disease and guaranteed protection thereafter from a more lethal infection. Vaccination, on the other hand, which was first introduced by the English physician Edward Jenner (1749–1823) at the end of the eighteenth century, was performed with a small dose of cowpox and gave the vaccinated person immunity without submitting them to smallpox itself.

Like the development of spas and water cures, the introduction and diffusion of inoculation involved complex processes of cultural exchange and negotiation rather than any single moment of 'discovery'. These exchanges occurred between different nations as well as between different social and ethnic groups. In Boston, Massachusetts, the Calvinist minister and physician Cotton Mather (1663–1728), who was an early convert to inoculation, seems to have learned about the practice from black African slaves who exposed their own children to the infection in order to guarantee later immunity. During the 1720s, physicians noted similar practices among country people from as far afield as Poland, Scotland and Italy. However, in western Europe inoculation was principally adapted from procedures observed in the Middle East.

It first gained wide publicity in England following the return to London of Lady Mary Wortley Montagu (1689–1762). While in Turkey with her husband, the ambassador to the Ottoman Empire at Constantinople (Istanbul), she had followed local practice in having her son inoculated. Back in smallpox-ravaged London in 1721, she instructed the surgeon Charles Maitland (1677–1748), who had attended on her family in Turkey, to inoculate her 3-year-old daughter. News of the inoculation rapidly spread among the *cognoscenti*, including members of the College of Physicians and the Royal Society, some of whom petitioned King George I (1714–27) for permission to conduct experimental trials into inoculation. In August 1721, they were allowed to inoculate six condemned prisoners. Five caught a mild dose of smallpox and recovered; the sixth was found to have had the disease already. Crucially, repeated exposure to smallpox was found to leave all five unaffected. Thereafter, the process was widely publicized in the press and some English physicians began to inoculate during periods of high smallpox mortality. In 1722, the procedure received the seal of royal approval – the Prince and Princess of Wales had their two children inoculated.

Despite such eminent support, inoculation remained highly controversial and did not become a general practice. For one thing, it was risky – on occasions the inoculated person died. Moreover, some saw the idea of introducing a fatal disease into the body of an otherwise healthy person as impious. In 1722, for example, the London clergyman Edmund Massey (1690–1765) preached a thunderous sermon (much reprinted) against inoculation. Others argued that it was contrary to the office of a physician deliberately to expose a patient to such a dangerous infection. Lastly, some suggested that the procedure actually helped to spread the disease because of the increased danger of infection from inoculated people. Partisans of the practice thus had to build a case for its use.

The manner in which these claims were debated reveals much about the development of medicine in the eighteenth century. In particular, the controversy surrounding smallpox inoculation provides an early example of what we might anachronistically term the statistical evaluation of new therapies. A leading advocate of this approach was James Jurin (1684–1750), who, as secretary to the Royal Society, was a noted enthusiast for the use of mathematics in medicine. In his research, Jurin compared the proportion of people who died as a result of smallpox inoculation with those who were killed by 'natural' smallpox. Using among other things the London bills of mortality, he concluded that one in fifty died from smallpox induced by inoculation, whereas one in fourteen died from 'natural' smallpox. He then revised these figures, pointing out that many infants died before they were exposed to the disease, to show that the risk of dying from 'natural' smallpox was even greater. Inoculation, he concluded, would save lives (for an example of the methods which Jurin used to accumulate data and publicize his evidence, see 'Medical statistics and smallpox in the eighteenth century', Source Book 1, Reading 11.7).

In the event, neither Jurin's calculations nor his case histories were sufficient to produce general support for his conclusions. Across Europe, clerics, medics and the public remained divided on the merits of inoculation. In France, for example, the medical establishment was generally hostile. There, inoculation was usually promoted by those who advocated self-consciously 'modern' methods in science and medicine and the culture of improvement associated with the Enlightenment. One of the most eloquent of the **philosophes**, Voltaire (1694–1778), was typical in writing in favour of the practice (see 'Voltaire on smallpox inoculation', Source Book 1, Reading 11.8).

So far I have been writing about 'inoculation' as though it were a single, unchanging practice. In fact, over the course of the eighteenth century, it evolved in various different ways. Up to the 1750s, inoculators generally inserted pus from smallpox pocks into a cut in the patient's arm. Most were physicians, and they customarily advised would-be patients that they should prepare for the procedure by undertaking a lengthy course of medically supervised purging. Although they treated smallpox as a specific disease entity in a manner of which Sydenham would have approved, inoculation had been turned into a highly individualized and expensive course of treatment. Consequently, it was far too costly for general use among the poor. Between 1755 and 1761, the Suffolk surgeon Robert Sutton (1707–88) developed a new form of inoculation. This involved a simple procedure in which lymph taken from the early stages of a smallpox pustule was introduced into a simple scratch. It involved no preparatory regimen and produced a much milder form of the disease (it was actually much closer to the form of inoculation practised in Turkey). During the course of the 1760s, Sutton and his son Daniel (1735–1819) built up a substantial practice based on their ability to inoculate safely.

Their renown reached as far afield as Russia. In the mid-1760s, the Empress Catherine II (the Great) (1762–96) was acutely aware that she had never contracted smallpox and that her son, Paul, was similarly at risk. She was understandably alarmed by an epidemic in Moscow and St Petersburg, particularly when one of her ladies-in-waiting fell sick of the disease. In regular correspondence with Voltaire on this and other matters, Catherine resolved to be inoculated. Approaches were made to the Suttons, and when these were unsuccessful the empress's advisers persuaded another English inoculator, Thomas Dimsdale (1712–1800), to come to St Petersburg. He arrived in 1768 and in that year both the empress and her son were successfully inoculated. She had, reported Voltaire, with typical salacious anticlericalism, 'been inoculated with less fuss than a nun taking an enema' (Alexander, 1989, p.148). The procedure made Dimsdale rich and hugely enhanced his reputation, but it is unclear how far the practice spread beyond Russian courtly circles. Certainly many nobles followed Catherine's example and the empress sponsored inoculation in Moscow's Foundling Hospital, but it is unlikely that it became widely diffused in her vast domains.

Inoculation may have had a limited impact in Russia, but the procedure pioneered by the Suttons and used by Dimsdale on Catherine now offered an unprecedented opportunity for changing the susceptibility of whole populations to devastating diseases such as smallpox. Dimsdale himself showed the way forward by offering the state a new and powerful incentive to promote population growth and wealth. As Dimsdale wrote following his return to England:

> To preserve the lives and health of the inferior part of mankind has been an object carefully attended to in all civilized and well regulated states, not only from motives of compassion, but because it has been plainly demonstrated that it is the interest of the wealthy in every nation to encourage population, and provide for the wants of the poor.
>
> (Dimsdale, 1776, sig.a)

Dimsdale's hopes had, to some extent, been anticipated by the actions of charitable hospitals earlier in the century. In 1744, the London Foundling Hospital had agreed to inoculate all children in its care in order to save young lives. Two years later, a smallpox hospital had been established in the capital which encouraged inoculation of the poor. In the late 1750s and 1760s, Suttonian inoculation was employed in a number of English parishes. In May 1766, for example, 487 inhabitants of the Essex town of Maldon were inoculated by Daniel Sutton. Two months later he inoculated hundreds more at Maidstone in Kent (Smith, 1987, p.47). Many of these initiatives represented local responses to periodic upsurges in the infection. However, in the 1770s and 1780s medical practitioners tried to make the procedure more systematic by sponsoring regional associations to promote general inoculation. At Chester, for example, around 1778, the physician to the local infirmary, Francis Haygarth (1740–1827), helped to create a philanthropic society which paid for a general inoculation of the city's poor. It also established a set of hygienic rules that all inoculated families were forced to follow in order to prevent contagion; financial rewards were offered for observing them. For the first few years of the enterprise, smallpox mortality in the city fell dramatically. The scheme received a good degree of press attention and reports emphasized the way in which the spread of inoculation was being emulated both in England and abroad.

Exercise

Read 'A newspaper account of inoculation for smallpox (1788)' and 'Smallpox and inoculation in a provincial town: Luton (1788)' (Source Book 1, Readings 11.9 and 11.10). What do these two extracts tell us about the way in which information about inoculation was communicated in late eighteenth-century England?

Discussion

Both extracts suggest that information about inoculation circulated in a variety of ways. Stuart's letter indicates that informal channels and personal correspondence were important for passing on information about the practice. Both sources, however, reveal the importance of the press in publicizing inoculation. Although Sir William Fordyce was a fellow of the Royal Society, he chose to make use of a non-professional publication in order to achieve the widest possible publicity for the cause of inoculation. Likewise, the report in *The Times* was aimed at a wide reading public.

Evidently, discussion of inoculation was not confined to medical or specialist journals. The story in *The Times* does, however, attest to the communication of information within medical circles across national boundaries. The Genevan inoculation was, it seems, inspired by Dr de la Roche's translation of Haygarth's account of the Chester society.

The decentralized nature of the English schemes of inoculation is in stark contrast to events elsewhere in Europe where central government played a greater role in introducing systematic policies of inoculation as part of a general programme of improved medical care and population growth. In France, for example, where medical and ecclesiastical opposition had been overcome by the 1770s, the government initiated a programme of inoculation in *hôpitaux généraux* in 1786. The precise demographic consequences of inoculation, however, remain a matter of some controversy. For our purpose, its impact or extent is less significant than the ambitious nature of the schemes and the various statistical and administrative methods that were now applied to understanding eighteenth-century society. As you will see in the final section, such initiatives are best understood as part of wider schemes for the reform of medicine, the environment and society in general.

11.5 Changing places? Hygiene and improvement

After she had been inoculated, Catherine the Great proclaimed that her objective had been 'through my example, to save from death the multitude of my subjects who, not knowing the value of this technique, frightened of it, were left in danger' (Alexander, 1989, p.147). Her adoption and advocacy of inoculation thus had an ideological dimension. It was linked to Catherine's interest in developing her state and her desire to promote the general health of her subjects. This was also evident in other reforms initiated by Catherine. In 1763, she was instrumental in establishing a Collegium Medicum to oversee medical training and practice in Russia. In the same year, she founded the first public hospital in Moscow, and in 1764 she encouraged the creation of a foundling and lying-in hospital in the city. In 1775, she implemented administrative reforms that divided Russia into provinces (*guberniia*), which in turn were sub-divided into districts (*uezdy*). Significantly, Catherine proposed that every district should hire a doctor, surgeon and assistants for public service. In the same year, plans for rebuilding Moscow were drawn up which laid down that the city's public hygiene and water supply should be improved (Alexander, 1974, 1980; Raeff, 1983).

Catherine was unashamedly adapting ideas developed elsewhere in Europe. A Collegium Medicum with powers to supervise medical practice had, for instance, been established in Brandenburg-Prussia in 1685. As Foucault has argued, underlying these projects was the ideal of the well-ordered polity which drew its strength from the efficient management of its human resources and the maximization of its people's health. The concept of 'police' permeated many of these discussions and proposals. In the early modern period it encompassed much more than its modern-day usage (crime prevention and detection; crowd control) suggests. The term was central to an emerging language of statecraft and could almost be translated as 'policy'. Rulers and their officials set out to produce prosperity and to establish and maintain order by decree and regulation. In many early modern Protestant kingdoms of central Europe, ordinances prescribed detailed rules governing areas of life ranging from trade to transport and from forestry to fire prevention. By the early eighteenth century the notion of 'police' was systematized and taught as a university subject. In the 1720s, for instance, professorships in *polizeiwissenschaft*, or the science of police, were established at the universities of Halle and Frankfurt an der Oder in order to instruct young men destined to serve the fledgling Prussian state. A century later, their remit was so extensive that in a handbook on the subject Günther Heinrich von Berg could write that:

> *Policey* is like a well-intentioned genius who carefully levels the way for those committed to his care; cleans the air that they breathe; secures the villages ... in which they dwell, and the streets along which they walk ... Its watchful eye is ubiquitous.
>
> (Tribe, 1984, p.274)

During the late seventeenth and eighteenth centuries, the idea of police began increasingly to incorporate medical matters as governments, under the influence of notions of political arithmetic, reassessed their human resources. By the late eighteenth century, some writers were referring to the concept of 'medical police', by which they expressed a desire for greater professional supervision of medical practice and an eradication of threats to public health. The term appears to have been coined by the Austrian physician Wolfgang Thomas Rau (1721–72), but was most fully elaborated by another Austrian doctor, Johann Peter Frank. Educated at Heidelberg, Frank completed the first volume of his monumental *System einer vollständigen medicinischen Polizey* [A Complete System of Medical Police] in 1779. It received immediate international acclaim and gained Frank the valuable patronage of another self-styled enlightened ruler, Joseph II of Austria. He subsequently held a succession of university chairs in medicine, including those at Pavia, St Petersburg and Vienna. His ideas on the subject of 'medical police' were elaborated in a further six volumes (two of which were published after his death) which set out a comprehensive programme of state-sponsored medical intervention in more or less every aspect of life. Frank's concerns ranged from the dangers of celibacy to the supervision of food supply, but one of the most striking aspects of his work, and other work in this field, was the preoccupation with place, especially the need to regulate and clean up the environment in order to make it healthy.

Exercise

Read 'Cleanliness and the state in eighteenth-century Europe' (Source Book 1, Reading 11.11).

1   What did Frank understand by the term 'cleanliness' in relation to health?

2   How did he use ideas of 'civilization' to justify his plea for the strict supervision of public health?

1   Frank's understanding of cleanliness was both capacious and rigid. His standards were far more rigorous than those of other groups and his attitudes towards other hygienic practices were often chauvinistic. However, he clearly saw an integral link between lack of cleanliness and disease. This was not just a matter of street cleaning or personal hygiene. Frank argued that the whole environment needed close supervision and regulation if the health of the people was to be guaranteed.

2   Frank recognized that different individuals and cultures had different mores with regard to cleanliness. However, he implicitly argued for a model in which cleanliness increased with civilization. He presented what he thought of as poor hygiene as 'animal-like' and thus implied that the cleaner a culture, the more civilized its government, and vice versa.

Many of Frank's recommendations can be seen as an intensified campaign to implement changes that had long been mooted and pursued – as for example in earlier measures to combat miasma and the plague. Unlike these, however, eighteenth-century attempts to promote medical police were not formulated as a direct response to epidemics. Here, Hippocratic medicine and medical police combined in order to effect permanent transformation of environments that were seen as pathological. Doctors and officials were no longer engaged in seeking simply to stave off disease; now they sought to eradicate it entirely by transforming the environment in which diseases were born and spread. The first attempts to introduce new forms of hygiene generally took place in restricted and controllable spaces, which were more readily subjected to medical discipline. One good example of this is the organization of military encampments and barracks advocated by the Scottish physician Sir John Pringle, which you encountered in Chapter 10. Another is the experimental use of ventilators to alter the atmosphere in prisons and hospitals. These were pioneered in England by Stephen Hales. After conducting experiments into the amount of air that seemed to be consumed by combustion and respiration, he became convinced that air would become 'vitiated' if it was not allowed to circulate freely, and would thus foster diseases. In 1752, therefore, he prevailed upon the City of London authorities to allow him to build a windmill on the roof of its notoriously unhealthy Newgate prison (Figures 11.6 and 11.7). This remarkable machine powered ventilators which drew stale air from the wards of the prison and, so he claimed, greatly reduced mortality rates in the institution. Shortly thereafter he advocated their use in hospitals (see 'The use of artificial ventilators in hospitals', Source Book 1, Reading 11.12).

In some ways, improving the atmosphere of a prison or a hospital was a relatively simple task. After all, the inhabitants of such places had little power. It is striking, however, that late eighteenth-century doctors began to reorder much more public and socially contested parts of the urban environment, even to the point of intervening in, and recommending the reform of, popular customs. One of the most celebrated of these episodes centred on the closure of the Cimitière des Saints-Innocents (Cemetery of the Holy Innocents) in Paris between 1785 and 1787.

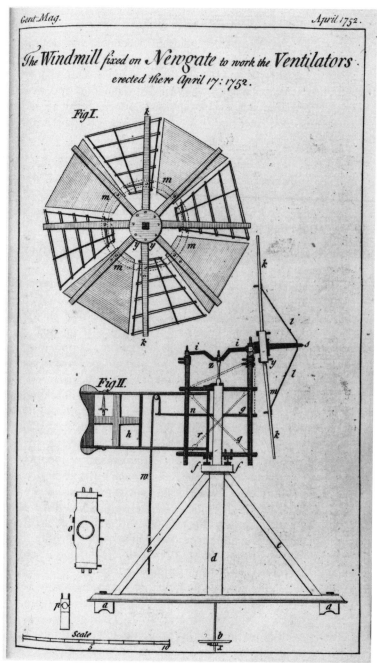

Figure 11.6   This engraved diagram of the windmill erected on the roof of Newgate prison in London by Stephen Hales was more than ornamental. By publishing in *The Gentleman's Magazine* the project was being given maximum publicity. But publication was also intended to encourage emulation and the construction of similar engines. As you can see, the design is to scale and all the constituent parts are marked with letters that were fully explained in a lengthy description of the engine that accompanied the illustration. *The Gentleman's Magazine*, 22 April 1752, facing page 180. © The British Library

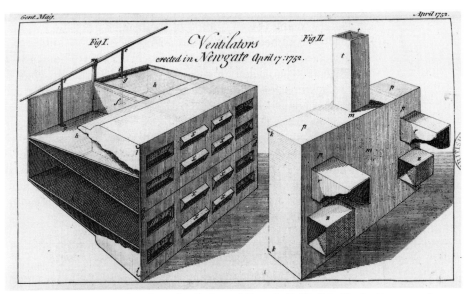

Figure 11.7 Less precise than the design of the windmill, this illustration reveals further details about the entire atmosphere of Newgate prison. It could be ventilated and the air changed through the valves marked v and x in the diagram on the left. *The Gentleman's Magazine*, 22 April 1752, facing page 181. © The British Library

During the eighteenth century, between 1,800 and 2,400 people a year were buried here. By modern standards, it was clearly full. The gravedigger of the cemetery told an inquiry in the 1760s that when digging pits there he sometimes encountered 'bodies that have not been consumed' (Ariès, 1981, p.57).

The odour of decomposing bodies thus hung around the cemetery and was periodically denounced as a health hazard. In 1737, local inhabitants complained to the *parlement* of Paris about the stench; the *parlementaires* commissioned a report from prominent Parisian medics who recommended that there should be improvements in its drains and greater care in the conduct of burials. Between 1763 and 1765 a second controversy resulted in an ordinance which forbade interments in city churches and intra-mural cemeteries, but the order was not implemented. Matters came to a head, however, in the winter of 1779–80 when mephitic matter began seeping into the cellars of buildings adjoining the cemetery and an epidemic began (described in 'Public health measures in Paris on the eve of the Revolution: the Cemetery of the Holy Innocents', Source Book 1, Reading 11.13). In the summer of 1780 the cemetery was closed for burials. So too were other city-centre cemeteries in the ensuing years. The Société Royale de Médecine now investigated and recommended that the site be closed permanently. The cemetery was cleared and all human remains were reinterred in an extra-mural burial ground. During the winter months of 1785–7, thousands of cartloads of bones and cemetery soil imbued with the remains of generations of Parisians were carried out of the city.

This episode was rooted in the local history and culture of Paris, but the closure of the Holy Innocents was not an isolated phenomenon. During the eighteenth century, many voices warned of the danger from the mephitic exhalations of the dead, recommending that interments should no longer be carried out within churches or city-centre graveyards. In 1745, for instance, a canon of Caen in Normandy published an essay denouncing burials in churches and near human dwellings because of the 'pestilential vapours' that tombs emitted. In a series of articles published in the ***Encyclopédie*** in the following decade, the *philosophe* Jean le Rond D'Alembert (1717–83) warned of the dangers presented by the practice and recommended the establishment of extra-mural cemeteries in order to preserve the public's health. Such hygienic developments were not confined to France. In 1775 it was commanded in Prussia that burials should only take place outside towns and cities; other German states followed suit, and similar orders were issued in Tuscany between 1777 and 1784. Concerns over hygiene were helping to redraw the boundaries of city space.

11.6 Conclusion

As you will see in the next two chapters, medical men intervened in many other areas of the environment during the eighteenth century, often through the auspices of institutions such as the Société Royale de Médecine. There are striking links between their views about the proper role of medicine in society and the intellectual content of their work. As Ludmilla Jordanova stresses in 'Environmental medicine in late Enlightenment Europe' (Source Book 1, Reading 11.14), the approach to disease synthesized in the late Enlightenment drew extensively on many of what we might now describe as the environmental sciences – climatic studies, geography and so on. The responses to disease advocated and developed by eighteenth-century medics often stressed the concept of hygiene and used it both as a basis for, and as a legitimation of, attempts to remould society in ways that made doctors important agents in the state.

Their proposals had far less impact on the ground than the ambition of their proposals might suggest. Ventilation, for instance, was no universal panacea and did not sweep hospitals into perfect health. If one looks back from the vantage point of nineteenth- or twentieth-century public health, then the impact of these developments was comparatively modest. However, it is dangerous to be so present-minded. The scale of the intellectual developments that occurred in terms of approaches to disease and the role of medicine in society between 1500 and 1800 is remarkable. Studying the nature and articulation of these developments also highlights the tension between coercion and social improvement and the dangerous overlap between public health and social control that continue to bedevil health policy today.

References

Alexander, J.T. (1974) 'Catherine II, bubonic plague, and the problem of industry in Moscow', *American Historical Review*, vol.79, pp.637–61.

Alexander, J.T. (1980) *Bubonic Plague in Early Modern Russia: Public Health and Urban Disaster*, Baltimore: Johns Hopkins University Press.

Alexander, J.T. (1989) *Catherine the Great: Life and Legend*, Oxford: Clarendon Press.

Ariès, P. (1981) *The Hour of Our Death*, Harmondsworth: Penguin.

Bergman, T. (1784) *Physical and Chemical Essays*, translated by E. Cullen, 2 vols, London: J. Murray.

Brockliss, L.W.B. (1990) 'The development of the Spa in seventeenth-century France' in R. Porter (ed.) *The Medical History of Waters and Spas*, *Medical History*, Supplement 10, pp.23–47.

Brockliss, L.W.B. and Jones, C. (1997) *The Medical World of Early Modern France*, Oxford: Clarendon Press.

Burton, R. (1968) *The Anatomy of Melancholy*, 3 vols, London: Everyman.

Christian Jr., W.A. (1981) *Local Religion in Sixteenth-Century Spain*, Princeton: Princeton University Press.

Cipolla, C.M. (1992) *Miasmas and Disease: Public Health and Environment in the Pre-Industrial Age*, translated by E. Potter, New Haven and London: Yale University Press.

Cunningham, A. (1989) 'Thomas Sydenham: epidemics, experiment and the "good old cause"' in R. French and A. Wear (eds) *The Medical Revolution of the Seventeenth Century*, Cambridge: Cambridge University Press, pp.164–90.

Delumeau, J. (1977) *Catholicism between Luther and Voltaire*, translated by J. Moiser, London: Burns & Oates.

Dimsdale, T. (1776) *Thoughts on General and Partial Inoculations*, London: W. Richardson.

Erasmus, D. (1992) *The Correspondence of Erasmus: Letters 1356–1534 (1523–1524)*, translated by R.A.B. Mynors and A. Dalzell, vol.10, Toronto: Toronto University Press.

Erasmus, D. (1997) *Colloquies*, ed. by C.R. Thompson, Toronto: Toronto University Press.

Findlen, P. (1994) *Possessing Nature: Museums, Collecting and Scientific Culture in Early Modern Italy*, Berkeley and London: University of California Press.

Forster, M.R. (2001) *Catholic Revival in the Age of the Baroque: Religious Identity in South-West Germany, 1550–1750*, Cambridge: Cambridge University Press.

Franklin, A.L.A. (1891) *La Vie privée d'autrefois*, vol.9, Paris: Plon, Nourrit.

Graunt, J. [1662] (1973) *Natural and Political Observations made upon the Bills of Mortality* in P. Laslett (ed.) *The Earliest Classics*, Farnborough: Gregg.

Hamlin, C. (1990) *A Science of Impurity: Water Analysis in Nineteenth-Century Britain*, Berkeley: University of California Press.

Harley, D. (1990) 'A sword in a madman's hand: professional opposition to popular consumption in the waters literature of southern England and the Midlands, 1570–1870' in R. Porter (ed.) *The Medical History of Waters and Spas*, *Medical History*, Supplement 10, pp.48–55.

Hippocrates (1923) *Airs, Waters, Places and Epidemics*, translated by W.H.S. Jones, 4 vols, Cambridge, MA: Harvard University Press.

Johansen, J.C. (1997) 'Holy springs and Protestantism in early modern Denmark: a medical rationale for a religious practice', *Medical History*, vol.41, pp.56–69.

Johnson, T. (1996) 'Blood, tears and Xavier-water: Jesuit missionaries and popular religion in the eighteenth-century Upper Palatinate' in R.W. Scribner and T. Johnson (eds) *Popular Religion in Germany and Central Europe 1400–1800*, Basingstoke and London: Macmillan, pp.183–202.

Lodge, T. (1963) *The Complete Works of Thomas Lodge*, 4 vols, New York: Russell & Russell.

Lonie, I.M. (1985) 'The "Paris Hippocratics": teaching and research in Paris in the second half of the sixteenth century' in A. Wear, R.K. French and I.M. Lonie (eds) *The Medical Renaissance of the Sixteenth Century*, Cambridge: Cambridge University Press, pp.155–74.

Mackaman, D.P. (1998) *Leisure Settings: Bourgeois Culture, Medicine and the Spa in Modern France*, Chicago: University of Chicago Press.

Nutton, V. (1989) 'Hippocrates in the Renaissance', *Sudhoffs Archiv*, vol.27, pp.420–39.

Owen, H. (1949) *Additional Letters of the Morrises of Anglesey (1735–1786)*, London: Honourable Society of Cymmrodorion Record Series, vol.49, part 2.

Palmer, R. (1990) '"In this our lightye and learned tyme": Italian baths in the era of the Renaissance' in R. Porter (ed.) *The Medical History of Waters and Spas*, *Medical History*, Supplement 10, pp.14–22.

Park, K. (1999) 'Natural particulars: medical epistemology, practice and the literature of healing' in A. Grafton and N. Siraisi (eds) *Natural Particulars: Nature and the Disciplines in Renaissance Europe*, Cambridge, MA: MIT Press, pp.347–67.

Raeff, M. (1983) *The Well-Ordered Police State: Social and Institutional Change through Law in the Germanies and Russia, 1600–1800*, New Haven and London: Yale University Press.

Razzell, P. (1993) 'The growth of population in eighteenth-century England: a critical reappraisal', *Journal of Economic History*, vol.53, pp.743–71.

Riley, J.C. (1986) 'Insects and the European mortality decline', *American Historical Review*, vol.91, pp. 833–58.

Rusnock, A.A. (2002) *Vital Accounts: Quantifying Health and Population in Eighteenth-Century England and France*, Cambridge: Cambridge University Press.

Short, T. [1767] (1973) *A Comparative History of the Increase and Decrease of Mankind in England and Several Countries Abroad*, Farnborough: Gregg.

Smith, J.R. (1987) *The Speckled Monster: Smallpox in England, 1670–1970, With Particular Reference to Essex*, Chelmsford: Essex Record Office.

Sydenham, T. (1848–50) *The Works of Thomas Sydenham*, 2 vols, London: Sydenham Society.

Tribe, K. (1984) 'Cameralism and the science of government', *Journal of Modern History*, vol.56, pp.263–84.

Van Andel, M.A. (1913) 'Public hygiene in a medieval Dutch town', *Janus*, vol.13, pp.626–34.

Walsham, A. (1999) 'Reforming the waters: holy wells and healing springs in Protestant England' in D. Wood (ed.) *Life and Thought in the Northern Church, c.1100–1700: Essays in Honour of Claire Cross*, Studies in Church History, 12, Woodbridge: Boydell & Brewer, pp.227–55.

Wotton, H. (1968) *The Elements of Architecture by Sir Henry Wotton*, Charlottesville: University Press of Virginia for the Folger Shakespeare Library.

Wrigley, E.A. (1983) 'The growth of population in eighteenth-century England: a conundrum resolved', *Past and Present*, vol.98, pp.121–50.

Source Book readings

A. du Laurens, *A Discourse of the Preservation of the Sight: Of Melancholike Diseases; of Rheumes; and of Old age ... Translated out of French into English ... by Richard Surphlet*, London: Felix Kingston, 1599, pp. 58-60 (Reading 11.1).

M. Todd, *The Culture of Protestantism in Early Modern Scotland*, New Haven and London: Yale University Press, 2001, pp.205–7 (Reading 11.2).

H. Eyre, *An Account of the Mineral Waters of Spa, Commonly called the German Spaw: Being a Collection of Observations from the most Eminent Authors who have wrote on that Subject*, London: J. Roberts, 1733, pp.14–15, 21–4 (Reading 11.3).

L. Brockliss and C. Jones, *The Medical World of Early Modern France*, Oxford: Clarendon Press, 1997, pp.637–8 (Reading 11.4).

T. Sydenham, *The Whole Works of that Excellent Physician Dr Thomas Sydenham. Wherein Not Only the History and Cures of Acute Diseases are Treated of, after a New and Accurate Method; But also the Shortest and Safest way of Curing most Chronical Diseases. Translated from the Original Latin, by John Pechy, MD of the College of Physicians in London*, London: Richard Wellington & Edward Castle, 1696, sigs A2r–A3r (Reading 11.5).

M. Foucault, *Power/Knowledge: Selected Interviews and Other Writings 1972–1977*, ed. by C. Gordon, Brighton: Harvester, 1980, pp.170–2, 175–6 (Reading 11.6).

A.A. Rusnock, 'The weight of evidence and the burden of authority: case histories, medical statistics and smallpox inoculation' in R. Porter (ed.) *Medicine in the Enlightenment*, Amsterdam and Atlanta, GA: Rodolpi, 1995, pp.289, 292–3 (Reading 11.7).

Voltaire, *Letters Concerning the English Nation*, ed. by N. Cronk, Oxford and New York: Oxford University Press, 1994, pp.44–7 (Reading 11.8).

The Times, 25 April 1788, p.3c (Reading 11.9).

W. Stuart to Sir William Fordyce, 1 March 1788 in *The Gentleman's Magazine*, vol.58, April 1788, pp.283–4 (Reading 11.10).

J.P. Frank, *A System of Complete Medical Police: Selections from Johann Peter Frank*, ed. by E. Lesky, Baltimore, MD: Johns Hopkins University Press, 1976, pp.183–4, 195 (Reading 11.11).

S. Hales, *A Treatise on Ventilators ... Part Second*, London: Richard Manby, 1758, pp.13–25 (Reading 11.12).

M. Thouret, *Rapport sur les Exhumations du Cimitière et de L'Eglise des Saincts Innocents; Lu dans la Séance de la Société Royale de Médecine, tenue au Louvre le 3 Mars 1789*, translated by Mark Jenner, Paris, 1789, p.5 (Reading 11.13).

L.J. Jordanova, 'Earth science and environmental medicine: the synthesis of the late Enlightenment' in L.J. Jordanova and R. Porter (eds) *Images of the Earth: Essays of the Environmental Sciences*, Chalfont St Giles: British Society for the History of Science, 1979, pp.127–9, 132–3, 148–50 (Reading 11.14).

12

Medicine and Health in the Age of European Colonialism

Andrew Wear

Objectives

When you have completed this chapter, you should be able to:

- appreciate the significance of the biological impact of European diseases upon colonized populations;

- assess how European medicine was a factor in enabling overseas settlement to take place;

- understand the nature and extent of the exchange of medical knowledge and remedies between Europeans and the indigenous peoples they encountered.

12.1 Introduction

In the late fifteenth century, Europeans began to spread across the globe. Today, the tide of overt European colonization has receded, but the result of the centuries-long process of exploration, commerce and settlement has changed the political geography of the world. The period from the late fifteenth to the seventeenth centuries saw the European settlement of America and the rekindling of European contact with the Far East. Portuguese, Dutch, French and British interests extended to the Indian and Pacific Oceans. During the course of the eighteenth century, India began to come under British rule and this process accelerated in the nineteenth century. At the same time, Australia and New Zealand were 'discovered' and subsequently colonized. Africa remained the 'dark continent' and 'white man's grave' until the mid-nineteenth century, when it started to be 'opened up' to European colonization. In this chapter, I shall focus mainly on America, as this is predominantly where large-scale European colonization took place in the period before 1800.

Central to European colonialism was the response of European settlers to those peoples already present in the 'new world' and elsewhere. Contact, conquest and settlement had implications for the health, medical knowledge and medical practice of both the indigenous peoples and the new arrivals.

In the first part of this chapter I discuss the catastrophic consequences of contact with Europeans for the indigenous peoples of America and, indeed, for those of other continents. I then turn to English North American settlers' perceptions of health and new environments to show the links between European medical theories and colonization. For prospective settlers, health was an important issue. Once settled in a new place, they could either recreate the medical provision and knowledge that existed in their home country or adapt and change with what later came to be called the 'frontier spirit'. The tenacity of European 'medical baggage' and the adaptability of Europeans to new situations are pivotal to our understanding of the medical care systems that were created in the Spanish and English colonies. I discuss these in some detail, as well as their impact on the exchange of medical knowledge between Europeans and indigenous peoples.

The history of European medicine in foreign places is linked much more obviously to power – here, power over other people and their cultures – than is usually the case in histories of early modern European medicine. This showed itself in the meeting of radically different medical cultures. When the Spanish encountered Aztec medicine in New Spain, Europeans retained their medical theories and denigrated those of the people they colonized, though they did appropriate some of their remedies.

While European medicine was sometimes imposed upon the indigenous peoples in Spanish America, it was the African slaves brought to America to work the settlers' plantations who were systematically forced to experience it. Even so, and despite white opposition, they managed to preserve some of their own medical culture. In discussing this process, I shall foreground the context of power in which medicine was applied.

12.2 The biological effects of European colonialism

The mere presence of Europeans in America and the Pacific killed enormous numbers of indigenous peoples. America and the southern Pacific did not share in the old world 'disease pool'. Although it is often not possible to translate early modern disease descriptions and names into equivalent modern diseases, we can usually make an informed guess. The original inhabitants of America and the South Pacific died in far larger numbers than Europeans when exposed to diseases such as smallpox, influenza, mumps, measles, chickenpox, typhoid, scarlet fever and other old world diseases. Europeans, unlike the indigenous peoples, had been exposed for centuries to these diseases, and had thereby acquired a degree of immunity. **Virgin soil epidemics**, it is now argued, greatly helped Europeans to conquer America and much of the South Pacific (Crosby, 1986) (Figure 12.1).

The 'disease exchange' between Europe and America was unequal. It is thought that only the 'French disease', or the pox (probably syphilis), came from America to Europe, though even this has been questioned. Although the pox produced horrific symptoms, especially in its early years in Europe, its mortality was probably not great. In contrast, as contemporary European accounts make clear, whole populations in parts of America were wiped out by successive epidemics of European diseases. Smallpox, especially, was recognized by Europeans as one of their own diseases that killed far more American Indians (Amerindians) than Europeans. It struck at the indigenous population as the Spanish established a colonial presence in America after Columbus's first voyage of 1492. One Spaniard reported that in the Caribbean 'in the past year of 1518 smallpox, until now

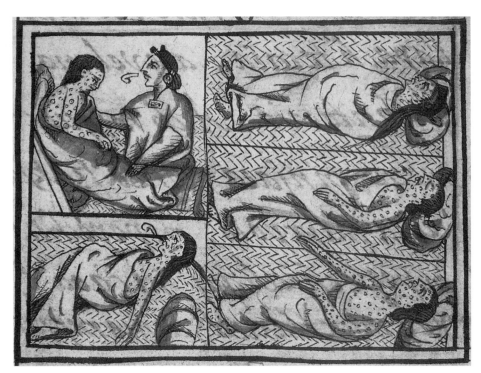

Figure 12.1   American Indian smallpox sufferers. Note the absolute prostration of the figures on the right. The figure on the lower left is drawn as if in pain, while only the figure on the top left is being given any help. The overall impression conveyed here is one of despair. These images come from the Florentine codex produced by Bernardino de Sahagún around 1578–9, but they are based on work he began on his arrival in New Spain in 1529. Sahagún wrote in Nahuatl, which he learned in New Spain. He also provided a translation in Spanish. Significantly, the images are in the part of the codex that records the Spanish conquest of Mexico. Smallpox was clearly seen by Sahagún's informants as presaging the conquest. Biblioteca Medicea Laurenziana. Photo: Microfoto srl

unknown by them (the American Indians), was ignited among them as flocks infected by contagious vapours' (Cook, 1998, pp.60–1).

Smallpox spread rapidly from the Caribbean to Mexico and Peru, facilitating the process of conquest. By 1521, Hernando Cortés (1485–1547) had destroyed the Aztecs of central Mexico, and in 1533 Francisco de Pizarro (d.1541) sacked Cuzco, the capital of the Incas in Peru. Two complete civilizations had fallen in the space of a few years to groups of Spaniards who were numbered in their hundreds. Virgin soil epidemics were highly significant in reducing resistance to the Spanish, and the burden of illness and death made it easier for the Spanish to dismantle American Indian cultures. Such epidemics also helped to confirm to Europeans that their culture and religion were superior. In North America a century after the Spanish conquests, John Winthrop, the governor of the new English colony of Massachusetts, saw through his puritan eyes God's providence at work when he wrote in 1634:

> But for the natives ... God's hand hath so pursued them as, for three hundred miles' space, the greatest part of them are swept away by the smallpox, which still continues amongst them. So as God hath hereby cleared our title to this place ...
>
> (quoted in Emerson, 1976, p.119)

Utilizing evidence such as this, Alfred Crosby has put forward the thesis that whenever Europeans encountered isolated indigenous communities, European microbes, viruses, plants and animals successfully competed with native organisms and thereby created 'neo-Europes' (see 'Ecological imperialism and the impact of old world diseases on the Americas and Australasia', Source Book 1, Reading 12.1). This is, however, a controversial argument. Social historians are generally wary of arguments from 'nature' or biology, and argue instead that contact with European material culture and the imposition of European social and economic practices was just as likely to destroy indigenous societies.

In the opinion of Captain James Cook (1728–79), writing of the Tahitians in 1773:

> We debauch their morals already prone to vice and we introduce among them wants and perhaps diseases which they never before knew and serve only to disturb that happy tranquillity they and their forefathers had enjoyed. If anyone denies the truth of this assertion let him tell what the natives of the whole extent of America have gained by the commerce they had with Europeans.
>
> (quoted in Moorehead, 1966, pp.55–6)

Cook was also aware that the Tahitians were losing their culture. The process of deculturation meant that they were forgetting their traditional skills, such as making stone tools and axes, and were coming to rely instead on European iron tools (Moorehead, 1966, p.70). The near extinction or the sharp decline in the numbers of American Indians, Polynesians, Australian Aborigines and New Zealand Maoris following contact with Europeans is an acknowledged historical fact. Disease clearly played an important role in this process. Alongside European rule, with its wholesale appropriation of land, the introduction of forced labour and the imposition of Christianity, disease eroded native resistance and paved the way for the systematic destruction of indigenous cultures.

12.3 Climate, place and health

It was widely believed in the early modern period that going abroad could be dangerous, and that strange climates and places to which the body was not accustomed were potentially pathological. How did medical writers and non-specialists come to this conclusion? As explained in the previous chapter, they argued that a place and its climate shaped the humoral constitution or balance of the body, so that when the body was placed in a different climate it was no longer in harmony with its natural environment and thus became susceptible to illness.

Such thinking, based as it was on the notion of the four qualities, was as accessible to ordinary colonial settlers as it was to philosophers and physicians. In relation to climate and place, the four qualities were constantly referred to in everyday language. Climates, like places and bodies, might be described as mixtures of hot, cold, wet and dry. The accessibility of such views to the general public partly explains why discussions of health, climate and place pervade the European accounts of new discoveries and settlements. Moreover, climatological theories of health and disease continued to shape colonial thinking to the end of the nineteenth century, long after the demise of humoral theories of disease associated with Galenism. That these ideas were sustained for so long was probably due to a number of interrelated factors. First, experience showed that Europeans continued to die at a far greater rate when they were in the tropics than at home. Second, there was the essentially agricultural nature of European colonization. The notion of 'planting a colony' was to be taken literally, and applied to people as much as to plants and animals: if European plants and animals were able to survive and flourish in alien climates, so too might human beings. Adaptation, it was believed, was always possible, but only if new settlers heeded the considerable body of medical advice that linked climate and place with health.

Early modern Europeans attached great importance to regimens or rules of health, and these rules were themselves shaped by, among other things, the place or climate in which one lived. There was a long tradition of medical writing on this subject dating back to the time of Hippocrates (see Chapter 11). Books on regimen typically discussed places that were inimical to health and how one should adjust one's lifestyle to cope with such dangers. Not surprisingly, this approach was also extended to medical writings concerned with health in the colonies. By the eighteenth century, these consistently warned prospective settlers of the dangers of foreign places, the hot and humid tropics being viewed as especially harmful to Europeans. In time, a genre of medical writing on the subject was created which became known in the nineteenth century as medical topography.

An example of this approach is the work of the naval surgeon James Lind, whom you encountered in Chapter 10. In 1768, he published his *Essay on Diseases Incidental to Europeans in Hot Climates* in which he mapped the world in terms of health and disease and provided travellers and settlers with advice on places to avoid and/or how to make them healthy (Figure 12.2). In customary vein, Lind warned against exposure to disease-making damp and putrid miasmatic fogs. As shown in Chapter 6, medical writers in sixteenth- and seventeenth-century Europe had routinely invoked such environmental factors as the cause of diseases such as the plague. Lind now took this model of disease and applied it to the humid tropics. He thus advised:

> The best preservative against the mischievous impressions of a putrid fog, a swampy, or of a marshy exhalation, is a close, sheltered and covered place; such as the lower apartments in a ship, or a house in which there are no doors or windows facing these swamps.
>
> (Lind, 1768, p.136)

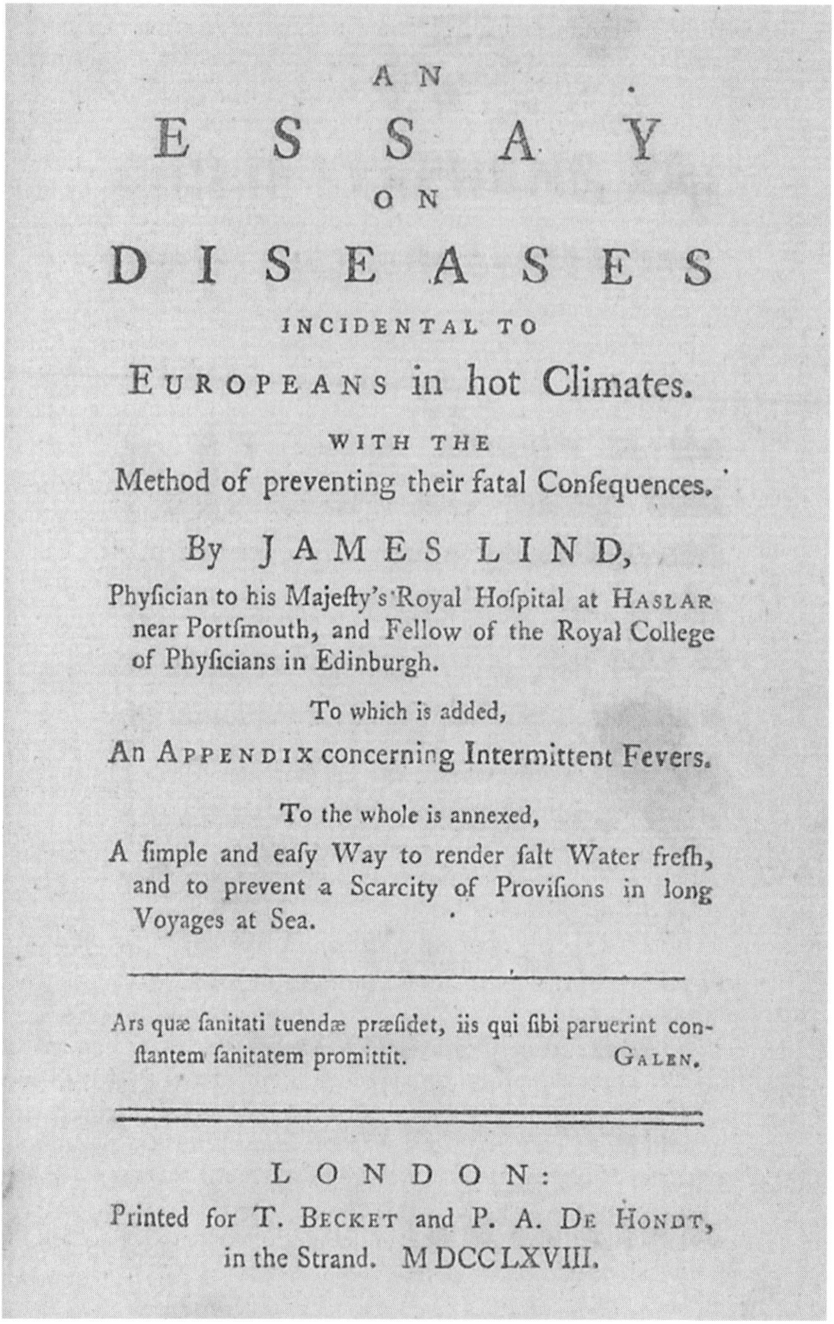

A N

E S S A Y

O N

D I S E A S E S

INCIDENTAL TO

EUROPEANS in hot Climates.

WITH THE

Method of preventing their fatal Confequences.

By J A M E S   L I N D,

Phyfician to his Majefty's Royal Hofpital at HASLAR
near Portfmouth, and Fellow of the Royal College
of Phyficians in Edinburgh.

To which is added,

An APPENDIX concerning Intermittent Fevers.

To the whole is annexed,

A fimple and eafy Way to render falt Water frefh,
and to prevent a Scarcity of Provifions in long
Voyages at Sea.

Ars quæ fanitati tuendæ præfidet, iis qui fibi paruerint con-
ftantem fanitatem promittit.   GALEN.

L O N D O N:

Printed for T. BECKET and P. A. DE HONDT,
in the Strand. MDCCLXVIII.

Figure 12.2   Title page to James Lind's *An Essay on Diseases Incidental to Europeans in Hot Climates* (1768). Note the link between diseases and climates, and how the title page conveys optimism. It promises that Lind will provide the means of preventing such diseases, or preventing their worst effects. Lind, who had been a naval surgeon and is well known for *A Treatise of the Scurvy* (1753), had been appointed in 1758 to be the head physician to the new and very large Haslar Hospital near Portsmouth, which the navy had built. He had also devised a way of distilling drinking water from sea water using a coal-fired apparatus. The title page indicates Lind's concerns with enabling his readership – Europeans and the navy – to survive the tropics and long voyages. Wellcome Library, London

Alternatively, the environment could be engineered to suit European bodies:

> Marshes could be drained to prevent putrid air from rising up from the ground, and 'noxious woods', such as those found in West Africa, which held stifling damp and illness-making air, should be cut down 'for the admission of wholesome and refreshing breezes'. Lind wrote disapprovingly of 'such an uncultivated swampy country as Guinea' in West Africa, and promoted the idea of 'improvement', which he associated with the introduction of European systems of cultivation. He thus declared that: 'If any tract of land in Guinea ... was as well improved as the island of Barbadoes, and as perfectly freed from trees, shrubs, marshes, etc. the air would be rendered equally healthful there, as in that pleasant West Indian island.'
>
> (Bewell, 1999, pp.37–8)

Changing the environment to make it healthy for European bodies had the effect of 'Europeanizing' it, and so making it, as it were, belong to Europeans. It can be argued that medical advice books such as Lind's, by justifying this 'improvement' and European-style cultivation of the land in the name of health, helped to encourage and legitimate the process of colonization.

More generally, it is clear that medical writings on health abroad helped to enable colonization to occur in the first place. Adapting one's way of living to the new climate, and 'seasoning' or acclimatization were possible strategies. A knowledge of medical geography might also help for as Lind put it: 'there is hardly to be found any island, or any large extent of continent, that does not contain some places where Europeans may enjoy an uninterrupted state of health during all the seasons of the year' (Lind, 1768, pp.192–3). Such places were generally located on high ground, and were ventilated by breezes, as for example in the hill stations of India. European medicine may have been pessimistic in pointing to the high mortality rates for Europeans in the tropics, but by providing positive advice on how best to live in alien places it became one of the factors that enabled European colonization to take place.

12.4 Perceptions of health and new environments in the early English settlements of North America

The prelude to English colonization in North America came with Sir Walter Ralegh's failed attempt to establish a colony at Roanoke Island, off the coast of North Carolina, in 1585. An attempt to resurrect the colony was made in 1587, but it too failed, for when it was visited again in 1590 there was no trace of the immigrants. The first viable English colony was Virginia, which was established on the mainland with its principal settlement of Jamestown in 1607. Between 1610 and 1630, attempts were made to colonize Newfoundland to the north, and further success was forthcoming in New England following the arrival of the Pilgrim Fathers aboard the *Mayflower* in 1620.

How did the early English settlers in North America judge and make sense of the health of their new lands? The answer to this question was of vital importance to the success or failure of the colonial enterprise. Without a positive vision of the health and climate of the North American continent, it would have been difficult to attract colonists and investors for the various enterprises that sprang up in the late sixteenth and early seventeenth centuries. Columbus, it should be noted, had adopted an equally positive pose in portraying his Indies to the Spanish back home as idyllic, with gentle breezes, sweet smells and possessed of gold.

In the early accounts of North America, health was often viewed as if it was a commodity – one to be shared rather than traded among the new settlers. It was mentioned alongside descriptions of its soil, minerals, plants and animals. Riches and health often went together. In other words, health formed part of the prospectus. An account of the Bermudas in 1609 described the islands as 'one of the sweetest Paradises that be on earth ... a safe, secure, temperate, rich, sweet and healthful habitation' (Jourdain, 1613, sig. A3). The Puritan minister Thomas Welde of New England, writing in 1632 to his former parishioners in old England, also associated health with prosperity: 'Here I find those great blessings, peace, plenty and health in a comfortable measure.' He went on to commend the place since it 'well agreeth with our English bodies [which] were never so healthy in their native country'. Colonists who could not get rid of headache, toothache and coughs in old England were now free from them, 'and those that were weak are now well long since'. In addition, Welde noted that New England was so rich that even 'the poorest have enough', the Indian corn was 'pleasant and wholesome food' and their cattle 'do thrive and feed exceedingly' (Emerson, 1976, p.96).

How did the early colonists come to the conclusion that a place was healthy? There seem to have been two major components for such a judgement. One was empirical, the other theoretical. At a time when the science of statistics was unknown, experience allied to simple arithmetical-based trials were commonly used as evidence to discover the healthiness of a place.

Exercise

Read 'Health and the promotion of colonialism: Thomas Hariot (1588)' (Source Book 1, Reading 12.2). How did Hariot try to convince his readers that 'Virginia' was healthy?

Discussion

Hariot used a typical method for convincing the reader back in England that America was healthy. He wrote that despite the hardships of the expedition, such as drinking strange water and eating strange plants and having to live all winter in the open air, the wholesomeness of the air in Virginia was attested to by the fact that there were only four deaths in the whole company of 108 men. Moreover, all four were previously of a sick disposition in England. For Hariot, the mere fact that the majority of settlers had remained healthy for a long period of time was evidence enough of its healthy state.

The native Indians could be brought in as evidence for the healthiness of a place. In 1602, John Brereton claimed that both natives and settlers benefited from the climate of the northernmost part of Virginia:

> And truly, the holsomenesse and temperature [humoral constitution] of this Climat, doth not onely argue this people to be answerable to this description, but also of a perfect constitution of body, active, strong, healthfull, and very wittie ... For the agreeing of this Climat with us ... we found our health and strength all the while we remained there, so to renew and increase, as not withstanding our diet and lodging were none of the best, yet not one of our company (God be thanked) felt the least grudging or inclination to any disease of sicknesse, but were much fatter and in better health than when we went out of England.
>
> (Brereton, [1602] 1983, p.159)

Judging the health of a place by the health of its inhabitants was, as we have seen, common practice. However, such links were not always consistently made. Indians might be portrayed as noble savages, but when their lands were sought by European settlers they became transformed into unhealthy, degenerate beings, unworthy of admiration or pity.

Surviving in American air and on American food was, then, experimental proof that the place was healthy. The emphasis on experience is easily understood. In the absence of official bodies whose opinions had privileged status, everyone's testimony carried equal weight as long as it was reliable and experienced. What, though, constituted the theoretical basis for the healthiness of North America for 'English bodies'? As we have seen, contemporaries firmly believed that there was an intimate correspondence between a person's constitution or humoral balance and the climate of the country of their birth. Karen Kupperman has pointed out that English settlers to America were anxious about breaking this link. William Vaughan, the Welsh writer and unsuccessful colonist of Newfoundland, asked in his *Directions for Health* (1617), 'What is the best Ayre?' He answered:

> That which is a man's usuall soyle, and Countries ayre is best. This by the Philosophers is approved in this principle: Every mans naturall place preserveth him which is placed in it.
>
> (quoted in Kupperman, 1984, p.215)

The connection between an individual and their country of birth was expressed in various ways. Native herbs were considered best for curing the diseases specific to that country and were most suitable for the people born there. William Harrison, in his *Description of England* (1577), attacked the use of exotic, foreign drugs for English constitutions and diseases. American Indian remedies took much longer to work for Europeans:

> With them also the difference of the clime doth show her full effect. For where as they [the Indians] will heal one another in short time with application of one simple etc, if a Spaniard or Englishman stand in need of their help, they are driven to have longer space in their cures and now and then also to use some addition of two or three simples at the most.
>
> (Harrison, 1994, p.267)

To counter such bad publicity, many of the reports coming back from the new settlements took special care to point out that American remedies were as efficacious as English ones (Figure 12.3). Richard Whitbourne, the promoter of Newfoundland, stressed in his *Discourse and Discovery of New-Found-Land* (1622), that 'many Physical [medicinal] herbs and roots' had cured 'many of our Nation' (Whitbourne, [1622] 1982, p.120).

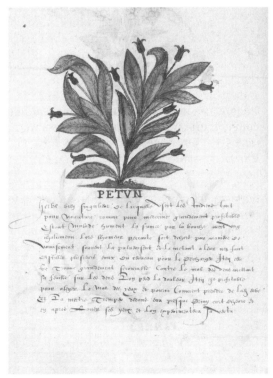

Figure 12.3   A picture of tobacco from the *Histoire Naturelle des Indies*, a late sixteenth-century French manuscript that describes the products and people of the southern parts of America. The medical uses of tobacco were a source of controversy in early modern Europe. The smoking of tobacco quickly became a popular social habit, and the product became commercially valuable. In the description of tobacco below, note how, as in Europe, a plant could be both a food and a medicine.

> PETVN (TOBACCO) A special herb which the Indians use for food as well as an extremely beneficial medicine; when they are sick, they breathe in the smoke by mouth with a straw; soon the ill humour escapes by vomiting. They often pulverize it and, putting it in their noses, it distils several drops of water from the brain to discharge it. It also is found very helpful for toothache; laying its leaves on the teeth, the pain disappears; it is also beneficial for alleviating eye problems and, for this [purpose], it is advisable to take the herb and steep it in water about half of a quarter of an hour and then wash one's eyes and one will experience its benefit.

Image: 29.2 × 20 cm. MA3900, f.4v. The Pierpont Morgan Library, New York, NY. © Pierpont Morgan Library/Art Resource. Description (translation) from *Histoire Naturelle des Indies* (1996), p.253

The usual strategy employed to convince people of the healthiness of the new settlements was to argue that New England, Virginia and even freezing Newfoundland were suited to English bodies because they had the same constitution, essentially the same air and climate, as the mother country (though sometimes the Scots were seen as best fitted for Newfoundland). North America was presented on medical and patriotic grounds as home-from-home. It was presumably this sort of reasoning that was employed to calm the fears that gripped the Plymouth Brethren as they debated whether or not to leave Holland and go to America. They were reported by William Bradford (1588–1657), one of the first governors of the Plymouth colony, to be afraid that the 'chang of aire, diate and drinking of water, would infecte their bodies with sore sicknesses and greevous diseases' (Bradford, 1982, p.47). As this example suggests, in the days before the discovery of bacteria, parasites and viruses, the environment and climate were widely believed not only to indicate the healthiness of a place but to be the actual cause of disease. Sites near swampy ground and humid, stagnant air were thus commonly thought to induce illness (Wear, 2000, pp.190–3). In foreign lands, such places were doubly dangerous, given the additional risk of living in a place to which one's body was not accustomed.

William Strachey's account of Jamestown in Virginia in 1610 illustrates how the early settlers drew upon popular old world ideas relating to health and the environment:

> this our Fort or James Towne, as yet seated in some what an unwholesome and sickly ayre, by reason it is in a marish [marshy] ground, low flat to the River and hath no fresh water Springs serving the Towne but what wee drew from a Well sixe or seven fathom deepe, fed by the brackish River owzing into it, from whence I verily beleeve, the chiefe causes have proceeded of many diseases and sicknesses which have happened to our people, who are indeede, strangely afflicted with Fluxes [diarrhoeas] and Agues [intermittent fevers].
>
> (Strachey, [1625] 1906, vol.19, pp.58–9)

One way of presenting the health of the American settlements in a positive light was to describe the country as a paradise or Garden of Eden. The image of the garden or countryside as a place of health in contrast to the crowded, stinking city, where mortality rates were higher and illness abounded, was well known in England. Behind such images lay a vision of paradise, where death and illness were unknown. Christianity taught that illness and death first appeared on earth after the Fall of Adam and Eve and their expulsion from the Garden of Eden. References to America as paradisaical combined the idea of a lost yet hoped-for land with that of a healthy land. Columbus had referred to the existence of an earthly paradise. John Winthrop, one of the leading figures in the Massachusetts Bay Colony, described America to his wife in similar terms (Emerson, 1976, p.320).

Certainly, there was an element of idealization in such descriptions. Thomas Dudley, deputy governor of New England, wrote after the killing winter of 1630 of 'letters sent us from hence in England, wherein honest men out of desire to draw others to them wrote somewhat hyperbolically of many things here' (Emerson,

1976, p.75). In Virginia, the early settlers were forbidden to write negatively about the colony; a third offence was punishable by death. Nevertheless, we should not undervalue the appeal of sensory, qualitative images and metaphors based on the paradisaical garden in early modern colonial discourse. In an age that lacked sell-by dates, sanitary and food inspectors, and institutions capable of monitoring the quality of food, water and the environment, people had to be their own judges. In such cases, the paradisaical garden represented the ideal against which all else might be judged.

The reality of life and health in the new colonies was, however, often in stark contrast to this ideal. George Percy, who became President of Virginia in 1609, described the terrible ravages of the previous year in what became known as 'the starving time':

> Our men were destroyed with cruell diseases, as Swellings, Fluxes, Burning Fevers and by warres ... for the most part they died of mere famine. There were never Englishmen left in a forreigne Countrey in such miserie as we were in this new discovered Virginia.
>
> (Percy, 1969, p.144)

In New England the deaths of 1630 were often attributed, as befitted a Puritan colony, to the providential intervention of God. The deaths in swampy Jamestown, however, produced a less fatalistic response and led the colonists to build a new settlement on higher, healthy ground. Historical demographers are now confirming the truth of the propagandistic claims of the early settlers. The northern American settlements did, in fact, enjoy a more favourable expectation of life than old England (Dobson, 1989).

In the second half of the seventeenth century, accounts of the health of North America became less idealistic and more matter of fact, a reflection perhaps of greater experience and the influence of the observational methodology of Baconian natural history. At the same time, it was realized that a period of gradual 'seasoning' or acclimatization was necessary (helped by avoiding the mid-day sun, keeping in the shade, avoiding hard manual labour, etc.) if English settlers were to adjust to the different constitutions of the American colonies. This was especially so in the hotter, southern colonies such as the West Indies, South Carolina and Maryland.

Here, 'fevers', including what we now call falciparum malaria and yellow fever (imported with the slave trade from West Africa), were more prevalent, as were dysentery, diarrhoeas and typhoid. It was a popular saying that 'Carolina is in the spring a paradise, in the summer a hell and in the autumn a hospital' (Dobson, 1989, p.272). Under such circumstances, settlers were forced to alter their day-to-day behaviour. Clothing became lighter, and houses were designed for maximum ventilation and often built on hills rather than on the coast. Such practices were dictated by both the demands of comfort and medical theory, which perceived the heat and humidity as dangerous to health. Medical theory and cultural responses meshed and gave settlers confidence that they could survive in an otherwise hostile environment.

Read 'Medicine and acclimatisation' (Source Book 1, Reading 12.3).

1   Why were English settlers so anxious about the great heat of the southern colonies of North America?

2   How did they mitigate these fears?

1   Anxiety about the climate of these colonies was rife among English settlers because of the high death rate and related fears about the dangers of living in such an alien climate.

2   Adapting and changing one's food, clothing and housing gave people a sense of control over their environment. By changing their accustomed lifestyles they felt that they could keep the heat of the sun and its pathological effects at bay. Such changes did not require specialist knowledge. The heat, cold and damp of a climate was experienced by everyone, so that all were able, in theory at least, to effect changes to their way of living. The belief that one could exert some control over one's environment gave settlers the confidence that they might survive even when the mortality figures seemed to indicate otherwise.

12.5 Systems of medical care in the Spanish and English colonies

European settlers in foreign parts adapted their lifestyles in order to fit their bodies to their new environment, but what changes, if any, did they make to the way in which they organized their systems of medical care? To what extent did they retain the 'cultural baggage' of European medicine that they brought with them? Or did they prefer to adapt and change their models of medical organization to suit their new environment? To some extent, national systems of government were replicated in the colonies, and national medical systems followed suit. However, the link between mother country and colony (or centre and periphery) was sometimes tenuous. A colony's particular needs and interests, which were often shaped by local concerns and the presence of indigenous cultures, might create special circumstances that allowed deviation from the 'central model'. New, hybrid models of government and organization often developed in European colonies and gave them a distinct identity and character.

Medicine in Spanish America

The Spanish had a centralized system of government which they exported to the Americas. The Spanish crown quickly established a bureaucracy and judicial system in America which it tried to control from Spain. In medicine, a similar process of bureaucratic centralization was attempted. In Spain, the *protomedicato*, a tribunal named after the *protomedico* or royal physician who oversaw it, was usually composed of two physicians and two surgeons who were responsible for examining and licensing medical practitioners as well as supervising apothecaries and the quality of their wares. In New Spain (Mexico), similar institutions were quickly set up. Mexico City appointed a *protomedico* to examine practitioners in 1525. And in 1575 the Spanish crown appointed Francisco Hernández (1517–87) as *protomedico* to regulate medicine throughout the whole of New Spain. The lack of university-educated physicians placed a practical limit on the *protomedicato*'s powers. Empirics were more readily accepted, as were *curanderos*, originally the traditional healers of old Spain, who often used magic and folk remedies. In New Spain, they employed a mix of Indian and Spanish medicine and catered to the poor of both groups. Nonetheless, a key part of the Spanish medical system had been transplanted across the Atlantic. Other elements of the domestic system were also imported. Many hospitals were soon founded in the Spanish colonies, serving religious, philanthropic and therapeutic purposes. Likewise, medical education in the form of university medical faculties was introduced in the sixteenth and seventeenth centuries, though the number of graduate physicians was always small.

Exercise

Read 'The introduction of European medicine to New Spain' (Source Book 1, Reading 12.4).

1   To what extent did medical practice and organization in New Spain deviate from that in the mother country?

2   How does Risse account for different approaches to medical care and organization in New Spain?

Discussion

1   At first glance it appears that the Spanish in America copied much of what existed in Spain. New universities, with medical faculties, were established, and the role of the *protomedicato* was reaffirmed in the new colonies. However, this is a matter of degree. In two key areas – hospitals and the reaction to native medicine and medical practitioners – deviation from the home model is apparent.

While hospitals were built in large numbers in both old and New Spain, serving a similar purpose in addressing the medical needs of the poor, and guided by philanthropic and religious motives, there were also differences. Hospitals in Spanish America were built to express the imperial benevolence of the Spanish to the people they had conquered, to instil Spanish culture in them, and to convert them to Christianity (though note Risse's reference to a precedent here in the case of attempts to use hospitals to convert the Moors in old Spain). Hospital building also took place on a much larger scale in Spanish America. Many were specifically built with conversion in mind, and as with medical missionary work in the nineteenth century it was hoped that gratitude for Spanish benevolence and the acculturation of the indigenous population would result.

Curanderos, or illicit medical practitioners, existed in both old and New Spain, where they provided medical assistance for the great majority of the population. However, in the colonies they also played a vital role in preserving American Indian culture and medicine. Despite attempts by the authorities to dismiss native medicine as superstitious, magical and therefore illicit, the *curanderos* of New Spain managed to combine aspects of Spanish medicine with native traditions and thus create a new hybrid medical culture.

2   These developments were the product of the different practical and ideological circumstances under which medicine operated in New Spain. In practical terms, the medical schools of New Spain produced very few graduate or learned physicians. Unlicensed practitioners, or *curanderos*, were therefore allowed greater freedom in New Spain, where the role of the *protomedicato* was severely circumscribed. The ideological role of medicine in the Spanish colonies of the new world was also slightly different, particularly where the authorities sought to impose the religious and cultural norms of the mother country upon the native population. In particular, the provision of hospital care encouraged acceptance of Spanish rule and assisted the process of acculturation.

Medicine in New England

As with Spain and its colonies, old England provided the model for medical organization and practice in the Americas. There were few effective forms of medical regulation in England and, on the whole, medical practice in New England was similarly unregulated. There were very few university-trained physicians in the colonies, and the informal system of medical care that was characteristic of the mother country – centred on family, neighbours, skilled women and clergymen – was replicated in America. There were some professional practitioners in New England. However, the hierarchical distinction between physicians, surgeons and apothecaries that officially existed in England, but was largely ignored in practice, elided into the New England 'doctor', who combined all three roles and was usually trained by apprenticeship.

England had few hospitals up to the end of the seventeenth century. New England had none. The first was the Pennsylvania Hospital, founded in 1751. The first medical faculty – that of the College of Philadelphia – was not set up until 1765. Only in 1783 did Harvard create its medical school (the college itself was founded in 1636). The New England colonies took the deregulated, non-institutionalized English model of medical practice to an extreme. Indeed, for most of the eighteenth century an American physician could become learned in medicine only by travelling to Europe (most were attracted to Edinburgh).

12.6 Remedies and medical contact between the old and new worlds

Both the Spanish and the English believed and hoped that new herbs and drugs might be found in the new world that would prove valuable both commercially and therapeutically. In the sixteenth century, some Europeans became increasingly aware that the herbal remedies of northern Europe differed from those found in the Mediterranean region, the source of the plant remedies of classical medicine. They were also becoming familiar with exotic drugs from the Middle and Far East. Moreover it was widely held that a merciful God had placed in each country remedies that would cure the diseases native to that country. America held out the promise, therefore, that the *materia medica* of Europe would be further enriched.

Remedies for the pox, for instance, were urgently sought. This disease produced despair and immense suffering when it first arrived in Europe with, as it was thought, Columbus's sailors. Guaiac wood (*Guaiacum officinalis*), which was found in the West Indies, became a favoured remedy. The Spanish had observed the Caribbean Indians using decoctions of guaiac wood against the disease. This appeared to confirm the idea of a merciful and providential God, who provided 'medicines out of the earth' (Ecclesiasticus 38:4). By 1508, the Spanish had introduced guaiac into Europe, and for a time, until it was no longer seen as efficacious, it replaced the standard mercury treatment whose side effects were often as horrific as the disease itself. Guaiac was extremely profitable, and what had been seen as a local remedy for a local disease crossed cultural and geographical boundaries. Some writers complained that the cost of the new exotic drugs put medicine in Europe out of reach of the poor, though such opposition could not suppress the commercial drive to introduce foreign remedies into European medicine. In time, other drugs and remedies were imported from the new world and were readily integrated into humoral medicine (see 'The reception of American drugs in early modern Europe', Source Book 1, Reading 12.6).

Other remedies from America included sarsaparilla (*Smilax aristolochiaefolia*), which was used by the Aztecs as a diuretic, as well as being employed by Europeans as a cure for the pox. In the seventeenth century chinchona bark, or quinine, an Inca remedy, was thought by Europeans to be effective against intermittent fevers, including malaria (wrongly, as it happened, in the case of non-malarial fevers).

These new remedies did not create a new American medicine, but were seen as additions to the exotic range of remedies already available. Moreover, like other plant-based remedies, they were easily integrated into the learned medicine of the time and given qualitative characteristics (hot, cold, dry, wet), which explained their therapeutic powers. Nicolas Monardes (*c.*1493–1588), a physician from Seville in Spain, played an active part in this process of assimilation with the publication of his influential treatise, *Dos Libros. El Uno Trata de Todas las Cosas que Traen de Nuestras Indias Occidentales* [Two Books. One which Deals with All Things that are Brought from our Western Indies], which appeared in three parts between 1565 and 1574. The book, which publicized the virtues of American remedies, was translated into French and German and abridged into Latin. There was also an English version with the evocative title, *Joyfull Newes out of the New Founde Worlde* (1577). The new remedies represented commodities for European traders and useful resources for settlers far from the remedies of their home countries. Indigenous medical beliefs, however, had little impact upon elite European medicine after its arrival in the Americas.

12.7 The exchange of medical knowledge

Today we know a little of Aztec medicine. A few pre-Colombian codices, or manuscripts, of Aztec pictographs have survived. We also have the evidence of those few Spaniards who recorded Aztec practices and beliefs, most notably the Franciscan friar Bernardino de Sahagún (d.1590). Inevitably, however, they often described and recorded the Aztec world through Spanish and Christian lenses (Figures 12.4 and 12.5).

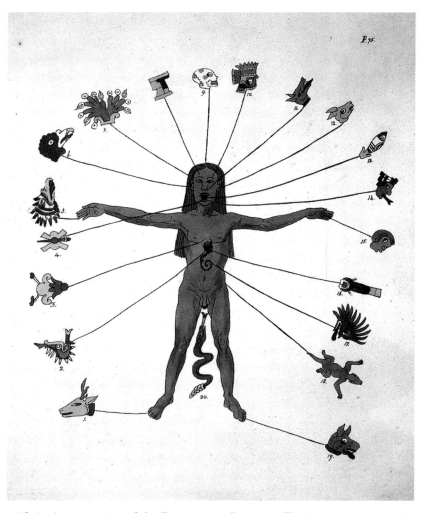

Figure 12.4 Aztec version of the European zodiac man. This image is very similar to the European 'zodiac man' in which different parts of the body are assigned different signs of the zodiac, each sign having influence over its particular body part. Here, parts of the body are linked to the twenty Aztec 'day' signs (the solar year was divided into eighteen segments of twenty days plus five 'unlucky days'). There is no evidence that the Aztecs envisaged the body in this way. The image, which was painted around 1566–89, 'reflects the Europeanizing tendency in the Early Colonial Period' (Ortiz de Montellano, 1990, p.135). Wellcome Library, London

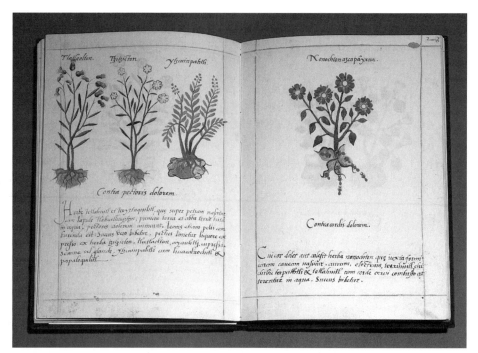

Figure 12.5   Aztec medicinal plants. These pictures come from the Badianus codex written in Nahuatl by the Aztec doctor Martin de la Cruz. The codex was translated into Latin by Juan Badiano. It was sent to the royal court in Spain some time after 1552, but had no influence in shaping European understanding of Aztec culture until the twentieth century. The plants on the left were intended to relieve chest pain; those on the right are for pain in the heart. While the Aztec names and uses were given, the plants themselves were drawn in the style that was common in European herbals, which would have made the codex more recognizable to European eyes and therefore more acceptable. Wellcome Library, London

In contrast to Aztec remedies, Aztec medical knowledge had little influence on European medicine. Why was this? A combination of factors was probably responsible for the poor reception of Aztec medical beliefs in the Spanish world. Much of Aztec medical culture was alien to the newcomers. It was also in the nature of the colonial enterprise to subvert and destroy those aspects of the indigenous culture that threatened European supremacy and authority. As a result, there was little regard in Spanish circles for Aztec medical knowledge, which was rarely discussed in those works published in Europe describing the new world.

Superficially, Aztec medicine shared much in common with European medicine. The Aztecs reasoned that illness came from a continuum of religious, magical and natural causes. Like Christians, they believed that illness was often sent as divine punishment. The supreme god, Tezcatlipoca or Titlacuhuan, like the Christian God, sent plagues to punish whole communities. Sorcerers, as in Europe, were widely believed to be able to bewitch others with illness. The Aztecs also thought that heat, cold and phlegm were disease-making (Ortiz de Montellano, 1990, pp.131, 155–61). However, Aztec religion was polytheistic, and not monotheistic as in

Europe. A whole galaxy of gods, goddesses, spirits of the woods and rivers were thought capable of inducing illness, and of taking it away if presented with suitable supplication and gifts. Like religion, magic also played a role in both European and Aztec medicine. In Europe, however, its practice was illicit, and governing elites and the church authorities, both Protestant and Catholic, punished those found guilty. In contrast, magic was integral to Aztec society and government. Another aspect of Aztec culture for which educated Spaniards expressed distaste was the cult of human sacrifice.

> *Xipe Totec*, the flayed God, so called because he was covered by the skin of one of his victims, was responsible for exanthematic diseases [rashes], boils, scabies and eye ailments. Patients with exanthema and skin infections used to march in the front of the processions during the god's festivities *tlacaxipehualiztli* in the second Aztec month, also covered with skins from human sacrifices, to appease the god and obtain a cure.
>
> (Guerra, 1966, p.320)

Spanish observers of Aztec medicine based their condemnation of Aztec culture and, by extension their medicine, on Christianity and European norms of reason. To have accepted Aztec medical theories and beliefs, the Spanish would have been required to reject some of their own deeply held religious and cultural values. Moreover, as colonizers it was in the interests of the Spanish that their own culture and medicine should appear superior to those of the peoples they conquered. We should also note that very few works which described Aztec medicine were available in Europe, except as manuscripts locked away in a few royal libraries and in the Vatican. An exception was the work of Francisco Hernández, which was published posthumously in the seventeenth century (discussed further below). The early modern European reading public therefore had little inkling of Aztec medical beliefs. There was no meaningful exchange of medical knowledge though this did not prevent, as we have seen, the import of foreign remedies and drugs.

Exercise

Read 'The Europeanisation of native American remedies' (Source Book 1, Reading 12.5). To what extent can Hernández be said to have 'Europeanized' the description of the Aztec herbs?

Discussion

Hernández usually kept the Aztec name for the herbs and he often noted the Aztec uses for them. For instance, *Tzocuilpátli* was reported to restore 'lost mobility'. The settlers were, however, beginning to give Mexican herbs their own names. Hernández noted of *Cihuapatli* that the natives called it the hemionitic cihuapatli, 'but the Spanish women of New Spain call it "mother's herb"'. These medicines became fully Europeanized when Hernández turned from naming and describing them to discussing how they worked.

Knowledge of their effects may have been derived from Aztec experience but the theory of why they cured was Galenic. Hernández was concerned to demonstrate the herb's Galenic qualities. He thus wrote of *Tzocuilpátli* that the root was 'hot and dry in the fourth degree'. As illnesses were cured by medicines made from contrary qualities, this was a suitable cure for easing colds and evacuating phlegm from the head. Likewise, *Tepetlachichicxíhuitl*, 'hot and dry in the third degree', was useful in ridding the body of excess 'phlegmatic and bilious humors'.

The result of such Europeanization of American drugs was to enhance their value as commodities for sale in Europe, their 'exotic' origins advertised in order to increase the price. In addition, they served the Spanish settlers as substitutes for European drugs. The globalizing tendency of Galenic medicine is shown by the way that its adherents took on board new medicines from America and the Far East while remaining impervious to the medical theories of non-Europeans.

When the British established first a commercial and then a military presence in India in the eighteenth century, they too were on the lookout for efficacious drugs. However, in contrast to the Spaniards in the Americas, they found the Hindu medical systems of **Ayurveda** – the 'science of life', based on classical Indian texts – to be not too dissimilar to their own, as both used the language of qualities and humours. The Muslim medical system of **Unani-tibb** was based on Greek medicine transmitted through the Arabic medical compendium of Avicenna's *Canon* (begun 1012 CE), and was even more familiar to European doctors than the Hindu system. By the end of the eighteenth century, the fashionable preoccupation with 'orientalism' in Europe, with its esteem of ancient Indian knowledge and civilization, made India's medical systems even more congenial to the British. It was not until the nineteenth century that British medical men and government agencies began positively to campaign against non-European forms of medicine.

12.8 Medicine and slavery

No account of colonial medicine can ignore slavery. Slaves were one of the largest groups of migrants to the Americas. The best estimate of the total number of slaves that were transported from Africa to the Americas between 1500 and 1870 is around 9,000,000 (Klein, 1999, pp.210–11; citing Curtin, 1969 and Eltis, 1989). Slaves were brought from Africa to provide the heavy labour on plantations. White settlers were not willing to undertake such work and the indigenous Indians could not as, in the West Indies especially, they were ceasing to exist. Moreover, in the late eighteenth century new white immigrants to the Caribbean died at four times the rate of newly arrived slaves (Curtin, 1990, p.81). It was simply economically more viable to import black slaves rather than white servants. The difference in death rates also helped to create the view among white slave owners that the constitutions of black people were more suited than whites to working in the heat of the West Indies. Slaves were brought from Africa to provide, if they survived the Atlantic crossing, heavy labour on the plantations (Figure 12.6; Plate 10).

In this final section, I discuss two specific aspects of medicine and slavery. First, in what way was white medicine part of the system of colonial slavery? And second,

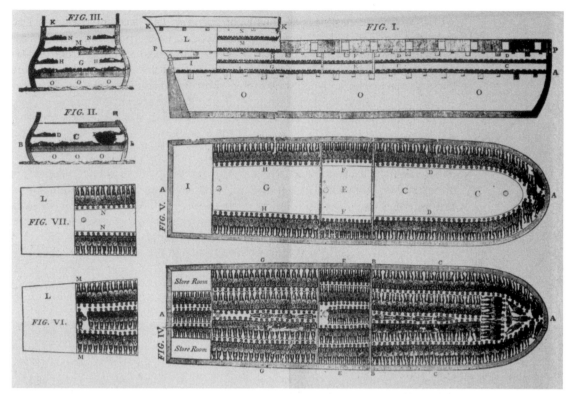

Figure 12.6   Sectional view of a slave ship. William Wilberforce, who campaigned against the slave trade, used this picture to shock his readers. On the 'Middle Passage' from the west coast of Africa to America, slaves were packed like 'herrings in a barrel', as Sir William Dolben put it when he introduced 'Dolben's Act' of 1788. This Act regulated the slave trade and awarded ships' surgeons an extra £50 if mortality among the slave cargo was less than 2 per cent, or £25 if mortality was no greater than 3 per cent. Mortality on the passage declined from 23.5 per cent in 1680–8 to between 9.5 per cent and 2.5 per cent in the late eighteenth century. Despite the financial incentives to keep slaves healthy, surgeons could do little when outbreaks of smallpox or dysentery broke out. Mortality could then be as high as 50 per cent (Sheridan, 1985, pp.123, 121, 110). Wilberforce House, Hull City Museums and Art Galleries, UK/Bridgeman Art Library

what happened to the slaves' medical knowledge and practices that they brought with them from Africa?

Power, slavery and medicine

Slaves were property. They belonged to their owners and could be sold or hired to others. The sale of a slave emphasised his or her status, and medical practitioners were often involved in the transaction. At every sale, the 'soundness', and hence the value, of a slave was assessed. Doctors were frequently asked to judge a slave's health and his or her strength, to predict whether they were liable to illness, and to estimate the length of their working life. In so doing, white medical practitioners were acting as cogs in the system of slavery. They were responding to the economic interests of the owner or buyer rather than considering the interests of the slave (Fett, 2002, pp.20–5).

When slaves were ill, it was the owner or overseer who decided whether or not to call a doctor. The slave had no say in the matter. Slavery was, to use the language of sociologists, a 'total institution'. As in prisons, and to a lesser extent hospitals, decisions about all aspects of an individual's everyday life were made by others. For instance, treatments could be forced upon slaves against their will. The ethical requirement of early modern European medicine that patients, with the exception of children and the insane, should consent to treatment was ignored in the case of slaves. At best there was a tripartite negotiation between doctor, slave owner and slave (Fett, 2002, pp.145–7).

The decision as to whether a slave should be treated with European medicine was often an economic one. In the British West Indies especially, a high mortality among slaves was accepted as the consequence of the profit motive (Sheridan, 1985, p.322). The owner would calculate whether the cost of treatment and hence the possibility of cure was cheaper than buying a new slave. The more valuable the slave, the more likely it was that he or she would be treated. Slave owners and overseers had a greater financial incentive to seek medical attention for sick, valuable slaves such as young adults, domestic slaves and those engaged in trade and crafts. The old, who could no longer work, were given the least medical attention (Higman, 1984, pp.270–2). In the American South, both before and after Independence, where, unlike the British West Indies, slave reproduction was encouraged, there was more of a birth-to-old-age society. Todd Savitt has pointed out that pregnant women, children and the old, despite being less productive, had a measure of protection. They were excused hard work and were provided with food and medical care (Savitt, 1978, pp.96, 115–17, 201–7).

Despite the minimal and often unenforced protection of the slave laws in the islands of the British West Indies and the American South, the power of the slave owners and overseers over their slaves was virtually absolute. White medical practitioners tacitly accepted this fact, and it becomes more readily apparent when we consider that the type of medical treatment regularly offered to slaves was frequently feared and disliked by them.

White medical treatment of slaves

Slaves were treated by a variety of white practitioners. In the American South lay medical practice was common and slave owners and their wives often treated slaves as they did their own families. In serious cases a medical practitioner might be requested. In the British West Indies, where absentee owners were the norm, overseers dealt with minor illnesses and injuries. John Baillie testified, perhaps a little idealistically, to a parliamentary select committee in 1832 that in his Jamaican plantation the overseer examined each patient daily in the plantation hospital and noted their illnesses in a book. Baillie stated that 'if it is a trivial complaint – we are all more or less Doctors – we order them a Dose of Salts or Oil [which act as purgatives] or an Emetic: these are common things; a Negro who has the Superintendence of the Hospital administers them.' Only if the illness was serious was the doctor sent for, but, he continued, 'the universal Practice is for the Doctor to visit the Estate twice a Week. The Book is open to him and he prescribes for the sick accordingly in that Book' (Sheridan, 1985, p.294).

The quality of care reflected the oppressed position of slaves and the economic imperatives that controlled their lives. In the British West Indies slaves were given a watered-down version of the medicine offered to whites. A crucial difference was that while a physician charged his patients on a fee-per-patient visit basis, when he treated slaves he was contracted to do so by the plantation owner and was paid yearly. The contract specified the number of visits per week to the plantation (usually one or two), but he was not paid according to the number of slaves that he happened to treat on any given day. Moreover, the visit was often short, especially when the physician had to visit other, perhaps distant, plantations. There was little incentive to enquire closely into the health of all slaves or to treat many of them. While attending white patients, physicians were expected to offer them courteous and considerate treatment in order to keep their custom. They were under no such necessity in the case of slaves. In the American South, the contract system was not universal, and in the nineteenth century, following pressure from the newly emerging medical societies, it was phased out for a fee-per-patient service. This tended to produce better standards of care for slaves (Sheridan, 1985, pp.292–320).

Medical treatment often took place in the dilapidated huts and shanty houses of the slave quarters. In the larger plantations in the West Indies and the American South, owners built hospitals or 'hot-houses' of varying sizes. Contemporary descriptions were often coloured by politics. Abolitionists pointed to the poor, slum-like conditions inside plantation hospitals. Pro-slavery writers, on the other hand, pictured them as airy and clean, and as symbols of the enlightened benevolence of the slave owners. What is clear, however, is that they were extensions of the system of total control exercised by owners over their slaves. The owner or overseer, rather than a doctor, was in charge, with day-to-day patient care being undertaken by other slaves, usually elderly women. The plantation hospitals often had barred windows. They were sometimes installed with stocks to immobilize patients who required treatment, as well as to punish recalcitrants. The dual function of the hospital as both a place of medical treatment and a jail indicates how the medical treatment of slaves was essentially an instrument of coercion and control (Fett, 2002, pp.120–3; Savitt, 1978, p.162; Sheridan, 1985, pp.268–87).

The treatments administered to slaves by white doctors, overseers, owners and slaves under orders from whites, were those of white medicine. They consisted of the usual bleeding, purging, vomiting, sweating and blistering of European medicine, which was designed to evacuate noxious humours. They were carried out on an even more heroic scale than was normal for whites. Eighteenth- and nineteenth-century white racial thinking held that black people had stronger constitutions than whites, making them less sensitive to white medical procedures and drugs. White medicine, with the exception of some herbal remedies, was, not surprisingly, feared and disliked by slaves. It was often painful, and slaves often feared that they were being poisoned by the drugs they were forced to take. Moreover, when slaves could not speak English, there was no communication, no description, no explanation of symptoms or of treatment, between slave patient and practitioner. Nor could agreement to treatment, if allowed, be given. Sometimes, as Sharla Fett points out, purgatives were used to punish and dehumanize slaves (Fett, 2002, pp.147–50; Savitt, 1978, pp.149–50; Sheridan, 1985, pp.330–1).

Exercise

Read 'Medicine and slavery' (Source Book 1, Reading 12.7). In your view, to what extent should historians pass moral judgements on the actions of slave owners and doctors with regard to the medical care of their slaves?

Discussion

Historians such as Richard Sheridan write about the demographic and biomedical aspects of slavery while at the same time expressing concern for the ways in which contemporaries viewed their own actions. In this passage, Sheridan's debt to biomedical thinking is obvious. He uses modern-day knowledge to make a retrospective evaluation of white medicine. It may well be unhistorical to condemn slave owners for not possessing our modern understanding of the effects of their treatments on black patients. At the time, many whites believed humoral medicine and its accompanying cathartics were the best type of medicine. They used it, after all, upon themselves. Some historians, however, believe demographic and biomedical history should be avoided because it distorts the past through the use of hindsight, and thus prevents us from understanding the past in its own terms. Nevertheless, biologically, white medicine may have been harmful, and if we are concerned with the health, illnesses and deaths of slaves it is useful to know this – as long as we do not criticize people at the time for not possessing our present-day knowledge, and as long as it does not stop us from grasping the medical beliefs of past peoples on their own terms.

The forcible treatment of slaves can, however, be condemned. There is a moral dimension to this history that is worthy of consideration. Sheridan's judgmental tone, in my opinion, comes from his dislike of slavery. Most historians share this dislike. But should we apply modern standards of morality to the past? In the eighteenth and nineteenth centuries the moral condemnation of slavery was by no means universal; today it is. Do we risk distorting our understanding of the past by invoking such moral outrage? My own view is that all historians make moral judgements, though they often hide them in order to appear 'objective'. The case of slavery represents such an extreme evil that I welcome the fact that modern historians express a moral stance on the subject, and use it to uncover the true horrors of slavery.

Black medicine

Medicine, as we have seen, was not independent of the relationships of power and resistance that ran through the institution of slavery. White medicine was fully integrated into the institution of slavery. However, slaves did have recourse to an alternative medicine – black medicine – which was often invoked in the context of resistance to white medicine, white culture and white power.

Slaves brought their own cultures, complete with medical knowledge and practices, from different parts of Africa. Just as European medicine in America came into contact with the medicine of the Aztecs and Incas, so too did it encounter African medicine.

Black herbal medicine

Black herbal medicine and conjuring medicine (called Obeah medicine in the West Indies) provided medical resources to which slaves eagerly turned. Black herbal medicine constituted a gentler alternative to the 'heroic' remedies of white medicine, though sometimes purgatives were prescribed by both male and female black 'root doctors' or herbalists. Unlike conjuring medicine (discussed below), black herbal medicine was relatively porous to outside influences. Some of its plants were brought by the slave trade to America. African grasses and plants like liquorice and okra were used as medicines and food. Black herbalists borrowed remedies from whites, and also sought medicinal plants in the American countryside. At the same time whites were interested in black herbal remedies. Moreover, the African techniques of inoculation against yaws and smallpox were employed by black practitioners, and then taken up by the whites in the early eighteenth century.

Exercise

Read 'The survival of African medicine in the American colonies' (Source Book 1, Reading 12.8). Why do you think that black herbal knowledge crossed racial, cultural and geographical boundaries?

Discussion

As Fett makes clear, travel and trade across continents created an exchange of plants as well as peoples and their diseases. This globalizing process continues today. Once people were settled in a new continent they were always likely to make use of local plants as they adapted to their new surroundings. The familiarity of black slaves with the natural environment led them to recognize local American plants and to identify their therapeutic properties. In the process, they created a new hybrid pharmacopoeia.

Remedies, as opposed to medical theories, were more likely to cross racial and cultural barriers. Remedies were at one level simply products with therapeutic powers. As products, they were exchanged between neighbours and friends, while commerce made remedies into commodities that were then traded within and between continents and cultures. Many societies have viewed foreign remedies as valuable therapeutic substances while at the same time divorcing them from their spiritual and religious connotations. Whites clearly did this when they borrowed from black slave herbal knowledge.

Conjuring medicine

Conjuring medicine contrasts strongly with white medicine. Its popularity among black slaves indicates how culturally alien white medicine must have appeared to them. The conjuring doctor reflected African beliefs about how illness was caused and how it might be cured. As Fett has shown, conjuring medicine was based on a relational or social view of disease. As in Africa, slaves in America often believed that illness was the result of social interactions which had resulted in enmity. A person's enemy could, through magical powers, make one ill. This view of illness was part of a pluralistic system of belief that was comparable to that which prevailed in Europe before the eighteenth century and the erosion of magical and religious explanations of disease. Moreover, like their European counterparts, black slaves did not believe that all illness was the result of conjuration. A slave might suspect that he or she was conjured or bewitched only if they suffered from a sudden, inexplicable illness, a wasting disease, paralysis, mental illness or other ailments that could not be cured by herbal remedies.

In such a situation the 'conjure doctor' was consulted. As in Africa, this role was double-edged: he or she could either harm or cure. Someone who wished an enemy or rival ill went to the 'conjure doctor', as did the sufferer who sought relief:

> Sufferers expected 'conjure doctors' to answer several critical questions: who had placed the hoodoo spell? Would the 'conjure doctor' be powerful enough to overcome the spell and cure the victim before it was too late? Would the doctor turn the affliction back against the person who sent it? Each of these questions revolved around the conjurer's power to intervene in the pharmacosm by initiating processes of healing and harming. The fact that many 'conjure doctors' could be hired to either 'cure or kill' served only to increase their stature as healers.
>
> (Fett, 2002, p.95)

Fett also points out that the materials used in the 'conjure packet' by 'conjure doctors' in the American South to place illness on a person were similar to those employed in Africa. The processes of divination, used to discover who had instigated the illness, were also similar to those traditionally used in Africa (Fett, 2002, pp.95, 101–3). In other words, conjuring medicine helped African slaves in America to make sense of their illnesses and, like African-American herbal medicine, provided a link to their African past. Despite the enormous inequality between themselves and their white owners, slaves succeeded in retaining their medical culture and beliefs. They preserved this cultural space despite the fierce resistance of the slave owners. Conjuring doctors and Obeah men in the West Indies were believed by whites to exert control over blacks and thus appeared to threaten white control. They were often associated by whites with rebellion and insurrection, and were suppressed by planters and governments. In 1748, Virginia enacted a law forbidding slaves from practising medicine (Savitt, 1978, p.175). In Jamaica, following the 1760 rebellion, legislation was passed against Obeah medicine and 'witchcraft'. Many Obeah practitioners were hanged, but Obeah continues today in the West Indies (Sheridan, 1985, pp.77–8).

Slave owners or white physicians might sometimes make use of the knowledge of slave herbalists, but there was no meeting of minds when it came to European medicine and African conjuring medicine. White medical practitioners considered conjuring medicine to be superstitious and irrational. Moreover, white medicine was the medicine of the dominant group that was intent on retaining power over its slaves. White doctors and slave owners together asserted the supremacy of their culture and knowledge, and attempted to suppress those aspects of black slave culture that they saw as threatening their dominance. Conversely, as you have seen, a part of the American slaves' African culture, conjuring medicine, was kept alive and intact by slaves.

White medicine and white power were thus inextricably linked. Both were imposed on unwilling slaves but neither could suppress the African-American slave medicine. As with the *curanderos* of New Spain, non-European medical knowledge and practice survived, though it often led a precarious underground existence.

12.9 Conclusion

European medicine was an enabling factor in the process of colonization and settlement. It provided guidance as to where healthy settlements might be established, and its learned practitioners proffered helpful advice as to how European bodies might become accustomed to hostile and alien climes through the processes of seasoning or acclimatization. As a result, English settlers adapted their lifestyles to the heat and disease of North America and the Caribbean. Others appropriated the cures of native peoples and created a new medicine – most notably in New Spain, where the *curanderos* administered their hybrid medicine to both the Spanish and the Indian poor. On the whole, however, the medical exchange between the old world and the new was uneven and unequal. The medical knowledge of native cultures was largely ignored or dismissed as superstitious, and only selective remedies were approved. The mere presence of Europeans in the Americas brought new diseases and mass mortality of the indigenous peoples. Medicine was, then, an instrument of colonial power and oppression – a fact most evident in the treatment of slaves on the new plantations.

References

Bewell, A. (1999) *Romanticism and Colonial Disease*, Baltimore: Johns Hopkins University Press.

Bradford, W. (1982) *Bradford's History of Plymouth Plantation*, ed. by W.T. Davis, New Jersey: Barnes and Noble.

Brereton, J. [1602] (1983) 'A briefe and true relation of the discoverie of the north part of Virginia' in D.B. Quinn and A.M. Quinn (eds) *The English New England Voyages 1602–1608*, London: Hakluyt Society.

Cook, N.D. (1998) *Born to Die, Disease and New World Conquest, 1492–1650*, Cambridge: Cambridge University Press.

Crosby, A.W. (1986) *Ecological Imperialism: The Biological Expansion of Europe, 900–1900*, Cambridge: Cambridge University Press.

Curtin, P. (1969) *The Atlantic Slave Trade: A Census*, Madison, WI: University of Wisconsin Press.

Curtin, P. (1990) *The Rise and Fall of the Plantation Complex*, Cambridge: Cambridge University Press.

Dobson, M. (1989) 'Mortality gradients and disease exchanges: comparisons from Old England and Colonial America', *Social History of Medicine*, vol.2, pp.260–79.

Eltis, D. (1989) *Economic Growth and the Ending of the Transatlantic Slave Trade*, Oxford: Oxford University Press.

Emerson, E. (ed.) (1976) *Letters from New England: The Massachusetts Bay Colony, 1629–1638*, Amherst: University of Massachusetts Press.

Fett, S.M. (2002) *Working Cures: Healing, Health, and Power on Southern Slave Plantations*, Chapel Hill: University of North Carolina Press.

Guerra, F. (1966) 'Aztec medicine', *Medical History*, vol.10, pp.315–38.

Harrison, W. (1994) *The Description of England*, ed. by G. Edelen, New York: Dover.

Higman, B.W. (1984) *Slave Populations of the British Caribbean 1807–1834*, Baltimore: Johns Hopkins University Press.

Histoire Naturelle des Indies (1996) translated by R.S Kraemer, New York: Norton.

Jourdain, S. (1613) *A Plaine Description of the Barmudas*, London: W. Stansby.

Klein, H.S. (1999) *The Atlantic Slave Trade*, Cambridge: Cambridge University Press.

Kupperman, K.O. (1984) 'Fear of hot climates in the Anglo-American colonial experience', *William and Mary Quarterly*, vol.41, pp.213–40.

Lind, J. (1768) *An Essay on Diseases Incidental to Europeans in Hot Climates*, London: T. Becket and P.A. de Hond.

Moorehead, A. (1966) *The Fatal Impact: An Account of the Invasion of the South Pacific 1767–1840*, London: Hamish Hamilton.

Ortiz de Montellano, B. (1990) *Aztec Medicine, Health and Nutrition*, New Brunswick: Rutgers University Press.

Percy, G. (1969) 'Observations gathered out of a discourse of the plantation of the Southerne colonie in Virginia' in P.L. Barbour (ed.) *The Jamestown Voyages under the First Charter 1606–1609*, Cambridge: Hakluyt Society.

Savitt, T.I. (1978) *Medicine and Slavery: The Diseases and Health Care of Blacks in Antebellum Virginia*, Urbana, IL: University of Illinois Press.

Sheridan, R. (1985) *Doctors and Slaves, a Medical and Demographic History of Slavery in the British West Indies 1680–1834*, Cambridge: Cambridge University Press.

Strachey, W. [1625] (1906) 'A true reportorie of the wrack, and redemption of Sir Thomas Gates, Knight ... July 15. 1610' in S. Purchas (ed.) *Hakluytus Posthumus or Purchas His Pilgrimes*, Glasgow: James MacLehose, pp.5–72.

Wear, A. (2000) *Knowledge and Practice in English Medicine, 1550–1680*, Cambridge: Cambridge University Press.

Whitbourne, R. [1622] (1982) 'A discourse and discovery of New-Found-Land' in G.T. Cell (ed.) *Newfoundland Discovered: English Attempts at Colonisation, 1610–1630*, London: Hakluyt Society.

Source Book readings

A.W. Crosby, *Ecological Imperialism. The Biological Expansion of Europe, 900*–1900, Cambridge: Cambridge University Press, 1986, pp.196–216 (Reading 12.1).

T. Hariot, *A Briefe and True Report of the New-found Land of Virginia ... Directed to the Adventurers, Favourers, and Welwillers of the Action, for the Inhabiting and Planting there*, London, 1588, sigs F2v–F4r (Reading 12.2).

K.O. Kupperman, 'Fear of hot climates in the Anglo-American colonial experience', *William and Mary Quarterly*, 41, 1984, pp.213–40 (Reading 12.3).

G.B. Risse, 'Medicine in New Spain' in R.L. Numbers (ed.) *Medicine in the New World: New Spain, New France, and New England*, Knoxville: University of Tennessee Press, 1987, pp.29–45 (Reading 12.4).

The Mexican Treasury. The Writings of Dr Francisco Hernández, ed. by S. Varey and translated by R. Chabrán, C.L. Chamberlin and S.Varey, Stanford: Stanford University Press, 2000, pp.138, 139, 140 (Reading 12.5).

A. Wear, 'The early modern debate about foreign drugs: localism versus universalism in medicine', *Lancet*, 354, 1999, pp.149–51 (Reading 12.6).

R.B. Sheridan, *Doctors and Slaves: A Medical and Demographic History of Slavery in the British West Indies, 1680–1834*, Cambridge: Cambridge University Press, 1985, pp.329–31, 335–6 (Reading 12.7).

S.M. Fett, *Working Cures: Healing, Health, and Power on Southern Slave Plantations*, Chapel Hill and London: University of North Carolina Press, 2002, pp.62–9 (Reading 12.8).

13

Organization, Training and the Medical Marketplace in the Eighteenth Century

Laurence William Brockliss

Objectives

When you have completed this chapter you should be able to:

- understand how the organization and practice of health care developed in the eighteenth century;

- appreciate how the growth of educational opportunities and training for surgeons undermined the privileged status of the physician, and helped to blur distinctions between the two groups;

- assess the extent to which medicine operated according to the principles of the marketplace in eighteenth-century Europe.

13.1 Introduction

As you will recall from earlier chapters, the treatment of the sick in the sixteenth and seventeenth centuries was broadly the province of two different types of practitioner. On the one hand, a small but growing number of educated and licensed practitioners ministered generally to the social elite. On the other, a large and indeterminate battalion of unlicensed, unqualified and often casual healers – mountebanks, Ladies Bountiful, clerics, wise women, executioners, farriers and so on – looked after the urban poor and the peasantry. Although the distinctions were blurred on the edges – many unqualified healers were licensed by the authorities, for instance, and some educated doctors did treat the poor – there was an economy of healing that largely mirrored the division of society into rich and poor.

In this chapter you will be introduced to the changes that occurred in the provision of medical care in the eighteenth century. This was a period in which most parts of Europe experienced sustained – and in Britain's case permanent – economic growth after a century of relative stagnation. It was also the heyday of the absolute state, in which the unrepresentative governments of Continental Europe intruded ever further into the lives of their subjects in the hope of creating more productive taxpayers and building more effective armies. Above all, the eighteenth century was the age of Enlightenment. This was a movement of intellectual emancipation which broke with the traditional Christian belief that life was a vale of tears and preached the possibility of moral and material progress. Everything now became possible, provided that knowledge was gained by experience and not accepted on the word of authority, and that the state ensured the conditions in which individuals could fulfil their potential untrammeled by the constraints of legal and corporate privilege.

First, you will read in Section 13.2 about the developments that took place over the century in the organization of licensed medical practice. In Section 13.3, you will learn about the expansion in the number of licensed practitioners and the changing pattern in their geographical distribution. Then, in Section 13.4, you will discover how the training of physicians and surgeons began to converge over the century, under the influence of Enlightenment ideas about the value of practical institutionalized learning. And finally, in Section 13.5, you will find out about the ways in which the traditional division between licensed and unlicensed medical practitioners was breaking down completely, with the emergence of a single medical marketplace in which doctors of all kinds competed with one another for custom, and rich patients increasingly chose the practitioner they preferred irrespective of his other qualifications. In consequence, by the end of the chapter, you will understand why many learned practitioners came to believe that the provision of medical care had descended into anarchy and demanded that the organization of the profession be put on a new footing.

Voluntary
hospitals are
discussed in
Chapter 6.

The modern social history of eighteenth-century medicine is still in its infancy. We know a great deal about Britain thanks to the pioneering work done by the late Roy Porter and his associates in the field of medical practice, and to the recent studies of the new voluntary hospitals and medical schools, especially in Edinburgh and London (e.g. Bynum and Porter, 1985; Lawrence, 1996; Porter, 1989; Porter and Porter, 1988, 1989; Risse, 1986). The situation in France, too, has been reconstructed in detail by several historians, while others have begun to leave their mark on German-speaking Europe and the Italian peninsula (e.g. Brockliss and Jones, 1997; Gelfand, 1980; Gentilcore, 1998; Keel, 2001, especially Chapters 5 and 7; Lindemann, 1996; Ramsey, 1991). Most of Europe, however, remains largely a closed book.

In the following pages, you will be introduced to the fruits of this historiography. Inevitably, the examples used in the text and the exercises reflect our present limited knowledge. You will find that France is given even greater attention than Britain, but this makes sense. France in the eighteenth century was the richest, most powerful state in Europe, with a population of 27 million in 1789, second only to that of Russia. It was also the centre of the Enlightenment, and its court set the cultural tone for the rest of the Continent. Britain had begun her rise to world dominion but in this period was still an up-and-coming power. When reading the chapter, however, you should always bear in mind that despite France's political, economic and cultural predominance, the French model was not necessarily replicated throughout Europe. For example, we know that there were significant differences between Britain and France in the field of medical care. We know, too, that across Europe there was a wide diversity in the way licensed medical practice was organized.

13.2 The organization of licensed medical practice

In earlier chapters, you learned that from the late Middle Ages, licensed medical practitioners in Europe (excluding Russia and the Ottoman Empire) were divided into three distinctive groups – physicians, surgeons and apothecaries. Physicians, who dealt with the diagnosis and cure of disease, were trained in university faculties, principally in medical theory. Surgeons and apothecaries, on the other hand, who performed manual operations and prepared drugs, trained as apprentices, usually had little formal instruction and were considered inferior to the physicians whose orders they carried out. You also learned that in the course of the sixteenth and seventeenth centuries, those licensed medical practitioners who were based in towns became increasingly organized into guilds and colleges with a wide variety of privileges, most importantly the right to a local professional monopoly and the right to co-opt members by examination. Finally, you were told that the system never worked perfectly, even in the large towns where most licensed practitioners were to be found. There were always many more surgeons and apothecaries than physicians, with the result that the 'subordinate' medical professions were continually involved in the practice of medicine as well as carrying out the wishes of physicians.

In this section, I explore how the organization of health care developed in the course of the eighteenth century. Essentially, licensed medical practice continued to be corporatively structured around this traditional threefold division until the outbreak of the French Revolution in 1789. Even before then, however, as a result of growing state intervention, significant developments had occurred in the way the traditional structure was organized and policed. From the end of the seventeenth century, a number of absolutist rulers on the Continent began to take an interest in erecting a homogeneous and nationwide structure of licensed medical practice, and this concern only grew after 1750 as they and their advisers came under the influence of the Enlightenment and its programme of social reform. Few *philosophes* believed it was possible or even desirable to end the great division between rich and poor, but most felt that the state should provide basic education, health care and charity for all and replace the haphazard cover hitherto afforded by the church. These developments, it must be stressed, complemented rather than destroyed the traditional corporative organization of health care, but they did lead to the emergence of significant regional and/or national distinctions in the way health care was organized. On the eve of the French Revolution, three different models can be identified.

The British Isles

In Great Britain and Ireland, the existing rudimentary system of licensed medical practice had all but collapsed. Before 1700, separate medical corporations had only ever existed in London, York, Norwich, Glasgow, Edinburgh and Dublin, although in some English towns medical practitioners had formed part of other guilds. This continued to be the case throughout the eighteenth century, even though the urban population grew dramatically over the period, with the great expansion of overseas trade and the onset of industrialization after 1760. Europe's population rose from 100 to 187 million across the century, but on the Continent, the urban population rose no faster than the population generally. In Britain, between 1700 and 1780, the population rose by less than 50 per cent (6.9 to 9 million) but the urban population almost doubled (1.2 to 2.2 million). That no more medical corporations were created reflected the British establishment's distrust of corporate monopolies of all kinds. The British eighteenth-century state was run for the most part by **Whig** politicians, who were the ideological heirs of the opponents of the absolutist Stuarts and thought that guild monopolies were an affront to an Englishman's right to follow any career he chose. Moreover, unlike the other large European monarchies, Britain was also a constitutional state, whose rulers were responsible to a parliament full of landowners jealous of their local power and suspicious of central government interference. It was completely uninterested therefore in policing public health at national level, and even in maintaining the existing degree of organization.

Theoretically, anyone who wished to practise medicine outside the jurisdiction of the British and Irish medical corporations had to seek a licence from the local bishop. This requirement, though, was never enforced during the period. Nor, too, were the medical corporations able to maintain their professional monopoly. Perhaps not surprisingly, the Dublin King's and Queen's College of Physicians (founded in 1692) could never make good its right to license physicians throughout Ireland, but even the more prestigious London College of Physicians could not stop unlicensed physicians practising in the capital and its environs (Figure 13.1). Legally, only fellows of the Royal College or its licentiates (other physicians granted the right to practise, all of whom had to be Anglicans) could offer medical care in London, and in the seventeenth century interlopers had been continually hauled in front of the courts. All this changed, however, after 1704, when a London apothecary called William Rose challenged the college's monopoly in the House of Lords and won the right to practise physic without the college's licence

Exercise

Read 'Challenging the physicians' monopoly in London: the Rose Case (1704)' (Source Book 1, Reading 13.1). What were the arguments put by the two sides?

Discussion

The Rose Case was really a struggle between two corporate bodies: the Royal College and the Society of Apothecaries, the latter anxious to extend the rights of its members, the former to preserve its privileges. The two sides, though, defended their position very differently. The Royal College stood on its legal rights and warned of the danger of opening the floodgates to empirics of all kinds. The Society of Apothecaries, in contrast, played to the gallery, by claiming that its members were the doctors of the poor and that their involvement in the practice of physic was socially useful.

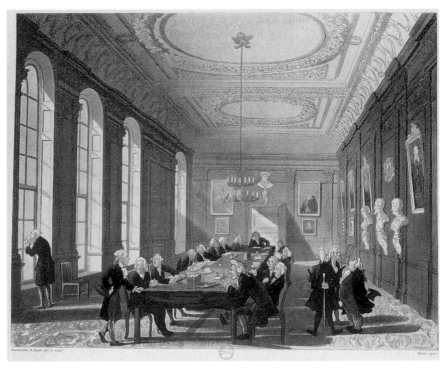

Figure 13.1   In this engraving of the London College of Physicians, a candidate stands, hands on table, and is quizzed, while other members chat and look out of the window. T. Rowlandson and A.C. Pugin, colour engraving, from Rudolph Ackermann, *Microcosm of London*, 1808–10. Bibliothèque Nationale, Paris, France/Lauros/ Giraudon/Bridgeman Art Library

The outcome of the case was ultimately governed by the dictates of party politics. In the reign of Queen Anne, the House of Lords was dominated by the constitutionalist Whigs. In Whig eyes, the Royal College was a stronghold of **Tory** privilege and tyranny, which had received its most recent charter from the deposed 'tyrant', James II (1685–8). Thereafter, the college continued to see itself and be seen as the pinnacle of the English profession and to award its licence to properly qualified physicians. By 1800, however, in the eyes of many of its critics, it was an irrelevant joke run by stuffy hangovers from an earlier age.

France

On the other side of the English Channel, in contrast, the traditional pattern of organization was broadly retained but subjected to partial homogenization and centralization. By 1700, the corporative organization of licensed medical practice in France was extensive. There were some 300 apothecaries' guilds, the same number of surgeons' guilds and 43 colleges of physicians, many of which were also faculties of medicine. In the course of the eighteenth century, the corporative map did not change (although there were additions, with France's annexation of the independent duchy of Lorraine in 1766). Rather, the practice of physic and surgery was more carefully policed by the state, as its guild organization became increasingly subject to governmental authority – a part of the absolute monarch's attempt to assert his authority over all corporate institutions for a mix of fiscal, ideological and enlightened reasons. First, the independent medical corporations were brought under the direct authority of the king or his chief medical officers, with the insistence from 1692 that each college or guild should contain an official *médecin* or *chirurgien du roi*, who would look after royal interests. Then, in 1707 and 1730, regulations were established for the organization of physic and surgery nationwide. From 1707, no one could legally practice medicine in the kingdom who had not studied for three years in a French faculty and obtained a medical degree after a proper examination. From 1730, all surgeons too had to seek a licence by passing an examination before a guild. At the same time, the content of the examination, the length of apprenticeship and other credentials were standardized.

Medical training is discussed further in Section 13.4.

In addition, the first steps were taken to bring physicians and surgeons (inside or outside the corporative system) under the overarching authority of umbrella institutions based in Paris. In 1731, the crown created the Académie Royale de Chirurgie, whose members twenty years later were given the specific remit of promoting surgical research. Thereafter, surgeons everywhere were encouraged to send in observations, take part in the annual prize essay competition, and covet the possibility of raising their status in the surgical profession by becoming a corresponding member of the academy. In 1776, the crown founded a similar institution for the physicians, the Société Royale de Médecine, which was under the control of the anatomist and doctor to the queen, Félix Vicq d'Azyr (1748–94). Initially set up as a 'committee of epidemics', subsequent to the **rinderpest** outbreak of 1774, it evolved into a research institute and an instrument of medical police. Its membership consisted of physicians practising in the capital, and again correspondents were appointed in the provinces to help with the task of collecting information about epidemics and therapies. At the same time, the society had the right to license new remedies and investigate the properties of mineral waters.

Exercise

Read 'The Académie Royale de Chirurgie and medicine in *ancien régime* France' (Source Book 1, Reading 13.2). Why do the authors call the academy an ***ancien régime*** institution?

Discussion

The French Académie Royale de Chirurgie did not accord with the modern concept of a national scientific academy. Its members were not the best and brightest surgeons in France, and the academy was really an offshoot of the Paris corporation of surgeons, who monopolized membership. Also, recruitment was ultimately in the hands of the king. Even more than the other Parisian academies, it was a partisan, privileged and elitist institution, and was, not surprisingly, closed by the revolutionaries. Admittedly, the academy did help to promote and organize French surgery, but it was very much an *ancien régime* institution, not a modern body.

Spain, Italy and Germany

In Spain and many of the states of Italy, the traditional corporative structure was shaken up even further by absolutist regimes anxious to extend their authority. In these parts of Europe, too, the corporative organization of medicine was well developed before 1700 – indeed, medical guilds had developed in the Italian peninsula earlier than elsewhere – but the eighteenth century saw the independence of the corporations steadily eroded by a state official, the *protomedico*. The latter was given the primary responsibility for granting a licence to practise, regardless of where a candidate intended to establish himself. In addition, this official was responsible for annually vetting apothecaries' shops, presided over a tribunal that pursued unlicensed healers and issued permits to quacks whose remedies seemed to be useful. In the Italian peninsula, admittedly, the position was frequently more honorific than powerful. For example, physicians were never under the *protomedico*'s control, certain towns might be outside his jurisdiction altogether and he was often little more than a government tax farmer who sold licences for a fee. Moreover, the *protomedico* did not sit on the local boards of health set up to combat the plague and other epidemic diseases, which were staffed by non-medical bureaucrats. In the Spanish kingdom of **Castile**, however, the position had real weight and the official controlled the whole medical system. Over time, the office developed into a licensing board with sub-committees all over the country, where candidates for the different branches of the profession were carefully examined. Traditionally, the board was run by physicians, but, from 1779, separate departments for medicine, surgery and pharmacy were established by the crown, and thereafter physicians were not involved in licensing members of the other two medical professions. In Spain, as in France, the crown was interested in promoting medical innovation and in 1734 set up a single academy for both medicine and surgery.

From the end of the seventeenth century, the state similarly began to take over the administration of medicine in Protestant northern Germany, where corporative medical bodies were far thinner on the ground. (Germany in the eighteenth century consisted of some 300 independent territories nominally owing allegiance to the Holy Roman Emperor. The northern part of the region was largely Protestant, the southern, Catholic.) A royal college of medicine was established by the **elector of Brandenburg** in 1685 to vet army doctors, but it soon became the licensing body for all medical practitioners in eighteenth-century Prussia and was given a general responsibility for medical matters. Prussia's Protestant neighbours quickly followed suit. The duke of Braunschweig-Wolfenbüttel, for instance, created his own Collegium Medicum, with an equally broad remit, in 1747. In the north German states, too, state medical officers were not just attached to existing colleges and guilds, as they were in France. Rather, each town and district had its independent, salaried *Stadt-* and *Land-arzt* (municipal and rural physician), who was a government bureaucrat and combined private practice with state service. Such officials had often existed from the late sixteenth century, but they had formerly been municipal appointees and, before the early eighteenth century, their duties were largely confined to providing legal reports on suspicious deaths. By the end of the century, however, they had become the local medical policemen. According to a handbook published by Johann Schwabe in 1786–7, the *physicus* (as he was called) was the local hygiene inspector, poor doctor, the official in charge of fighting epidemics and **epizootics**, the supervisor of local surgeons, apothecaries and midwives, and the scourge of unlicensed healers. The novel interference of the state in health care at the local level was a sign of the Protestant princes' commitment to the enlightened theories of state-building, developed in their territorial universities from the third decade of the century by **cameralists**, who stressed the importance of a healthy population for a prosperous state. Governments everywhere except in Britain could see the value in policing medicine more carefully in order to get the most out of the working population and ensure army recruits were fit and strong, but this was particularly the case in the smaller states of economically backward northern Germany. Not surprisingly, the evidence suggests that the *physicus*'s lot was not a happy one. Continually confronted by unhelpful colleagues and obstreperous officials, he had great difficulty in ensuring the orders on health policy sent down from the Collegium Medicum were ever carried out.

Exercise

Read 'Medicine and the state in eighteenth-century Germany: the plight of the *physicus* or state-physician' (Source Book 1, Reading 13.3). How does Spangenberg present himself? To what extent do you believe what he says?

Discussion

Spangenberg presents himself as a hard-working physician, frequently giving his services for nothing, who is weighed down by the poverty of the inhabitants and by his quarrel with the duke's representative, Heiland. The *Amtmann* (magistrate), it seems, pays no heed to the duke's medical ordinances. He allows local midwives to go unexamined and lets empirical healers practise in the district unhindered.

There is no reason to doubt much of what Spangenberg tells us. To a certain extent, the report seems balanced in that his is not a tale of relentless gloom: the surgeon, Siegfried Nezel, for one receives a very positive write-up. You should remember, however, that this is a report to the newly formed Collegium Medicum, or medical board. It is Spangenberg's chance to ingratiate himself with the leading physicians of the duchy. The author is no doubt anxious to present himself in the best light possible and to feed the board with the information he suspects they want. In his case, too, it is an opportunity to undermine and perhaps even force the removal of his local enemy. Heiland has clearly annoyed Spangenberg by not appointing or reappointing him (it is unclear whether he ever officially held the post) as *physicus* in the district when the former *Amtmann* died. Spangenberg's letter to the board gives him the chance to get his own back and emphasizes how easily physicians could be caught up in local power politics.

13.3 The distribution of licensed medical practitioners: the case of France

Having explored the way in which licensed medical practice was organized in the eighteenth century, I now turn my attention to the number and distribution of medical practitioners. Before 1700, it is only possible to know how many licensed practitioners there were per head of the population in the largest towns of Europe, where guild and college records survive and there were occasional demographic censuses. In the second half of the eighteenth century, in contrast, as states began to collect statistics about a wide variety of matters, it becomes easier, although still not straightforward, to construct a picture of the availability of professional health care. Plotting the distribution of the population against the provision of medical personnel really only becomes possible in most European states in the second half of the nineteenth century. This section concentrates on France, the state for which we have the most information in this regard.

The growth of statistical analysis is discussed in Chapter 11.

France, then as now, was a country of regions, so let us home in on one particular area – Brittany – a province with some two million inhabitants. This is a region about which we are particularly well informed thanks to the work of the historian Jean-Pierre Goubert (1974, Chapter 2). Using parish registers, a number of contemporary government estimates of the population and two administrative surveys of medical practitioners in 1750 and 1786, Goubert was able to produce a complex map of the provision of health care in the province. Concentrating primarily on physicians and surgeons, he established that there were 756 licensed medical practitioners in the province in the 1780s, of whom only 162 were physicians. Deciding that only 540 of these were available to care for the population all the year round, he concluded that there were 2.4 doctors per 10,000 Bretons, or, one doctor for every 4,074 inhabitants.

Goubert's ratio is extremely low, given the provision in European countries today. Britain in the 1980s had one **general practitioner** for every 950 inhabitants. It is clear, too, that his physicians and surgeons were very unevenly distributed across the province. To start with, seventeen of the forty-five administrative districts had no resident physician, while only three of the sixty-four physicians recorded in the 1786 survey were to be found in the countryside. Everywhere, urban dwellers had easier access to licensed health care than did their country cousins. There were only 0.9 doctors in rural areas for every 10,000 inhabitants against 7.7 in the forty towns that had more than 2,000 inhabitants. In the largest town – the port city of Nantes, which had 53,000 inhabitants – there were 9.2. Such findings, of course, are not surprising. Surgeons and physicians had invested heavily in their training in terms of time and money. They were unlikely to want to practise in a village where few people could afford their services or where they were distrusted as outsiders.

Broadly speaking, the picture described above pertained across France. Brittany, however, was a comparatively poor province and better rates of provision can be found elsewhere. When another French historian, François Lebrun, studied the 1786 survey of licensed medical practitioners in Anjou, a more prosperous region to the south, he discovered that there were seven practitioners per 10,000 inhabitants (one physician and six surgeons) (Lebrun, 1975, Chapter 6).

Everywhere, though, there were always more surgeons than physicians, and the towns were always better staffed than the countryside. It is also clear that it was not necessarily the largest towns which were the best provided. Look at Table 13.1.

You will immediately see that, with a few exceptions, the ratio of medical personnel to the population was much more favourable in towns under rather than over 30,000 inhabitants. Best of all was to live in a sleepy backwater, such as Villefranche-sur-Saône, where there were seven physicians for 4,500 people. The capital, Paris, was particularly poorly served. It might have boasted 480 licensed physicians, surgeons and apothecaries, but this still meant that it was no better supplied than the whole of Anjou.

The reason for this imbalance in provision lay in the corporative medical system. The most money was to be made in the large towns of France, so all things being equal, we would have expected them to have contained a higher proportion of licensed practitioners. The right to practise in these towns, however, was monopolized by the local medical corporations, who were anxious to keep the number of practitioners as low as possible so as to maximize their members' profits. In consequence, there was a tendency to admit new recruits only when a member died or moved away, unless candidates were sons of existing members. The most prestigious corporations largely maintained their closed shop by charging excessively high entrance fees to deter would-be recruits. Nobody could join the Paris college of physicians unless they had first taken their medical doctorate at the city's university. This required four years of study on the faculty benches, two years of rigorous examinations (see below), but above all, by the 1780s, the expenditure of some 7,000 *livres* (£280). This was a vast sum at a time when an artisan would be lucky to earn 250 *livres* (£10) per annum. It was also much more than the cost of an average medical degree in France, which could be had for 300 to 400 *livres* (£12–16). Arguably, then, most physicians and surgeons ended up plying their trade in small to medium-sized towns because they could not afford the fees charged in larger towns and cities, such as Paris. Their situation was not improved either by the fact that market forces were against them. In the course of the eighteenth century, the number of physicians, if not necessarily the number of surgeons, was steadily growing, as shown in Table 13.2.

The population of France grew over the century from 20 to 30 million, a rise of 50 per cent. There was a threefold expansion in the number of medical graduates over the same period, however. This was good news for ordinary people, who had a far better chance of consulting a physician in 1789 than in 1700, but bad news for many young physicians without contacts or means, who were condemned to earn a living in a small town.

France, it must be said, seems to have been particularly well supplied with licensed medical personnel. I have estimated from what we know about the annual number of medical graduates, adult lifespan, and the ratios of physicians to surgeons and surgeons to apothecaries in French towns (see Tables 13.1 and 13.2) that there were about 24,000 licensed medical practitioners in the kingdom in the 1780s, 3,000 of whom were physicians. At this date, the number of licensed practitioners in England, according to Simmons's *Medical Register* of 1783, was scarcely more than 4,000, of which 500 were physicians. Given that the population of England

Table 13.1 Number of physicians, surgeons and apothecaries in selected French towns in the 1780s

	Population	Physicians		Surgeons		Apothecaries	
		no.	per 10,000	no.	per 10,000	no.	per 10,000
Paris	660,000	153	2.3	192	2.9	135	2.0
Over 50,000							
Lyon	146,000	32	2.2	77	4.8	23	1.6
Bordeaux	111,000	16	1.4	88	7.9	22	2.0
Marseille	110,000	34	3.1	70	6.4	14	1.3
Nantes	80,000	12	1.5	40	5.0	?	
Rouen	73,000	9	1.2	39	5.3	8	1.1
Toulouse	53,000	40	7.5	32	6.0	17	3.2
Versailles	51,000	?		18	3.5	?	
Nîmes	50,000	12	2.4	22	4.4	11	2.2
Average			2.8		5.4		1.9
Over 30,000							
Orléans	48,500	10	2.1	16	3.4	14	2.9
Amiens	44,000	8	1.8	11	2.5	8	1.8
Metz	36,500	10	2.7	15	6.6	16	4.1
Rennes	35,000	10	2.9	18	5.1	?	
Nancy	33,000	14	4.2	15	4.5	7	2.1
Angers	32,000	12	3.8	20	6.3	10	3.1
Besançon	32,000	28	8.8	15	4.7	13	4.1
Caen	32,000	14	4.4	17	5.3	11	3.4
Clermont	32,000	10	3.1	10	3.1	5	1.6
Montpellier	32,000	34	10.6	36	11.3	13	3.9
Reims	32,000	7	2.1	8	2.5	9	2.8
Brest	30,000	6	2.0	15	5.0	?	
Average			4.0		5.0		3.0
(minus Besançon & Montpellier)			(2.7)		(4.3)		(2.4)

Over 20,000							
Montauban	29,000	6	2.1	11	3.8	18	2.8
Aix	28,500	14	4.9	19	6.7	?	
Troyes	28,000	5	1.8	8	2.9	?	
Arles	25,000	11	4.4	20	8.0	7	2.8
Grenoble	25,000	11	4.4	13	5.2	5	2.0
Dijon	22,000	10	4.5	12	5.6	6	2.7
La Rochelle	21,500	4	1.9	19	8.8	11	5.1
Arras	20,000	11	5.5	16	8.0	9	4.5
Béziers	20,000	6	3.0	7	3.5	2	1.0
Average			3.6		5.8		2.7
5,000–15,000							
Alençon	13,500	4	3.0	1	0.7	?	
Châlons s.M.	12,000	11	9.2	8	6.7	4	3.3
Auxerre	10,500	5	4.8	9	8.8	4	3.8
Cherbourg	10,000	7	7.0	2	2.0	1	1.0
Albi	9,000	1	1.1	2	2.2	?	
Pau	8,500	5	5.9	7	8.2	5	5.9
Soissons	8,000	4	5.0	7	8.8	5	6.3
Valence	7,500	5	5.3	2	2.1	6	8.6
Bourg-en-Bresse	7,000	4	5.7	5	7.2	4	5.7
Average			5.3		5.2		4.9
Under 5,000							
Villefranche-sur-Saône	4,500	7	15.6	5	11.1	2	4.4

(Brockliss and Jones, 1997, pp.522–3)

was then a little less than one-third of that of France, we would have expected the total to have been twice as large. Admittedly, the figures are not strictly commensurate: the first is a statistical manipulation and the second a notoriously incomplete contemporary survey of provincial doctors, compiled by a London doctor. Nevertheless, both totals underestimate the number of licensed practitioners, so the comparison is not invalid. It is virtually certain, too, that in both cases the number of physicians is fairly accurate. The number of physicians graduating each year in France can be calculated with some accuracy, so provided my estimate of the average length of service (twenty-five years) is sound, then the

Table 13.2 Number of physicians, surgeons and apothecaries in eighteenth-century France (estimated totals)

	Doctorates (p.a.)	Physicians*	Surgeons†	Apothecaries‡
1690–9	52.9	1,323	6,350	
1700–9	43.7	1,093	5,246	
1710–19	62.1	1,553		
1720–9	61.6	1,540		
1730–9	82.2	2,055		
1740–9	96.7	2,417		
1750–9	100.4	2,510	12,048	
1780–9	125.4	3,135	15,048	6,019

* Total based on an estimated average working career of twenty-five years
† Total based on a ratio of physicians to surgeons of 1:4
‡ Total based on a ratio of apothecaries to surgeons of 1:2.5
(Brockliss and Jones, 1997, p.520)

figure of 3,000 will be roughly right. Similarly, it can be assumed that the *Medical Register* records virtually all graduate physicians in England, who would have had the highest status among the medical practitioners in a county. Interestingly, the one part of England better supplied with licensed medical practitioners was the capital, where there were 960 medical practitioners serving a population of about 800,000, or one doctor for every 850 individuals (Bynum, 1985, pp.105–7). This was proportionally considerably larger than the number serving Paris, an indication presumably of the relative ease with which medical practitioners could establish themselves in a capital where the corporate system had broken down.

13.4 Medical training

The most important changes to the structure of licensed medicine across the eighteenth century occurred in the way in which practitioners were trained. Historically, one of the fundamental reasons why physicians had a higher social status than surgeons and apothecaries was their distinctive educational experience. Physicians had a lengthy formal education, which began with the study of the classical humanities and philosophy and concluded with the study of the science of medicine in a university faculty. Future surgeons and apothecaries, on the other hand, had only an attenuated classical education or none at all, and largely learned their profession on the job, first as apprentices and then as journeymen, often moving around the country. Physicians, then, were learned professionals; surgeons and apothecaries were literate artisans. In this section, you will learn how this distinction broke down after 1700, as surgeons in particular began to be given a more formal education and physicians took a greater interest in practical studies. You will also learn about the proliferation of private medical teaching in this era, which supplemented the institutionalized provision.

The education of physicians

Until the beginning of the eighteenth century, Europe's faculties of medicine primarily provided training in medical theory. Whether the content was determined by Galen or by the iatrochemical and iatromechanical theories that began to replace classical medicine in the second half of the seventeenth century made little difference in this respect. Professorial lectures were little more than *ex cathedra* dictations in Latin, with no visual aids, on some aspect of the five recognized sub-sciences of physiology, hygiene, semiotics, pathology and therapeutics. Although, from the mid-sixteenth century, a growing number of physicians, both inside and outside the faculties, began to insist on the importance of human anatomy and animal vivisection as the way to place physiology and pathology on firmer empirical foundations, their conviction was only gradually internalized by the wider profession. Instruction in practical anatomy was slowly introduced into most faculties after 1550, as were courses in practical surgery, botany (or the medical property of plants) and pharmacy (or the preparation of drugs, especially chemical ones). However, they always occupied a subsidiary position in the curriculum, and facilities, with the exception of those at Padua, Leiden and Montpellier, were unsatisfactory. It was usually felt that the chief reason a medical student might need to know something of these ancillary arts was to better supervise his subordinates, the surgeons and apothecaries. It might have been the case that Vesalius gained his interest in anatomy at Paris, but the Paris medical faculty made little effort to encourage the science. The faculty did not have a properly constructed anatomy theatre until 1749. The situation was only retrieved in the French capital by the fact that, from 1640, dissections were also performed in the Jardin du Roi. This was a botanical garden, which had been founded by the king. Entirely separate from the medical faculty, it had good facilities and, in the eighteenth century, provided tuition in botany, anatomy and chemistry.

From the beginning of the eighteenth century, however, it came to be accepted that instruction in the ancillary medical arts should constitute an important part of the medical curriculum. Presumably, the ever-growing number of anatomical discoveries (albeit, sometimes misunderstood) eventually made it impossible for faculty professors to deny the value of a detailed knowledge of the human body for the practising physician. The work of contemporary experimental physiologists, such as Albrecht von Haller at Göttingen, whose discovery of irritability you encountered in Chapter 7, can only have strengthened this belief. So must have, too, the groundbreaking achievements in pathological anatomy of Giovanni Batista Morgagni (1682–1771) at Padua, who pioneered the association of particular diseases with specific internal lesions (Porter, 1999, pp.263–4). From the mid-eighteenth century, moreover, professors were influenced by Enlightenment ideals that placed a much greater emphasis on underpinning medical science with empirical research. Whatever their theoretical starting-point – be they mechanists or vitalists – they accepted the Newtonian distinction between hypothetical theories and fact-based knowledge, and recognized that most of medical science had still to be built. At the same time, the eighteenth century saw an erosion of the traditional prejudice that the performance of surgical operations and the preparation of drugs were demeaning activities, and physicians were encouraged to become experts themselves in the arts of surgery and pharmacy. In part, this was a reflection of a broader cultural shift, again associated with the Enlightenment, which gave a new dignity to manual work. In the second case, though, this transformation was eased by the metamorphosis of the art of pharmacy into the science of chemistry around 1700. The subject was no longer just about the preparation of chemical drugs, but about the structure of matter, and it therefore began to have a potential relevance to physiology as well as to therapeutics.

As a result of this changing mentality, courses in the ancillary medical arts and sciences gained a new legitimacy in the curriculum and their number proliferated. Independent chairs were established in these disciplines where hitherto they had often been taught by one of the professors of theoretical medicine in his spare time. In the larger faculties, botany developed into natural history, chemistry and pharmacy (or *materia medica*, as it was called) became separate sciences, and physicians could even study obstetrics (admittedly, most of the chairs established in this subject were intended to offer instruction to midwives). In 1700, the only course in chemistry available at a French medical faculty was given at Montpellier. On the eve of the Revolution, in 1789, there were separate chairs at Paris, Caen, Toulouse, Nancy, Reims and Perpignan. Of course, we must not be too dewy-eyed about this development. Theoretical medicine always remained the core of the medical curriculum, the facilities often remained poor and the professors of the ancillary disciplines had a comparatively low status. Even when new chairs were established, the incumbent was not always paid. Nonetheless, the change from an earlier period was considerable. At Montpellier from 1738, it even became possible to take a special degree in surgical medicine for graduates who wanted to practise in both arts. It was definitely the case that no medical faculty could be established from 1730 which did not give an important place to the ancillary medical disciplines.

Exercise

Read 'Reforming the medical curriculum: Toulouse (1773)' (Source Book 1, Reading 13.4). What place was given to the ancillary medical arts in the curriculum?

Discussion

The new statutes adopted at Toulouse in the 1770s suggest that the ancillary medical arts had by then become an important part of the curriculum everywhere. According to the statutes, the faculty's students were expected to study the ancillary medical arts in all three years of the course. By the end of their studies, they would have devoted two years each to anatomy, chemistry, botany, pharmacy and surgery. Article V of the statutes seems to imply that students would also be examined on these subjects as well as on the traditional part of the curriculum if they wanted to take a degree, while an appended note reveals that several of them each year would have to act as laboratory assistants. On the other hand, the ancillary courses were studied alongside the traditional curriculum and were not obviously integrated with the study of physiology and pathology.

In the second half of the eighteenth century, furthermore, most faculties began to introduce practical training in patient care. Traditionally, a young graduate gained experience in treating patients by acting as an assistant to an established practitioner for a couple of years. The faculties did not consider it part of their remit to train practitioners. From 1700, however, a small but growing number of physicians called for a change of heart on the grounds that too many ill-prepared graduates were learning their craft at the expense of patients. Their opinion gradually gained weight, and across Europe courses were established in practical medicine. These courses were unlike modern courses in clinical medicine, in which students can observe a hospital patient's progress over a period of time. Rather, the faculty would run an outpatient clinic for the poor, once or twice a week, and the professors would diagnose in front of the students the complaints of those who presented themselves. Some professors, however, did establish a course around patients in a hospital ward. The first to do so was probably Hermann Boerhaave at Leiden, who, from 1715, set up a small clinical ward at the St Caecilia Hospital, where he would stand at the foot of each bed in turn and describe to the assembled students the patient's condition (Figure 13.2). Through Boerhaave's many pupils the practice then spread to other faculties, notably Edinburgh (only founded in 1725) and Vienna. In Edinburgh, John Rutherford (1695–1779) inaugurated clinical lectures at the new infirmary in 1749 (Figure 13.3); in Vienna, chairs of clinical medicine and surgery were established from 1754, first in the city's municipal and then in its Trinity hospital. Even by the 1780s, though, hospital-based faculty courses in clinical medicine were comparatively rare. In France, for instance, only the faculty at Strasbourg gave a hospital-based course in practical patient care. The fault did not necessarily lie at the faculties' door. In Catholic countries in particular, the hospitals were controlled by the regular orders, who did not want their patients treated as teaching aids or upset by rowdy students. As in earlier centuries, hospitals on the Continent continued to be refuges for the old and homeless, not just shelters for the sick poor. Hospital managers ran the institution for the benefit of all the inmates and did not prioritize the needs of the medical practitioners, who usually did not live on site and only visited patients irregularly.

The clinical courses that were established were structured in various ways. At Edinburgh there was no professor of clinical medicine as such. As at Leiden, the course was given in a small, specially created ward of at most twenty-nine beds, and students simply listened to the professor pontificate. There was no attempt to use the clinic as a research tool. The professors merely used the patients as exemplars to illustrate the conclusions taught in the course on theoretical pathology. At Vienna, on the other hand, from 1774, the whole hospital was opened up to clinical teaching and the course was much more interactive. Under Maximilien Stoll (1742–87), who held the clinical chair for eleven years, two wards were kept aside for students to diagnose patients. They then later discussed their

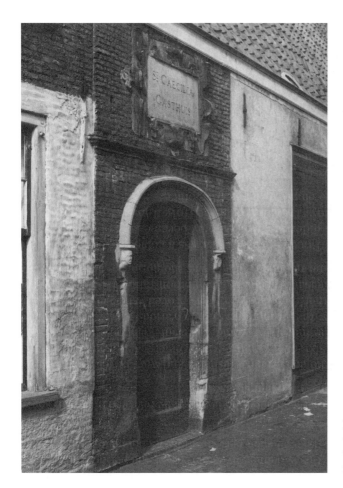

Figure 13.2   The ancient gateway of the St Caecilia Hospital, Leiden, as it appears today. PV Collection, City Archives Leiden, no.28403.2

conclusions with the professor and their peers in a debriefing session. Stoll also used the clinic as a forum to instruct his students in the new diagnostic techniques of **pulmonary auscultation**, which had been developed by his colleague Leopold Auenbrugger (1722–1809). Not surprisingly in an age in which learning through doing was praised more than learning through seeing, the approach of the Vienna faculty was the one that gained favour everywhere at the beginning of the nineteenth century. Later proponents of clinical teaching also approved of the way Stoll and his predecessor, Anton de Haen (1704–76), developed Morgagni's work on pathological anatomy and used the hospital clinic as a vehicle for gaining new knowledge about disease. In the next exercise, you can read what the French physician Philippe Pinel (1743–1826) had to say in 1793 about the organization and value of clinical teaching.

Exercise

Read 'The clinical education of the physician in late eighteenth-century France: Philippe Pinel (1793)' (Source Book 1, Reading 13.5). Did Pinel belong to the Leiden school or to the Viennese school?

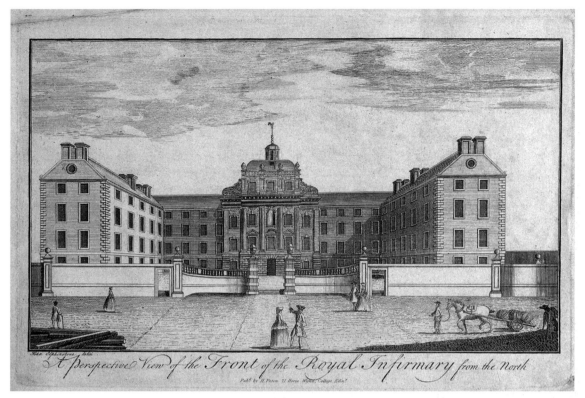

Figure 13.3   The Royal Infirmary, Edinburgh, 1741–1879. Wellcome Library, London

Discussion

The extract reveals that Pinel belonged squarely to the Leiden school. He showed no interest in clinical teaching as a means to a better understanding of disease. Although he appreciated that the clinic could be a source of sounder therapeutic knowledge, he was scornful of de Haen's readiness to introduce his students to obscure and complex cases. The clinic's purpose was to teach students how to recognize diseases and predict their outcome. The ward should only be filled therefore with patients with clear-cut diseases. On the other hand, Pinel appreciated certain aspects of the Viennese school. He thought that the clinical ward should be small, and he expected students to be assigned patients to look after.

These changes in the curriculum, it must be stressed, had little effect on the examination rubric. As in earlier centuries, most faculties demanded that candidates for a doctorate in medicine underwent one or more oral examinations and wrote one or more short dissertations, which they publicly presented. By and large, the oral examinations were perfunctory and concentrated on medical theory, while the dissertations concentrated on a limited repertoire of well-rehearsed themes and were occasionally ghost-written. By the end of the eighteenth century, only a handful of faculties subjected their graduands to a practical examination. Provided a student had followed the course laid down in the statutes, he was virtually guaranteed to pass. The failure to restructure the examination system and the ease with which medical degrees were granted reflected above all overcapacity in faculty provision. There were just too many medical faculties in Europe for the number of students, and only a handful – one or two per state, depending on its size – were really active as teaching centres. The others were degree factories, which lured graduands with the promise of cheap and quick-to-obtain doctorates.

While this situation pertained, it was impossible for the serious teaching faculties to be too demanding. Throughout the eighteenth century, the notoriously venal faculty of Reims, for instance, graduated twenty to thirty medical students a year from all over Europe, including the British Isles. Students merely had to pass through the town en route from Paris, Leiden or some other famous faculty, submit themselves to a perfunctory oral, pay the fee and collect their degree. The continual trickle of graduates towards Reims would have become a flood if standards had been uniformly raised in the major medical centres. Only faculties that deliberately wanted few graduates could bring the examination system in line with the curriculum. Paris, for instance, from 1730, expected its graduands to pass two week-long practical examinations in anatomy and surgery. But Paris doctors, as you will recall, gained an automatic right to practise in the capital and it was in the local college's interest to make the degrees both as difficult and as expensive as possible. The faculty was also, not surprisingly, unconcerned about how uncomfortable the experience might prove. When Nicolas Chambon de Montaux (1748–1828) – mayor of Paris in the early years of the Revolution – was examined in anatomy, he was asked to dissect, then demonstrate, the liver, while holding the viscera in his hand, of the most disgusting corpse he had ever encountered:

> At the moment I opened the lower abdomen, the room was filled with the most appalling stink. It hit my peers [i.e. the other candidates] with such violence that M. Corion, who had approached me to assist, ... fainted, was taken back home, and died in the space of 72 hours ... The examiners must have guessed what was going to happen for they covered their faces with their handkerchiefs soaked in eau de cologne.
>
> (Chambon de Montaux, 1813, no foliation)

The education of surgeons

Unlike medicine, the practice of surgery changed dramatically across the eighteenth century. Before the late seventeenth century, surgical knowledge was scarcely more advanced than it had been in the classical era, and, even in large towns, surgeons could perform few complex operations. A century later, the art had developed by leaps and bounds. Thanks to the dexterity and imagination of a handful of Paris and London surgeons in the early eighteenth century, notably Jean-Louis Petit, Henri-François Le Dran (1685–1770), Sauveur-François Morand (1697–1773) and William Cheselden (1688–1750), surgery became enriched with a series of new and successful techniques for amputating limbs, closing fistulas, extracting bladder stones, excising cancers, removing cataracts and so on. These developments encouraged the most prominent surgeons – usually those in the service of the prince – to think more positively of their art. Skilful surgeons resented the traditional subordination of surgery to physic, but recognized that the status of the profession would never improve while most of the brethren were ignorant barbers. For this reason, they began to demand that surgeons, just like physicians, should have a proper classical education and receive formal instruction. In this way, surgery in turn would become a learned profession, while the new surgical techniques would be effectively diffused throughout the surgical community.

Even before 1700 there had been an opportunity for many tiro surgeons to gain some formal instruction through the courses in anatomy and surgery given in a number of medical faculties. These might have been principally intended for medical students but they were usually delivered in the vernacular so that they could be followed by students of surgery as well. The faculties maintained this tradition in the eighteenth century and often provided a first-class introduction to the art. At the new faculty of Edinburgh, for instance, the courses in anatomy and surgery, given in English by Alexander Monro I (1697–1767) and Alexander Monro II (1733–1817), had a nationwide reputation and were attended by future surgeons or surgeon-apothecaries from all over the British Isles. The leading surgeons in Continental Europe, however, found the faculty courses either of too low a standard or inadequate in scope, and campaigned vigorously for the establishment of independent colleges of surgery. Their lobbying was often successful. Surgical colleges were founded all over Europe in the second half of the eighteenth century, especially in France where many of the new procedures had first been developed and tested (Figure 13.4).

The most important of the French colleges, and the first to be founded, was in Paris. The Paris surgeons' guild had tried to establish lecture courses for apprentices in the late sixteenth and early seventeenth centuries, but their efforts had been stymied by the Paris medical faculty, anxious to maintain its monopoly. In 1725, however, through the influence of two court surgeons, François Gigot de La Peyronie (d.1747) and Georges Mareschal (d.1733), a permanent surgical school was attached to the guild and funded by the crown. Initially, there were only five lecturers (in surgical principles, osteology and bone diseases, anatomy, surgical diseases and operations, and surgical therapy), but the number was gradually increased to nine with the addition of chairs in ophthalmology (1765), obstetrics (1774), chemistry (1774) and botany (1783). Initially, too, the professors gave a series of discrete courses: there was no surgical curriculum. From 1750, however, when the guild was permitted by the crown to call itself a college, a system of student registration was introduced and a three-year cycle of lectures was established, which students who intended to become Paris masters were obliged to follow. In 1784, the college curriculum was further refined. Students wishing to receive a certificate of attendance at the Paris college had henceforth to have completed the three-year course, which was specifically described as being divided in the manner of the faculty curriculum into physiology, pathology and therapeutics. Each year students had to follow a course in anatomy, surgical operations and obstetrics, and at some time during the three years study botany, ophthalmology and chemistry.

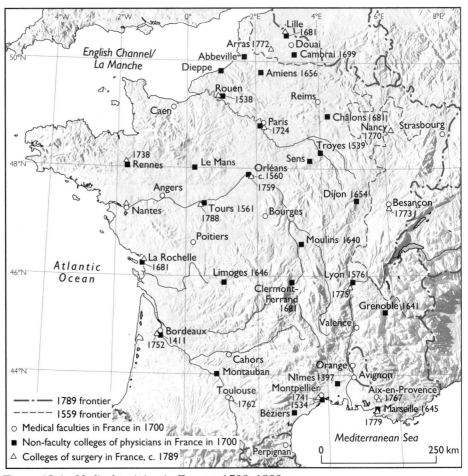

Figure 13.4   Medical training in France, 1700–1800

The Paris college of surgery became a formidable teaching institution, completely eclipsing the Paris faculty as a purveyor of surgical instruction. Its professors included most of the leading surgeons in the capital (and the country), such as Jacques Tenon (1724–1816), famous for his 1788 indictment of conditions at the city's largest hospital, the Hôtel-Dieu. In the third quarter of the century, the college had 700 to 900 students registered on its books, at a time when the faculty had only 100. Significantly, it was able to attract many foreigners, especially visitors from the British Isles. The courses, though consisting for the most part of practical demonstrations, were given in a traditional *ex cathedra* manner, there was limited interaction between professor and student, and students had little chance to gain practical experience themselves. From 1750, however, the college had a separate school of practical dissection, where every three months twenty students chosen by the professors had the chance to gain hands-on experience in anatomy and surgical dissection. From 1774, it also possessed its own hospice, where novice surgeons could follow the treatment of interesting surgical cases. The foundation of the hospice coincided with the college's installation in a completely new building, a neoclassical masterpiece designed by Jacques Gondoin, and from

1795 the site of the modern faculty of medicine. Once more, the Paris surgeons had the crown to thank for their good fortune. In 1769, Louis XV had allowed the surgeons to acquire one of the university's residential colleges and had provided funds for its refurbishment. His successor was just as enthusiastic in his support. Figure 13.5 shows Louis XVI laying the foundation stone for the new college in 1774, a relatively novel act for a prince.

It is not difficult to see why the French crown pandered to their surgeons' demands for separate educational institutions. Given the advances in the art and the state's need to recruit skilful army surgeons in an age of continuous warfare, fostering surgery made sense. It was for this reason, presumably, that the crown had erected an academy of surgery nearly half a century before it founded an academy of medicine. French surgeons knew, too, how to curry favour with the crown, as suggested by Figure 13.6, which is the frontispiece for the first volume of the academy of surgery's proceedings. In this case, the French crown swallowed the surgeons' propaganda completely. In 1772, surgery became a recognized liberal profession in France when the king abolished any need for surgeons to serve an apprenticeship. Instead, they all had to serve as pupils with a master surgeon for a

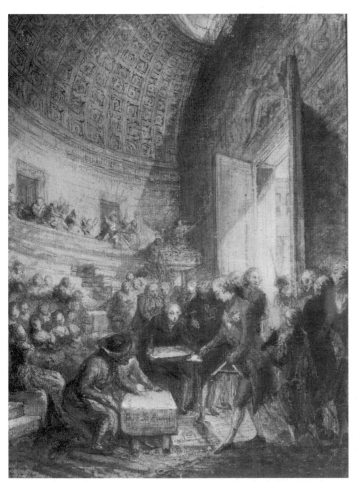

Figure 13.5 Louis XVI laying the foundation stone of the Paris college of surgery, 14 December 1774, by Gabriel de Saint-Aubin, gouache on paper, 1774. Louis stands centre right, holding a trowel. Musée de la Ville de Paris, Musée Carnavalet, Paris, France/Archives Charmet/Bridgeman Art Library

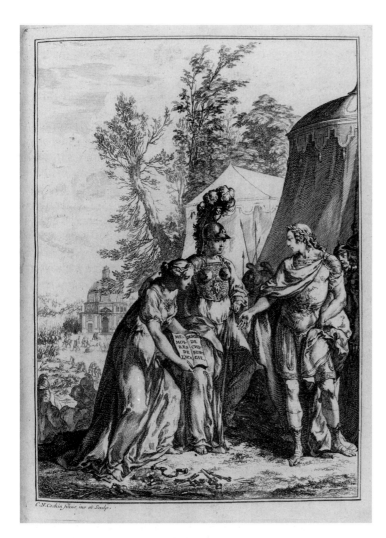

Figure 13.6 Surgery as the servant of the nation in war. In this engraving, surgery in the guise of a beautiful woman presents the volume to a martial Louis XV under the protection of Athena, goddess of wisdom and war and patroness of the craft guilds. In the background, the detritus of the battlefield is conveyed to the Invalides, Louis XIV's refuge for old soldiers. Wellcome Library, London

two- or three-year term, and spend one year (increased to two in 1784) in a surgical college.

Private courses

The faculties and the colleges of surgery lacked the facilities to give all but the fortunate few the chance to become adept in anatomy and surgery: usually students just listened and watched. In the case of surgeons this was not an insuperable problem. Most, whatever the legal position, continued to serve an apprenticeship and work as journeymen, and they could get practical experience as hospital assistants or dressers. For physicians, on the other hand, the absence of hands-on tuition in the faculties was felt acutely, especially given the Enlightenment's emphasis on the need to learn by doing. The problem was solved by the establishment of extracurricular teaching in practical anatomy and surgery, which was principally given by surgeons. In the course of the century, private courses in these subjects were created in capital cities and faculty towns across the Continent. Their continual expansion in numbers and the profits the professors evidently made, bore witness to the ever-growing demand.

Understandably, successful private instruction of this kind was first established in Paris in the second quarter of the eighteenth century, when the city was at the centre of surgical advance. The leading members of the city's guild of surgeons who held hospital appointments took pupils into their own homes, gave them access to bodies or body parts, and allowed them to assist at operations. For several decades, medical students visited the capital from all over Europe. Two of the most famous teachers were Le Dran and Morand, mentioned above, who both held appointments at the Hôpital de la Charité (Figure 13.7). This was a relatively small Paris hospital with only 200 beds, which was run by a special order of monks. Le Dran was an innovative lithotomist, whose pupils included Albrecht von Haller and his botanist compatriot, Johann Gessner (1709–90), both of whom left a diary of their stay in Paris. Morand, whose father was the chief surgeon at the Invalides and who had received, exceptionally for surgeons at this date, a good education in the classical humanities and philosophy, was particularly sought after by foreigners. In the period 1726–46, he purportedly had more than seventy pupils from abroad staying in his house, many of them English and Scots. The next reading is an account by Gessner of a typical day spent studying with Le Dran.

Exercise

Read 'Surgical instruction in early eighteenth-century Paris' (Source Book 1, Reading 13.6). Was Gessner learning by seeing or by doing?

Discussion

Part of the day was spent watching Le Dran operate, something which Gessner clearly still found fascinating and alarming, although he had been studying Paris surgeons at work for several months. While watching closely what was going on, the pain suffered by the patients worried him. The rest of the time was taken up by practical dissection, which by then had become routine. The extract emphasizes that anatomy students had to work on bodies in various stages of corruption. Such was the popular hostility to dissection that corpses in the eighteenth century were not easy to come by, and Le Dran's pupils had access only to the bodies of patients who died in the Charité. Gessner and his brother learnt by both seeing and doing. Although trained as physicians, they were also not too proud to act as surgeons, and when their cook all but sliced off his thumb during dinner, they had no qualms about binding the wound.

The leading Paris surgeons continued to attract a large clientele in the second half of the eighteenth century. So great was the demand from home students that a number of physicians set up as competitors, notably Antoine Petit (1718–94), the professor of anatomy at the Jardin du Roi, whose skills as a teacher were so outstanding that he could fill his lecture theatre even though he did not provide hands-on instruction. From 1750, too, French medical students began to come to the capital for private courses in the other ancillary medical disciplines, especially chemistry. It had been possible to gain private instruction in chemistry in several university towns in the second half of the seventeenth century – the philosopher John Locke (1632–1704), for one, had attended a course at Oxford. But at that date private tuition in the subject had been sought only by an enthusiastic minority. In the second half of the eighteenth century, in contrast, attendance became *de rigueur*. Few medical students who passed through Paris in the 1750s and 1760s, for instance, failed to attend the highly commended private lectures on chemistry given by the apothecary Guillaume-François Rouelle (1703–70). From the early 1770s, moreover, students were also seeking private clinical instruction in the French capital, something the Paris faculty still conspicuously failed to provide. No longer deeming it sufficient to be attached to an established physician for a couple of years, more and more medical students in the city paid a fee to accompany a hospital doctor on his tour of the wards. Initially, the students were simple spectators – they watched and listened – but on the eve of the Revolution hospital physicians had begun to offer their pupils the chance to care for patients themselves. In a memorandum written long after the Revolution, Chambon de Montaux, whom you have already met, left a graphic account of his approach in the 1780s at the Salpetrière, the city's chief hospital for women. The extract below

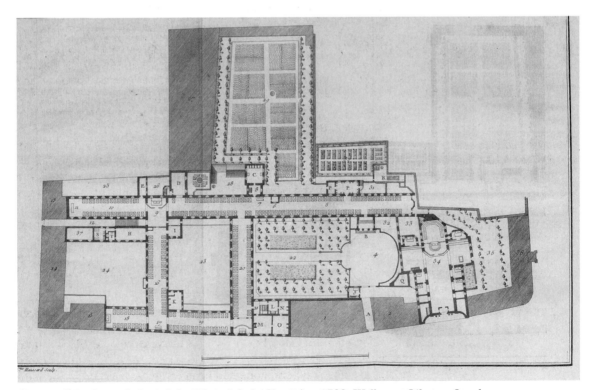

Figure 13.7   Ground-plan of the Hôpital de la Charité, *c*.1788. Wellcome Library, London

suggests that he was already employing the method promoted by Pinel in 1793, which you studied in Reading 13.5:

> Although my duties were totally limited to looking after the sick, I would eagerly seize any opportunity to help the studies of young men who showed the smallest desire to get to grips with the difficulties of their calling. I used to designate one or two patients each to a group of three or four young men, taking care first of all to choose diseases which were the easiest to distinguish and the simplest in their course. The young men would interrogate the patients, render an account of their present condition and its indications, and propose treatment; I would rectify the suggested therapy in making the students understand how it might be defective, insufficient, too active etc.; then I would press them for their reasons for preferring these remedies rather than others.
>
> (Chambon de Montaux, n.d., fol.8v)

As a result of these developments, medical students in Paris in the second half of the eighteenth century spent as much time attending private courses as they did in the faculty. Table 13.3 lists the programme of studies of Guillaume-François Laënnec, a Breton student and uncle of the inventor of the stethoscope, based on the letters he wrote to his father. Laënnec was in Paris from 1769 to 1772. As you can see from Table 13.3, he attended private courses of one kind or another throughout this period, including a number given by Petit.

After 1750, however, Paris was no longer the centre of private instruction in medicine, and the number of foreigners attaching themselves to the city's surgeons declined. Instead, the torch was passed to London, where some 200 physicians and surgeons are known to have given private lectures in medicine, surgery and pharmacy over the following 70 years. A number taught in their own homes or rented accommodation in imitation of the man-midwife William Hunter, who was the extremely rich proprietor of the Windmill Street Academy, founded in 1746. The majority, however, were physicians and surgeons with hospital posts who gave clinical lectures and practical demonstrations in the hospital buildings. At the beginning of the nineteenth century, all the most famous private lecturers were hospital-based, such as Astley Cooper (1768–1841, later knighted), who taught anatomy and surgery at St Thomas's and Guy's from 1797 to 1820, and William Babington (1756–1833), also of Guy's. Indeed, in the early nineteenth century, so many of a hospital's staff were offering permanent courses in some branch of medicine or surgery that a number of London hospitals had become *de facto* medical schools. Around 1815 there seem to have been about 400 students passing through their portals each year (Lawrence, 1996, p.111).

The reason for this explosion of private instruction in London lay in the peculiarly limited availability of institutionalized medical teaching in the British Isles. Apart from the Edinburgh medical faculty, there was no other functioning medical school in Britain and Ireland before 1800. While elsewhere in Europe colleges of surgery had been founded in some numbers, none had been created in Britain. In the mid-eighteenth century, trainee physicians, surgeons and apothecaries (and you will recall that in Britain the distinction between them was fluid) who sought formal

Table 13.3 Guillaume-François Laënnec's programme of extracurricular studies in Paris 1769–72

Year	Subject	Professor	Location
1769			
Spring	Experimental philosophy	Nollet	College of Navarre
	Botany	?	Private garden
	Surgery	?	College of surgery
Autumn	Philosophy	?	?
	Anatomy	Petit	Private theatre
1770			
Winter	Hospital visits*	Maloet/Thierry de Bussy	Charité
	Anatomy	Petit	Private theatre
	Practical anatomy	Sabatier	College of surgery
Spring	Surgical operations	Sabatier	?
	Anatomy/surgery	Petit	Jardin du Roi
Summer	Obstetrics	Petit	Private theatre
	Philosophy	?	?
	Practical midwifery	Solayrès	Private theatre
Autumn	Chemistry	Bucquet	?
	Female/child diseases	Petit	Private theatre
	Anatomy (relation to physiology and medical practice)	Vannier	Petit's theatre
	Surgical operations*	?	Hôtel-Dieu
1771			
Winter	Practical dissection	Sabatier	?
Spring/summer	Botany (× 2)	?	?
	Diseases	Petit	Petit's theatre
Autumn	Chemistry	Viellard	Collège royal
	Practical chemistry/ pharmacy	Mitouart	?
1772			
Winter/spring/summer	Chemistry	Bourdelin	Jardin du Roi

* Laënnec continued to visit patients at the Charité and attend operations at the Hôtel-Dieu thereafter.
(Rouxeau, 1926, pp.26–75)

instruction and private practical tuition usually went abroad, chiefly to Paris and Leiden. From the 1770s, Edinburgh rather than the Continent became the most popular venue for formal medical training, but the Scottish capital offered limited opportunities for hands-on study. London's entrepreneurial physicians and surgeons saw the potential demand and proceeded to fill it. The growing importance of the city's hospitals in providing this instruction reflected their recent foundation or reconstruction and their enlightened management. Newly built and run by lay patrons keen to promote medical knowledge and reform, the London hospitals were much easier to develop into sites of medical education than their mouldering sisters in France, which were controlled by the church. The fact that the staff had to pool the money they received from their private pupils only encouraged the attending physicians and surgeons to offer as many courses as possible in order to maximize their income.

Relations between physicians and surgeons

The growing similarity in the way in which physicians and surgeons were taught tended to erode the traditional distinctions between the two branches of the medical profession and inevitably led to tension. Well-educated surgeons in towns where medical practice was corporatively organized came to resent their inferior status and demanded the right to practise physic alongside the learned physicians. Physicians were equally determined to hold on to their monopoly and objected to the establishment of surgical colleges outside their control. The quarrel was particularly bitter between the two communities in Paris in the second quarter of the eighteenth century. The Parisian surgeons presented themselves as agents of Enlightenment fighting medical obscurantism, and successfully recruited under their banner the *philosophe* Denis Diderot (1713–84), the materialist physician Julien Offray de La Mettrie (1709–51) and the **physiocrat** François Quesnay (1694–1774), doctor to Louis XV's mistress, the Marquise de Pompadour. In general, though, the quarrel did not get out of hand, and even in a city such as London, where the corporative system had effectively broken down, members of the respective royal colleges usually stuck to their traditional last and worked with rather than against one another. Learned surgeons might argue in print in favour of uniting the two branches of the profession and ending the age-old distinction between physic and surgery, but in their professional behaviour they were more circumspect. Normally, if they wanted to practise physic in towns where there were resident physicians (incorporated or no), they regularized their position by taking a degree in medicine. In fact, in the second half of the eighteenth century, the physicians and surgeons had good reason not to push their differences too far. Whatever their mutual hostilities and jealousies, they had a novel need to demonstrate a common front in the light of the unprecedented challenge to their status, income and credibility from unlicensed outsiders.

13.5 The medical marketplace

In previous centuries, the activities of unqualified interlopers had caused licensed practitioners perennial concern, especially if they threatened their livelihood by finding clients among the rich, which they frequently did. Before 1700, however, the competition from quacks was a nuisance that the medical establishment had learned to live with: those who found favour at court usually sought to legitimize their position by purchasing a qualification or licence, while those who concentrated their attentions on the poor were largely ignored. In the eighteenth century, however, the competition stiffened considerably. The number of charlatans seeking custom among the well-to-do soared, while affluent patients were as ready to try the pills and potions of empirics as they were to follow the advice of educated and licensed practitioners. The traditional legal and moral rights of trained practitioners, especially physicians, were accorded less and less respect, and the learned and the unlearned came to occupy a common medical marketplace, where the patient called the tune. Understandably, the medical establishment felt threatened as never before and moaned long and loud about the cold wind of competition, especially as there were now many more graduate physicians trying to make a living than in previous centuries. Books had appeared in the past protesting against the ubiquity and insolence of empirics, but none matched the depths of outrage and despair evinced in works such as *L'Anarchie médicinale ou la médecine considérée comme nuisible à la société* [Anarchy in Medicine or Medicine Believed to Be Damaging to Society], which the Lyon physician and court doctor to the king of Poland, Jean-Emmanuel Gilibert (1741–1814), published in 1772.

One reason for the more positive attitude of the affluent towards empirical healers after 1700 lay in the new persona that many adopted. The majority of eighteenth-century quacks, whether they plied their trade in town or country, undoubtedly closely resembled their predecessors, and were indistinguishable from fairground barkers. Take for instance, 'Le Grand Thomas' (Figure 13.8), who earned a living extracting teeth on the Paris Pont-Neuf for three decades and was known as 'the pearl of charlatans' (Jones, 2000). All over western Europe, however, learned physicians and surgeons were also confronted by a new kind of empirical interloper – one who was a medical gentleman of the road, not a healer in rags or motley. Typical was one Buisson of Avignon, a locksmith by origin. His nefarious activities were reported in a letter of November 1786 written by the physician Esprit Calvet (1728–1810) to the secretary of the Société Royale de Médecine in Paris, Vicq d'Azyr. (Molière, mentioned below, was the pseudonym of Jean Baptiste Poquelin (1622–73), a French playwright of the reign of Louis XIV who satirized both the licensed and unlicensed branches of the medical profession in his comedies, especially *Le Malade imaginaire* of 1673.)

> [Buisson] has suddenly become a doctor by assuming Aesculapius's wand [i.e. the trappings of the profession]. He cures gout in three days, eye diseases in eight, the pox in fifteeen, all by his incomparable powders. I see this man in the morning dressed soberly in black, a ring on his finger [physicians were presented with a ring when they graduated], cane in his hand, doing the round of his patients. It is a spectacle which reminds me of a Molière comedy.
>
> (Brockliss, 2002, p.169).

Furthermore, besides dressing and behaving more decorously, this new breed of charlatan peddled his wares in a more acceptable fashion. Whereas the sixteenth

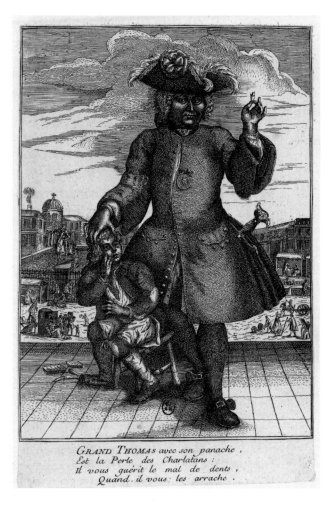

GRAND THOMAS avec son panache,
Est la Perle des Charlatans :
Il vous guérit le mal de dents,
Quand il vous les arrache.

Figure 13.8 *Le Grand Thomas*, c.1729.
Bibliothèque Nationale de France, Paris: D
269851

and seventeenth centuries had witnessed the creation and consolidation of the book trade, the eighteenth gave birth to the newspaper and the magazine as part of an ever-expanding and ever more accessible culture of print. Both served not simply to disseminate news, but also to disseminate goods, forging what Colin Jones has called 'The Great Chain of Buying' (Jones, 1996). Newspapers and magazines oiled the wheels of eighteenth-century consumerism through advertising a wide variety of wares and acting as mail-order catalogues. The new media were manna to the 'professional' charlatan: instead of vulgarly hawking his services in the street, he availed himself of the newspaper to announce his itinerary or sell his remedies to respectable clients. The more entrepreneurial among them even established a network of agents across a country, who acted as their surrogates, taking orders, giving medical advice and distributing their products. While Buisson of Avignon was no more than a local nuisance, the Ailhaud family in the neighbouring town of Carpentras was an international headache. In the 1730s, Jean Ailhaud (1684–1756) had begun to manufacture purgative powders, which, he claimed, were a panacea. His successor turned the business into a Europe-wide enterprise with agents in Paris, Strasbourg and Marseille, who themselves had their own sales representatives in neighbouring states. Sales were boosted by a twelve-volume pseudo-scientific publication called *Médecine universelle prouvée par le raisonnement et démontrée par l'expérience* [Universal Medicine Proved by Reason and Demonstrated by Experience] (1764–74), in which the virtues of the remedy were attested to by grateful clients. By the 1770s, Ailhaud's son was selling some 400,000 boxes (with 10 doses in each) every year. Table 13.4 reveals that his French patients were far from a bunch of ignorant yokels. Roughly 40 per cent hailed from large cities and 30 per cent from middling towns, while many clients were nobles or professional men. (The titles *noblesse d'épee* and *noblesse de robe* denote different classes of aristocrats and nobles.)

At the same time, the elite's willingness to be conned by unlicensed healers was encouraged by their raised expectations with regard to health. The booming consumer economy in most parts of western Europe after 1730, the concomitant growth in the standard of living of the middle and upper classes, and the dissemination of the Enlightenment belief in progress, all promoted the conviction that discomfort was the wages of poverty not affluence, and that disease, especially chronic disease, might be easily overcome. This new view of illness gave quacks a decided market advantage, in that they tended to offer painless, instantaneous and permanent cures for cash. Licensed practitioners, in contrast, frequently expected patients to suffer at length in return for their healing services, even to the extent of withdrawing from society for several months.

A growing lay scepticism, too, about the efficacy of learned medicine and the importance of therapeutic experimentation only helped to legitimize such apostacy. The French *philosophe* Diderot argued strenuously that there was much to be said for the empirical healer:

> I have sometimes thought that the charlatans who inhabit the suburbs of the large towns were not as pernicious as was supposed. It is empiricism which has given birth to medicine and it is only through empiricism that it can really expect to progress. An incurable patient at the centre of a family is like a dead tree at the centre of a garden, whose poisoned roots are fatal to all the bushes which surround them; the cares which tenderness and pity cannot refuse a sick old man [or] a languishing child, upset duty's routine and spread a blight on the day of those who proffer them; the bold empiric whom the patient summons when he is abandoned by the faculty physician either kills or heals him and gives back the joy of living to those who looked after him.
>
> (Diderot, 1875–7, p.499)

As a result of such views, learned, even supposedly expert, practitioners were often regarded with a great deal of suspicion, especially when patients felt themselves to be well informed about the medical art.

Table 13.4   Users of Jean Ailhaud's purgative powders, 1724–54

	No.	*%*
Location (*n* = 130)		
Cities over 50,000	25	19.2
Cities 20,000–50,000	26	20.0
Cities 5,000–20,000	37	28.5
Cities 2,000–5,000	13	10.0
Other locations	29	22.3
Gender (*n* = 163)		
Men	142	87.1
Women	21	12.9
Occupation (*n* = 128)		
Church	37*	28.9
noblesse d'épee	9†	7.0
noblesse de robe		
High	5	3.9
Middling and low	20‡	15.6
Professions		
Military	20	15.6
Medical	8	6.3
Law	5	3.9
Other	5	3.9
Business	12§	9.4
Foreign diplomats	4	3.1
High domesticity	3	2.3

* of whom six were women
† of whom one was a woman
‡ of whom two were women
§ of whom one was a woman
(Brockliss and Jones, 1997, p.654)

Exercise

Read 'Popular criticism of the medical profession: Tobias Smollett's *Humphry Clinker* (1771)' (Source Book 1, Reading 13.7). What does the extract reveal about the English gentry's attitude to educated medical practitioners in the second half of the eighteenth century?

The extract suggests that an English country gentleman in this period believed he knew as much about his own body and its ills as any doctor. Bramble has read widely about the virtues of the Bristol Hot Wells and is caustic about their medical value. When one of the physicians practising at the spa informs him he is dropsical, he treats the individual and the diagnosis with contempt. Bramble might be suffering from swollen ankles but he lacks the classic symptom of dropsy – a swollen belly – so the physician's judgement is dismissed as absurd. On the surface, the sturdy commonsensical tone of Bramble's letter invites the contemporary reader to take his side and agree that the eighteenth-century learned medical profession has little to recommend it. On the other hand, the more discerning would have understood that they were meant to be amused, not convinced by Bramble's critique. You will have noted that the letter is written to a medical practitioner, Dr Lewis, who was not only Bramble's friend but his medical crutch. Bramble was not as self-confident as he seemed and needed Lewis's confirmation that his view of the Bristol physician was correct. We do not know what Lewis replied, but it is likely that Bramble was civilly put in his place.

Furthermore, the learned physicians connived at boundary-breaking by often accepting that the science of therapeutics was far from perfect. Esprit Calvet of Avignon declared that even the handful of remedies known as specifics (drugs supposedly useful in curing particular diseases, such as quinine in the treatment of malaria) were of limited value:

> The small number of helpful drugs that we call specifics are not always so. We have shortened our life by remedies. What does a sick animal do? It lies down, it doesn't eat, it doesn't work, and either recovers or doesn't without joy or regret. A consultation by several doctors, especially for an important patient, is always dangerous, often deadly, but commonly laughable.
>
> (quoted in Brockliss, 2002, pp.151–2)

Calvet's convictions were shared by his contemporary, the vitalist professor of Montpellier, Paul-Joseph Barthez (1734–1806), who in his course of therapeutics delivered at the faculty argued that the science was still in its infancy. If he fell short of Diderot's faith in the art of the empiric, he certainly recognized that the learned physician did not have a monopoly in understanding the cure of disease. Medical training could dull rather than sharpen the ability to choose the right remedy, with the result that 'savages who have not had their faculties enfeebled by learning have their own natural resources which are more certain than ours' (Barthez, n.d., fol.16).

Empirical healers became even more acceptable to the extent that many licensed practitioners in search of lucrative clients began to ape the behaviour of the new professional interlopers. Recognizing the growing market for new wonder drugs, they developed their own specifics and puffed them in a variety of often spectacular ways. In 1773, for instance, the Paris physician Guilbert de Préval (*c.*1730–88) demonstrated the efficacy of his *prophylactique anti-vénérienne* (supposedly a lotion that prevented the user from contracting a venereal disease) by anointing himself with the substance, then having sex with a hideously diseased prostitute. Some licensed practitioners made vast fortunes from their entrepreneurial activities, especially in England where the commercial opportunities were much greater than elsewhere. Among London's many learned medical impresarios, none was more daring and imaginative than James Graham MD (1745–94), the owner of the Temple of Health in the Adelphi and later Pall Mall. Graham was a saddler's son born in Edinburgh, who studied at his home university, temporarily migrated to the American colonies, then practised in various English towns before setting himself up in the capital in about 1780. A passionate advocate of the powers of electrotherapy, he used saturation newspaper advertising to trumpet its efficacy and encourage the public to watch the maestro at work. His medical emporium was a box of delights where patients and visitors were treated to magical tableaux, sweet smells and enchanting sounds. Graham's *pièce de résistance* was his magnetized Grand Celestial Bed, where married couples could revive dampened physical ardour for a princely sum. Many of Graham's clients came from the cream of high society and included Georgiana, Duchess of Devonshire, who consulted him on her failure to produce a child after five years of marriage.

Exercise

Read 'Alternative therapies in Georgian England: James Graham's Celestial Bed' (Source Book 1, Reading 13.8). What does Roy Porter suggest were Graham's motives as a sex therapist?

Discussion

Porter cites other works by Graham to argue that the empiric was not selling exotic sex but believed his bed would play a part in regenerating the human species. In a later part of his analysis, he shows that Graham was alarmed by the frailty of the eighteenth-century physique and put this down to lacklustre sex. Too many males were wasting their precious seed in masturbation and too many couples had lost the ability to produce wholesome offspring – or any offspring at all. The sensual atmosphere in which the bed was placed and the enveloping magnetic effluvia would stimulate marital passion and ensure pregnancy by guaranteeing mutual orgasm (which some in the eighteenth century still believed was essential for conception).

Graham may have honestly believed in the message he peddled in his self-publicizing tracts, but he may simply have been manipulating the contemporary mood. All over Europe in the third quarter of the eighteenth century, governments and their advisers were told, quite wrongly, by the first demographers that the population was in free-fall. At the same time, a masturbation panic swept through the Continent, fired by the pamphlets of the Swiss physician Samuel Tissot

(1728–93) and the English Methodist John Wesley (1703–91), while killjoys lambasted the deleterious effects of taking coffee, tea and tobacco. Given the number of landed couples who found difficulty in this or any period of producing a male heir, it cannot have been too difficult for the unscrupulous practitioner to weave a convincing narrative from these different threads and entice the rich into his Celestial Bed.

Not surprisingly, the more conservative physicians and surgeons took umbrage at the activities of these medical entrepreneurs, whatever their background, accused them of charlatanism, and tried to ban their products or curtail their practice. Usually, on the Continent, they gained the support of the government. Keen to promote a healthy population, as we have seen, the prince and his advisers were normally nervous of a medical free-for-all, whatever their suspicions of traditional medicine. From the late 1760s in Brunswick, for instance, private agents were banned from distributing Ailhaud's powders and their sale became a government monopoly (Lindemann, 1996, pp.175–8). Frequently, though (and not just in London), it proved impossible to clamp down on the most successful quacks. Even more than in previous centuries, they had powerful protectors. In the new health-obsessed atmosphere of the eighteenth century, courtiers and female royalty frequently threw caution to the winds and continually undermined the valiant attempts of Continental governments to police the activities of medical interlopers.

13.6 Conclusion

From what you have read in this chapter, it should be evident that there was a growing discrepancy in the eighteenth century between the way in which health care was organized in theory and the reality on the ground. For a number of interrelated reasons – political, economic and cultural – the foundations of the traditional structure were seriously sapped. In many parts of the Continent, the corporative organization was subject to growing government interference, partly for fiscal and ideological reasons, but also in the hope of creating healthier subjects and fitter soldiers. In addition, in the more economically prosperous regions of Europe, the corporative organization was undermined by a new consumerism that bred unrealistic health expectations. However, the key agent of subversion was the Enlightenment. By emphasizing the possibility of moral and material progress and insisting that the state should promote the individual good, the *philosophes* helped to create a new mentality among Europe's educated elite, which made health a much more important public and personal issue. The Enlightenment impacted, too, on the traditional medical hierarchy by promoting an epistemology of science based on experimentation and experience, and privileging learning by doing and seeing, which in turn helped to erode the distinction between physicians and surgeons.

Nonetheless, on the eve of the French Revolution, the traditional corporate structure still held together, however fractured it had become. Indeed, even in Britain, a country where the system had only ever been half-heartedly imposed, the distinctions between physicians, surgeons and apothecaries, and between quacks and orthodox practitioners, continued to have meaning. By then, though, a number of learned physicians and surgeons, especially those associated with the

Continental academies who felt they were the government-appointed guardians of health care, had had enough of the way their position was being undermined by interlopers. Unlike Gilibert, they were not content to wring their hands but began to debate and publish reform plans. Moved by the humanitarian ideals of the Enlightenment, and confident that scientific medicine, whatever its deficiencies, was the only safe underpinning of medical practice, they sought to outlaw and isolate the charlatans and empirics by establishing a more national and inclusive health-care system, where trained practitioners would look after the whole population. The outbreak of the French Revolution and the subsequent abolition of all *ancien régime* institutions offered one nation the opportunity to place health-care reform firmly on the political agenda.

References

Barthez, P-J. (n.d.) *Cours de thérapeutique*, Bibliothèque Municipale Montpellier, MS 256.

Brockliss, L.W.B. (2002) *Calvet's Web: Enlightenment and the Republic of Letters in Eighteenth-Century France*, Oxford: Oxford University Press.

Brockliss, L.W.B. and Jones, C. (1997) *The Medical World of Early Modern France*, Oxford: Clarendon Press.

Bynum, W. (1985) 'Physicians, hospitals and career structures in eighteenth-century London' in W. Bynum and R.S. Porter (eds) *William Hunter and the Eighteenth-Century Medical World*, Cambridge: Cambridge University Press, pp.105–28.

Bynum, W. and Porter, R.S. (eds) (1985) *William Hunter and the Eighteenth-Century Medical World*, Cambridge: Cambridge University Press.

Chambon de Montaux, N. (n.d.) *Remarques sur le mode de l'enseignement de la médecine clinique*, Bibliothèque de la Faculté de Paris, MS 5143, separately foliated.

Chambon de Montaux, N. (1813) *Remarques sur les dangers auxquels les anatomistes sont exposés en disséquant*, Bibliothèque de la Faculté de Médecine de Paris, MS 5143, separately foliated.

Diderot, D. (1875–7) 'Plan d'une université pour le gouvernement de la Russie' in *Denis Diderot: Oeuvres complètes*, ed. by J. Assézat, 20 vols, Paris: J. Claye, vol.3, pp.429–534.

Gelfand, T. (1980) *Professionalizing Modern Medicine: Paris Surgeons and Medical Science and Institutions in the Eighteenth Century*, Westport: Greenwood Press.

Gentilcore, D. (1998) *Healers and Healing in Early Modern Italy*, Manchester: Manchester University Press.

Goubert, J-P. (1974) *Malades et médecins en Bretagne, 1770–1790*, Rennes: Université de Bretagne.

Jones, C. (1996) 'The Great Chain of Buying: medical advertisement, the bourgeois public sphere and the origins of the French Revolution', *American Historical Review*, vol.101, pp.13–40.

Jones, C. (2000) 'Pulling teeth in eighteenth-century Paris', *Past and Present*, vol.166, pp.100–45.

Keel, O. (2001) *L'Avènement de la médecine clinique en Europe, 1750–1815*, Quebec: Les Presses de l'Université de Montréal.

Lawrence, S. (1996) *Charitable Knowledge: Hospital Pupils and Practitioners in Eighteenth-Century London*, Cambridge: Cambridge University Press.

Lebrun, F. (1975) *Les Hommes et la mort en Anjou au XVII siècles*, Paris: Flammarion.

Lindemann, M. (1996) *Health and Healing in Eighteenth-Century Germany*, Baltimore: Johns Hopkins University Press.

Porter, R.S. (1989) *Health for Sale: Quackery in England 1660–1850*, Manchester: Manchester University Press.

Porter, R. (1999) *The Greatest Benefit to Mankind: A Medical History of Humanity from Antiquity to the Present*, London: Fontana.

Porter, R.S. and Porter, D. (1988) *In Sickness and in Health: The British Experience, 1650–1850*, London: Fourth Estate.

Porter, R.S. and Porter, D. (1989) *Patient's Progress: Doctors and Doctoring in Eighteenth-Century England*, Oxford: Polity Press.

Ramsey, M. (1991) *Professional and Popular Medicine in France, 1770–1830: The Social World of Medical Practice*, Cambridge: Cambridge University Press.

Risse, G. (1986) *Hospital Life in Enlightenment Scotland: Care and Teaching at the Royal Infirmary of Edinburgh*, Cambridge: Cambridge University Press.

Rouxeau, A. (1926) *Un étudiant en médecine quimpérois (Guillaume-François Laennec) aux derniers jours de l'Ancien Régime*, Nantes.

Source Book readings

Sir G. Clark, *A History of the Royal College of Physicians of London*, 2 vols, Oxford: Clarendon Press, 1964–6, vol.2, pp.476–9 (Reading 13.1).

L.W.B. Brockliss and C. Jones, *The Medical World of Early Modern France*, Oxford: Clarendon Press, 1997, pp.578–81 (Reading 13.2).

'Letter of Georg Spangenberg to the Collegium Medicum of Braunschweig (May 1747)' in M. Lindemann, *Health and Healing in Eighteenth-Century Germany*, Baltimore and London: Johns Hopkins University Press, 1996, pp.3–6 (Reading 13.3).

J. Barbot, *Les Chroniques de la Faculté de Médecine de Toulouse du XIIIe au XIXe Siècle*, 2 vols, Toulouse: Dirion, 1905, vol.1, pp.270–2. Translation by Elizabeth Rabone (Reading 13.4).

P. Pinel, *The Clinical Training of Doctors: An Essay of 1793*, ed. and translated by D.B. Wiener, Baltimore and London: Johns Hopkins University Press, 1988, pp.77–9, 85–93 (Reading 13.5).

J. Gessner, *Pariser Tagebuch 1727*, ed. and translated by U. Boschung, Bern: Hans Huber, 1985, pp.352–3. Translation by Rod Boroughs (Reading 13.6).

T. Smollett, *The Expedition of Humphry Clinker*, 1st edn 1771, Harmondsworth: Penguin, 1985, pp.51–3 (Reading 13.7).

R. Porter, *Health for Sale: Quackery in England, 1650–1850*, Manchester and New York: Manchester University Press, 1989, pp.161–2 (Reading 13.8).

Glossary

absolute state a European state in the seventeenth and eighteenth centuries where the will of the ruler was not legally checked by any representative assembly and where the prince was above the law. Absolute rulers were not tyrants: they believed they had to obey God's laws and rule for the general good. Nor were they as powerful as they wished to be, given that they all had to rule to a greater or lesser extent through the many corporative institutions established over the centuries which claimed a share in public authority.

absolutist see **absolute state**.

acute when used of a disease, it means coming to a crisis; it usually implies that the disease or injury is treatable and of finite duration, as opposed to **chronic**.

adepts scholars with a special expertise in a given field; exceptionally skilled operators or thinkers, whose knowledge was considered by some to be partly God-given.

ancien régime specifically, the social, political and administrative system of France in the seventeenth and eighteenth centuries. As an adjective, it has come to be used to describe any privileged or corporate institution of the **early modern** era.

Apocrypha those books of the Bible whose authenticity was not accepted by the Protestant reformers.

aqua vitae literally 'water of life', a strong distilled spirit.

archei see ***archeus***.

archeus the governing principle of bodily dysfunction. Originally devised by Paracelsus as a term to describe how disease and health were regulated in the various parts of the body, van Helmont elaborated the concept to include a specific chemical and spiritual function for the *archeus*. According to van Helmont, once disturbed, the *archeus* formed an 'idea' of disease that was transformed by the power of the **imagination** into a real physical ailment. Suitable medicines thus helped to pacify the *archeus*.

Arianism a fourth-century heresy, named after its founder, Arius, which questioned the divinity of Christ and the Trinity. It was revived in the sixteenth century by, among others, the physician Michael Servetus, who was executed for holding such views in Calvinist Geneva in 1553.

arterial relating to the arteries. In Galenic medical theory, arterial blood was blood mixed with ***pneuma***, which endowed the body with vitality via the arteries – a system of vessels entirely independent from the veins.

auricle literally something shaped like the lobe of the ear; the atriums of the heart were identified as the left or right auricles of the heart.

Ayurveda 'the science of life', based on classical Indian texts.

azygos Greek for 'without a pair'; in the **early modern** period, the azygos vein was believed to issue from the **vena cava** in the **thoracic** region.

Baconian during the first half of the seventeenth century, the English natural philosopher Francis Bacon (1561–1626) laid down a new approach to the study of nature, which emphasized the virtues of empirical observation and experimentation over book-learning, and argued that its underlying rationale was public utility. In the process, he was lauded as a the prophet of the 'moderns' in their struggle with the authority of ancient writers, thinkers and natural philosophers, whose works still formed the basis of most university curricula until the middle decades of the seventeenth century.

basilic vein part of the axillary vein (vein of the inner side of the arm); the right-hand basilic vein was believed to be connected to the liver, and the left-hand vein to the spleen.

Belvedere torso Roman statue of the first century CE, which came to light in 1503 and was believed to represent the body of Hercules. It was displayed in the Belvedere Gallery of the Vatican Museum, and quickly became one of the most famous fragments of antique sculpture.

bezoar a concretion found in the digestive organs of ruminant animals and supposedly effective against poisons.

bile in **early modern** medicine, a term used for either of two (out of the four) bodily **humours**; in modern understanding, it is a thick, bitter fluid secreted by the liver as an aid to digestion.

Black Death the name by which historians (contemporaries did not use it) refer to the plague epidemic that scourged Europe between 1348 and 1350.

blas the life force, which, according to van Helmont, oversaw the smooth running of all the parts of the body and regulated health.

bregma part of the skull where the frontal and the two parietal (side and top) bones join.

buboes plural of bubo, an inflammatory swelling usually located in the armpits or the groin, which was regarded as one of the main physical symptoms of the plague.

Byzantine relating to Byzantium, the name given to the eastern half of the Roman Empire, after it had been divided into two in 395. The Western Empire was in ruins within a century, but the Eastern (Byzantine) Empire continued until 1453, when it succumbed to the Ottoman Turks.

calendar reform the reform of the calendrical system, which was spearheaded by the church. The Julian calendar, which had been used in Europe since 46 BCE, had 365 days, with every fourth year designated a leap year (with one extra day in February). This resulted in the Julian year being approximately eleven minutes longer than the actual solar year; or a gain of about three days per 400 years. By the end of the fifteenth century, it was known that the slippage was such that the spring equinox was out of line from 21 March by about 10 days or so, and the Roman Catholic church had been asking astronomers to rectify this problem. The reform of the calendar was finally instituted by Pope Gregory XIII in 1582. It was not adopted in Britain until the eighteenth century.

cameralist an enlightened writer or *philosophe* with a specific interest in social policy. The term comes from the Latin word *camera* ('chamber') and refers to the room in the castle from which the prince or landlords managed their state/estates.

capillaries extremely small vessels that carry blood between the veins and the arteries. Capillaries form a fine network throughout the body's organs and tissues.

Castile in the eighteenth century, Spain consisted of two kingdoms – Castile and Aragon – that had united in the late fifteenth century. They did not always have the same institutions and there had never been a united *cortes*, or parliament.

cautery the therapeutic application of heated instruments to the skin.

chronic when used of a disease, it means deep-seated or long continued, as opposed to **acute**.

churching the service that took place when a woman went to church for the first time after giving birth. It has been interpreted as evidence of the belief that the woman needed purification, but also as signalling the conclusion of an all-female practice and the re-establishment of male hegemony.

city state an independent and ideally self-sufficient community that controlled both an urban centre and its agricultural hinterland.

complexion the particular balance of the **qualities** in an individual human body. Also called temperament or constitution.

compound fracture a fracture that breaks the skin and thus becomes liable to infection; also known as an open fracture.

comuni plural of *comune*, a small, self-governing territorial division; in medieval Italy, it comprised a city and the countryside immediately surrounding it, and was usually governed by councils of notable citizens (usually merchants).

consilium (plural *consilia*) literally 'letter of counsel'; a written report of an individual medical case, which usually included a description of it together with a prescription for its treatment.

constitution see **complexion**.

Council of Trent the church council called by Pope Paul III to reform the Catholic church; named after the place where it first met in 1545. Its decisions formed the cornerstone of the **Counter-Reformation**.

Counter-Reformation often referred to by historians today as the Catholic Reformation or the response of the Roman Catholic church to the spread of

Protestantism. The prime thrust of the movement was conservative and defensive. At the **Council of Trent** (1545–63), various measures were agreed, including the creation of an **Index** of prohibited books and the extension of the powers of the **Inquisition**. It also granted extensive supervisory powers to the order of the Society of Jesus (the Jesuits), particularly in relation to all aspects of education.

dissection   the act or art of cutting into parts the dead body of an animal or human, for the purpose of close examination.

doctrine of signatures   the belief that a plant that looks like a part of the body will be able to cure diseases incident to it. The idea was rooted in the concept, widely shared by Paracelsians, that the natural world was full of such correspondences, which provided evidence of the divine nature of the creation.

dura   outer membrane of the brain.

early modern   in Europe, this is defined by historians as the period from around 1500 to around 1800. Like all such periodization, its boundaries are flexible and to an extent arbitrary.

effluvia   minute particles that flow out of bodies, usually revealed by the presence of an odour, either pleasant or unpleasant.

eirenicist   as a result of the confessional disputes and wars of religion that tore Europe apart in the sixteenth century, there emerged in some quarters a growing belief in the need for some form of religious reconciliation (eirenicism), whereby the proponents of the various faiths might live in harmony with each other. Though such ideas proved especially attractive in central Europe, eirenicism remained an aspiration rather than a reality for much of the period, and religious conflict was the norm.

elector of Brandenburg   Brandenburg-Prussia was a composite state where the ruler had a variety of different titles; he only became king of Prussia in the early eighteenth century. The electors of the **Holy Roman Empire** were the princes who chose the emperor, an elective office.

electuary   a medicinal paste or conserve; could be produced with different substances, but usually included honey.

elements   according to Aristotle, the elements are: earth, air, water and fire. These four are the basic constituents of natural things beneath the sphere of the moon. Objects above the sphere of the moon were made of the fifth element, ether.

elixir vitriol   concentrated sulphuric acid.

empirics   healers without formal medical qualifications, who relied on experiential trial and error, rather than on mastery of causes and general principles, which characterized learned medical knowledge. 'Empirics' and 'quacks' were common names given to unorthodox healers, village wise-women or cunning-folk by learned physicians, who sought to control medical practice.

Encyclopédie a huge compilation of **Enlightenment** ideals and knowledge published in France in twenty-one volumes between 1751 and 1765.

Enlightenment an intellectual movement that emerged around the mid-eighteenth century. At its core was the belief that under the rule of reason and science, the economic and social conditions of humanity would steadily progress, and control over nature would be enhanced.

epizootics epidemic diseases affecting animals.

essentialist the idea that certain ideas or phenomena have remained unchanged in their essence over the centuries.

expectorant a medicine that helps to loosen phlegm in the chest.

femoral artery artery supplying the femur, or thigh bone.

fistulae plural of fistula, an abnormal passage between an organ (usually the anus) and the skin.

fomentation the application of a warm lotion to the body for medical purposes.

forceps a pincer-like instrument with two blades, for holding, lifting or removing.

gas van Helmont was the first to use the term 'gas', though he did so in a way that defies our modern understanding of the term. Rather than equating it with the atmospheric air, van Helmont invoked the term to describe a range of spiritual and chemical processes in the body that facilitated everyday bodily functions such as digestion.

gender a category introduced in the 1960s to discuss the multiple cultural and social meanings attributed to sexual difference (i.e. anatomical and physiological differences between the sexes) in different societies. Gender studies focus on the social and cultural factors that give shape to both male and female identity and roles. The assumption is that masculinity and femininity are highly complex and historically specific phenomena, which are defined in relation to each other.

general practitioner a state-salaried physician and first point of referral for sick members of the community.

gossips female friends who assisted and gave support to a woman in labour.

Habsburg the dynasty that since the thirteenth century ruled the territory of what is now Austria; in the **early modern** period, the dynasty also nominally ruled the **Holy Roman Empire**.

hagiographer a writer of saints' lives.

hermetic pertaining to the mythical sage Hermes Trismegistus.

Holy Roman Empire designation for the political entity that covered a large portion of Europe from 962 to 1806. The name was intended to revive the grandeur of the Roman Empire, which in 395 had been divided into two: the Western and the Eastern (**Byzantine**) Empires. The Western Empire was in ruins within a century. In 800, Charlemagne, the ruler of Franconia (parts of what are now France and Germany), received from the pope the title of emperor. Franconia itself later divided in two (the kingdoms of France and of Germany), but in 962, Otto I, ruler of the German kingdom, named himself as emperor of the Holy Roman Empire. The territorial limits of the empire varied over time, but it generally included Germany, Austria, Bohemia and Moravia, parts of northern Italy, present-day Belgium, and, until 1648, the Netherlands and Switzerland.

hôtel-dieu   the name given to the poor house established in most French towns in the **Middle Ages** to shelter the old and infirm. These ancient hospices still existed in the eighteenth century, although they were by then only one of several hospitals in the large cities.

Huguenot   name given to the French followers of the Protestant reformer Jean Calvin (1509–64); French Calvinists.

humanism   broadly speaking, the name given to the movement in learned circles during the **Renaissance** to revive the literary legacy of the ancient Greeks and Romans.

humours   the four fluids whose balance determined the bodily state: yellow **bile**, black bile, phlegm and pure blood. The blood in the veins was made up of the pure humour, blood, mixed with a lesser proportion of the other humours. Yellow bile (also known as red bile or choler) was believed to be found in the gallbladder, and to purify the blood. Black bile (also known as melancholy) was believed to be manufactured in the liver and received by the spleen, and to fortify the blood. Phlegm was a colourless or whitish secretion often associated with the brain. Each humour had a pair of **qualities** associated with it. The humours found expression in the **complexion** that marked an individual, and gave rise to different temperaments, with the predominant humour determining an individual's character. Thus people were classified as choleric (hot-headed and quick to react); melancholic (sad and low-spirited); phlegmatic (lethargic and apathetic); and sanguine (warm and pleasant).

hypochondrium   upper part of the abdomen.

hysteria   from the Greek word for uterus, it has been used since ancient times to define an allegedly typical female disorder. Descriptions of it have changed enormously over time, though the core symptoms included cramps in the abdomen, oppression and a sense of suffocation. In earlier times, these were thought to be linked to movements of the womb, and later, to uterine and menstrual disorders and the general weakness of the female nervous constitution.

iatrochemical revolution   iatrochemistry is the name given by scholars to the medical doctrine, promulgated in the sixteenth and seventeenth centuries, that emphasized the theoretical and practical benefits of medicines produced by chemical procedures. There were various schools of iatrochemical thought, including the Paracelsian and Helmontian, and the term is used in this book as a generic description of the practices and beliefs of these various groups. The term itself derives from the Greek word for physician, *iatros*.

imagination   van Helmont postulated an extremely close relationship between mind and body, arguing that one's mental condition and attitude to sickness played a crucial part in promoting health or causing disease. Many of his medicines were aimed at reinforcing the natural faculty of the imagination in preserving bodily health.

Index   the *Index Librorum Prohibitorum* [Index of Prohibited Books] was established in 1559 by Pope Paul IV as part of a rearguard attempt by the Catholic church to counter the threat of Protestantism and other heresies. Books placed on the Index were, in theory at least, proscribed in Catholic lands on pain of a range of ecclesiastical punishments.

indulgence   in the Catholic church, the remission given to repentant sinners of the punishments that were due to them.

infusion   the liquor obtained from the solution in water of an organic, usually a vegetable, substance.

Inquisition   an ecclesiastical tribunal originally established in the thirteenth century to fight heresies; after the **Reformation** it was reorganized and became one of the main weapons of the Catholic church for the discovery, repression and punishment of all kinds of religious dissent.

kirk sessions   parochial church courts of the Scottish Calvinist church or kirk. Composed of a minister and lay elders (usually substantial landowners or townsmen), they met at least once a week to oversee local ecclesiastical administration and moral discipline. Typically, they dealt with sexual offences, drunkenness, doctrinal error and profanation of the sabbath.

landgrave   princely title, equivalent to count, in Germany.

lay people   a term originally used to denote people who were not clergy in the church, but increasingly used (especially by historians) to refer to people who had no scientific training, or who did not have technical or professional qualifications in an area of specialized expertise, such as medicine.

liberal arts   seven subjects that made up a student's initial studies in a medieval university, before they proceeded to studies in the 'higher' faculties, such as law, theology or medicine. Students first studied the trivium (grammar, rhetoric and logic) and then the quadrivium (arithmetic, geometry, astronomy and music).

lithotomists   practitioners who specialized in cutting out kidney stones, a painful and extremely common ailment.

Lutheran Protestantism   the particular branch of Protestantism which followed the teachings of Martin Luther and Philip Melanchthon, and which, with its emphasis on faith, grace and the pure Word of God (i.e. the Bible, in the best translation from the best sources), was of paramount importance for Protestantism during the first decades of the **Reformation**.

materia medica   literally, 'the matter of medicine' – that is, the constituent parts of plants, herbs and other natural products, that were used in the composition of medicines. They could be used on their own, as 'simples', or could be mixed together to produce compounds.

medical semiotics   the theory and art of reading and interpreting bodily signs to make a diagnosis.

Methodists   founded by the Anglican preacher John Wesley (1703–91), the Methodists were an evangelical sect who rejected many of the established conventions of eighteenth-century religion and continued to believe in the existence of an active devil, witches and spirits.

Middle Ages   roughly, the period from the fall of the old Roman Empire (*c*.450 CE) to the onset of the **Renaissance** (*c*.1400).

morbific   disease-causing.

natural philosophy   a discipline created around the time when universities were founded in Europe, in the late twelfth century. Based on the writings of Aristotle, it was a Christian study of nature that dealt with subjects as diverse as the heavens, weather, the elements, motion, putrefaction and the soul. Fundamental to this discipline was the idea that nature was God's creation. Historians nowadays distinguish natural philosophy from both modern science (a wholly secular branch of study) and the ancient science of the Greeks (who practised a different form of religion).

Neoplatonism   the revival of the ideas of the Greek philosopher Plato (*c*.429–347 BCE) in the third century CE. It developed the mystical and religious aspects of Plato's thought, and placed them in a Christian context. In particular, it stressed the importance of spiritual forces in the universe and the intellectual capacity of the soul to aspire to divine wisdom.

Neoplatonic   pertaining to **Neoplatonism**.

Nestorian   relating to the teachings of Nestorius, a fifth-century patriarch of Constantinople, who claimed that the divinity and humanity of Christ were not united in a single personality.

ninety-five theses   the theses that Luther published for debate on 31 October 1517 and which have come to be seen as the beginning of the **Reformation**. In them Luther queried the claims of preachers to be able to remit sins, especially through the sale of letters of **indulgence**.

non-naturals   Galen listed six major causes that affected the **humours** all the time: surroundings (e.g. air); exercise (walks, riding, massages and sex); sleep (and waking); ingested substances (food, drink, medicine); those things that are eliminated or retained (secretions and excretions); and the 'passions of the soul' (emotional states such as anger, grief and envy). These six causes were given the name of 'non-natural' by Johannitius in his introduction to Galen's *Art of Medicine*, in order to stress the point that these causes were not internal to the human body. Managing the non-naturals was an important part of a Galenic physician's treatment.

occult sciences   the occult sciences – alchemy, astrology and natural magic – underwent an important revival in the **Renaissance**, when the rediscovery of various manuscripts purportedly written by an ancient seer, Hermes Trismegistus, became fused with the works of medieval, Jewish and Arab scholars. The result was an enormous upsurge of interest in these subjects as scholars sought to utilize this new wisdom in order to uncover the mysteries of the natural world.

ossicle   a small bone.

ostiola   literally 'little doors'; refers to the structures in the veins now known as valves, which were discovered by Fabricius, and which he believed functioned to delay blood flow.

oviparous   egg-laying.

Paracelsiana   one of the great problems surrounding Paracelsus and his legacy concerns the extent to which modern scholars have been able to attribute those works published in his name after 1560 to the Swiss physician. Much that circulated under Paracelsus' name was probably the work of his followers, or represents their interpretation of his manuscript writings. The problem is further compounded by the fact that Paracelsus himself often wrote in a deliberately esoteric and mystical vein, inventing new terms and phrases that often defy translation.

parlement **of Paris**   the senior legal body in *ancien régime* France. Among other things, it registered royal edicts and oversaw appeals from regional *parlements*. It should not be confused with the English/British Parliament in this period, since its political powers were severely circumscribed.

patristic   referring to the church fathers – that is, the early leaders of the Christian church in the centuries immediately following the death of Christ, whose writings were frequently invoked as authoritative in the **Middle Ages** and **Renaissance**. The two most cited were St Augustine and St Jerome.

pharmacopoeia   official publication of drugs, describing their ingredients and composition.

philosophe   an eighteenth-century intellectual, such as Voltaire or Rousseau, critical of the church and the social and legal system, who wanted to create a more egalitarian and secular society.

phlebotomy   from the Greek *phlebos*, meaning 'vein'; the practice of letting blood from the veins, using a small sharp knife called a lancet. Also known as **venesection**.

physiocrat   a *philosophe* with a particular interest in the mechanism of economic development. Unlike **cameralists**, who favoured state intervention, they promoted laissez-faire policies.

plethora   a state of excess blood in the body, which could lead to a variety of diseases.

pneuma   physical, very fine vapours that were taken from the air in the lungs into the arteries, and were considered to be a vehicle of life-giving heat.

post-Tridentine   term used to describe developments within the Catholic church in the decades after the **Council of Trent**.

Privy Council   the executive arm of monarchical government in England, which consisted of the monarch and his or her chosen ministers.

pulmonary auscultation   the technique of studying internal lesions of the lungs by striking the chest and listening to the vibrations.

purgative   also called purge; a substance that helps evacuation of matter from the body.

Quakers   Protestant sect founded in the 1650s by George Fox. They were widely feared for the subversive message of their radical preaching, which included attacks on established religion and the social and political hierarchy.

qualities   in Galenic medical theory, all parts of the human body were ultimately reducible to four qualities – hot, cold, wet and dry. These were associated with the four prime **elements** – earth, air, fire and water. The proportion in which the qualities occurred differed from person to person. An individual's particular mixture of qualities was called their **complexion**. The balance of qualities also affected the balance of the **humours** that existed within an individual's body. Galenic medicine involved countering the effects of particular qualities by prescribing treatments containing the opposite qualities, to restore the body's balance.

real   Spanish coin.

Reformation   the break-up of the Roman Catholic church in the sixteenth century, which gave rise to a variety of evangelical or Protestant churches.

regimen   means of maintaining or restoring health by management of the six **non-naturals**.

Renaissance   literally meaning 'rebirth'. Historians use this term to denote a period characterizing the revival of the learning of the ancient Greeks and Romans; more commonly it is used to denote the period from about 1400 to about 1600.

rinderpest   a virulent infection of cattle and other ruminants.

Rosicrucian movement   beginning in 1614, a group calling itself the Brotherhood of the Rose Cross, or the Rosicrucians, published a manifesto in Germany. It outlined a programme of moral, spiritual and political reform and included reference to an imminent revival of medicine and healing. Further publications appeared, generating a great deal of excitement in learned circles as to how and when this long-awaited process of regeneration might take place. It was particularly well received in alchemical and **hermetic** circles, though a number of more conservative scholars claimed that the whole episode was a hoax. Briefly, however, it did encourage a great deal of interest in Paracelsianism and iatrochemistry, especially in central Europe, where the outbreak of the Thirty Years War in 1618 and the revival of confessional conflict once again led to renewed hope in the imminence of the millennium.

Sack of Rome   the desecration and conquest of Rome by the troops of Emperor Charles V in 1527.

sacrum   a curved triangular section at the end of the backbone.

scapula   the shoulder bone.

scientific revolution   the term invented by an earlier generation of historians of science and medicine to describe the many new medical and 'scientific' discoveries of the seventeenth century.

serum   a watery liquid, especially that which separates from blood.

signature   see **doctrine of signatures**.

simples   see *materia medica*.

Spanish Inquisition   originally established in 1479 in order to expedite the forced conversion of the Jewish and Arab populations of Spain, it was increasingly used by the **Counter-Reformation** papacy to crush all forms of religious dissent in Spain and the Spanish Netherlands (modern-day Belgium).

'Spanish Road'   the main route along which Spanish troops travelled to the Netherlands during the Dutch Revolt/Eighty Years War.

spirits   subtle but material substances that in Galenic medical theory were thought to support bodily processes. Blood mixed with *pneuma* in the lungs to generate 'vital spirits', which endowed the body with heat (and thus life) via the arteries. Vital spirits were refined into 'animal spirits' in a net of nerves and vessels that were believed to exist at the base of the brain (later called the *rete mirabile*). These animal spirits were distributed through the nerves, and were regarded as instruments of sensation and movement. 'Natural spirits' conveyed nourishment to the veins to support growth. For Galen, these medical spirits were understood to be instruments of the soul.

suffocation of the mother   natural disease in which the womb was believed to move around and press on the other organs of the body in such a way as to produce various symptoms, including those associated with demonic possession and **hysteria**.

suppuration   the stuffing of wounds with all sorts of material in order to cause them to gather and evacuate pus.

terra sigillata   literally 'sealed earth'; a greasy clay containing various metals, out of which tablets were made. It was supposed to have drying and binding properties, and to be effective against poisons.

thorax   the chest – that is, the area between the neck and the diaphragm.

thoracic   pertaining to the **thorax**.

Tory   nickname of the supporters of the independent power of the king in late seventeenth and early eighteenth century England.

trepanation   operation to remove a piece of the skull; it was usually carried out to reduce pressure or remove a growth.

tria prima   according to Paracelsus, the three basic building blocks of life were salt, sulphur and mercury. In the process, he rejected the four Aristotelian **elements** – earth, fire, water and air.

Unani-tibb   'the medicine of Greece'; Muslim medicine based on earlier Greek forms with later Arabic and Indian additions.

United Provinces   modern-day Netherlands. It had come into existence in the late 1560s as a result of the secession of the northern (primarily Protestant) half of the Spanish Netherlands from the rule of the Catholic **Habsburgs**. The largest and most important of the provinces was Holland, which, along with its confederate neighbours, experienced an economic 'golden age' in the seventeenth century. It was also a haven for religious extremists, as well as a major centre of scientific and medical research.

uroscopy   diagnostic examination of urine.

vena cava   literally 'hollow vein'; in Galenic medical theory, the inferior vena cava carried blood from the liver to the lower part of the body, and the superior vena cava carried blood from the liver, via the heart, to the upper part of the body.

venesection   from the Latin *vena*, meaning 'vein'; the practice of letting blood from the veins, using a small sharp knife called a lancet. Also known as **phlebotomy**.

venous   relating to the veins. In Galenic medical theory, the venous blood was produced in the liver from digested food; its main function was to nourish each part of the body via the veins – a system of vessels entirely independent from the arteries. Some of the venous blood was mixed with *pneuma* to produce the **arterial** blood.

ventricle   one of the two lower chambers of the heart.

vernacular   languages spoken by the natives of a country, e.g. English, French, German. These were given a generic name to distinguish them from classical languages such as Latin, which in the **early modern** period was the language of most scientific and theological publications, and of elite higher education.

vesicle   a small globule or sac.

virgin soil epidemics   epidemic illnesses which hit populations that had not been previously exposed to them and so had not built up any immunity to them. In such epidemics mortality was very high.

viviparous   producing living young that have reached an advanced state of development before delivery.

vivisection   the act or practice of carrying out surgical operations on live animals for the purposes of physiological research.

voluntary hospital   virtually all of England's medieval hospitals run by the church were destroyed during the **Reformation**, except for a handful in London. In the eighteenth century, new hospitals were founded in ever growing numbers in the capital and the counties funded by voluntary donations and run by the donors.

Whig   nickname of the opponents of independent royal power in late seventeenth and eighteenth century England, who were the chief political beneficiaries of the Revolution of 1688.

women's history   a field of historical research that expanded in the 1970s in relation to the feminist movement; it focused on the collection of evidence and the interpretation of women's varied actions and experiences in the past.

Index

abortion 205

Africa 315, 321
   see also black medicine

age, and madness in early modern England 232

Agrippa, Henricus Cornelius 49, 50

Ailhaud, Jean 374–5, 378

air quality
   and health 286–8, 325
   and the miasma theory of disease 141, 285
   and the plague 285–6

Aix-les-Bains 292

Alberti, Leon Battista 20

Albucasis 12, 15

alchemy 112–13, 288

Alexander VI, Pope 2, 4, 20, 23

Allderidge, Patricia 249

almanacs, environmental themes in 286, *287*

alternative (complementary) medicine xiv, 27

Altötting, Bavaria, healing shrine at 245, *247*

Ambrose, St 60

American colonies 22, 315–41
   and the biological effects of European colonialism 316–18
   and herbal medicines 323–4, 329–30, 339, 340, 341
   hospitals
      New England 329
      plantation hospitals 337
      Spanish America xxiii, 328, 329
   New England 321, 322, 325, 326, 329
   Newfoundland 321, 325
   perceptions of health and environment 315–16, 321–7
   southern states
      and conjuring medicine 340
      health of colonists 326–7
      slavery and medicine 336, 337
   Virginia 321, 322–3, 325, 326, 340
   see also colonial medicine; slavery and medicine

American Indians (Amerindians)
   decline in numbers of 318
   herbal remedies 323–4
   smallpox sufferers 316–18, *317*
   and virgin soil epidemics xxiii, 316–18
   in Virginia 323

Amersfoort (Dutch town), plague in 285

amputations 44, *45*, 267–72, 282
   and artificial limbs 272, 273
   and cauterization 268, 272
   and gangrene 271
   ligature prior to 267, 268
   ointments and bandages after 271–2
   and the screw tourniquet *268*

anatomy
   classical anatomical theatres 74–5
   defining 5
   eighteenth-century 184–5
   and Fabricius 81
   male–female differences 196, 197–205, *199*
   and Malpighi's model of the body 176–81
   midwives and anatomical knowledge 218
   and Renaissance humanism 60, 61, 78
   and surgeons 46, 364, 367–8
   and university medical education 14, 49, 358, 359, 363
   and Vesalius
      anatomical drawings 73–4
      De Humani Corporis Fabrica 58, 74–9
      legacy of 79–80
      and the Reformation 86–8, 106
      Tabulae Anatomicae Sex 68–72
   see also dissections

ancient Greek medicine 4–11
   and Christianity 18–19
   and the human body 5–9
   and medical humanism 59–61
   and medieval medical education 12–18
   and medieval universities 15
   and Muslim medicine 334
   see also Galen and Galenic medicine; Hippocrates and Hippocratic medicine; humoral medicine

Andrews, Jonathan 249, 250, 251, 252

animalculism, and theories of procreation 212, 213

animals
   dissection and vivisection 77, 78, 168, 169, 172, *188*, 358

and the process of generation 208, 209–11, *211*

antimony, and Paracelsianism 111, *112*

Aphorisms (Hippocrates) 13

Apocrypha, and Helmontianism 125

apothecaries xviii, 27, 46–7
   education and training 17, 346, 357
   in England 118, 347
   in Florentine hospitals 151
   in France 348
      distribution of 353–5, 356
   in Germany 351
   guilds 30, 46
   licensing of 29–30, 346
   in Rome 3–4
   Society of 347

Arab philosopher-physicians 12, 13, 15, 18
   and bloodletting 67, 68
   and humanists 59, 60

Arianism 115

Aristotle and Aristotelian philosophy xxi
   and Christianity 18, 22
   Fabricius and the 'Aristotle Project' 81–2
   and Harvey's discovery of the circulation of the blood 171–2
   and humoral theory 7
   and male–female differences 197–8, 210, 223
   and medical education 12–13, 48, 86
   and new models of the body 166–7
   and Paracelsianism 110–11
   and the process of generation 107, 200, *207*, 207, 224
   and the status of medicine 50
   and Vesalius' *De Humani Corporis Fabrica* 75
   see also natural philosophy

armies *see* war and medicine

army surgeons xxii, 257–8, 260, 261, 282
   and amputations 267–72, 282
   chests for surgical instruments *269*
   and foot rot 275
   and gunshot wounds 263–5, *270*, 282
   pay of 270
   and shell shock 275

arquebus (firearm) 259

Arrighi, Stefano 140–1

arteries
femoral artery and amputations 268
in Galenic medicine 5
and Harvey's discovery of the circulation of the blood 169–71
Articella (Little Art of Medicine) 12, 13, 85
artificial limbs *272*, *273*, 273
astrology and medicine
and air quality 285
and bloodletting 63, *64*
environmental themes in 286, 287
and Helmontianism 122
and medieval medical education 13–14, 15, 86
and mental illness 241, 243
and physicians 52, 86
and popular medicine 33
in the sixteenth century 86
and syphilis 146, 147
zodiac man 63, *64*, *287*, *331*
asylums for the insane xxii, 228, 245–53, 254
Bethlem Royal Hospital (Bedlam) 245, *246*, 249–53, *250*
in Germany 238, 245–9, *248*
and the 'great incarceration' 229, 245, 254
St Luke's Hospital for Lunatics *251*, 251–2, 253
atoms, ancient Greek ideas of 7
Auenbrugger, Leopold 360
automata, and Descartes's image of the body 174, *175*
Averroës 12, 13
Avicenna 12, 23, 24
Canon 13, 22, 48, 334
Ayurveda (Hindu medical system) 334
Aztec medicine 316, *331*, 331–4, *332*

Babington, William 370
Bacci, Andrea 290
Bacon, Francis 295
Baconian theories 127, 128, 326
Badiano, Juan 332
Baener, Johann Alexander 122
Baillie, John 336
baptism
and Bugenhagen's church orders 101
midwives and emergency baptisms 85
Baptists 127
barber-surgeons 3, 269

and ancient Greek medicine 10
and bloodletting 15, 16, 45, 46, 65
Company of 46
in early modern London 43–6
shops 43–4
Barrough, Philip 237–8
Barthez, Paul-Joseph 376–7
Basil, St 60
Bath 292, *293*
Battie, William 251–3, *252*, 253–4
A Treatise on Madness 252–3
Belvedere torso 74
Benzi, Ugo 12, 13
'A medieval *consilium*' 11
Berg, Günther Heinrich von 306
Bergman, Torbern 295
Bethlem Royal Hospital (Bedlam) 245, *246*, 249–53, *250*, 254
bezoar 179
Bible
and Helmontianism 125, 126
Latin and Greek translations 60
and Paracelsus 110, 111
and the Reformation 106
Vesalius and Lutheran Protestantism 87
Biggs, Noah 124–6
Binns, Joseph 43, 46
biomedical history, and slavery 338
Biondo, Flavio 20
Black Death 99, 139, 144
black medicine xxiii, 338–41
conjuring medicine 339, 340–1
herbal 339, 340, 341
Blane, Gilbert 276
blistering 159, 192
blood
blood flow in Galenic medicine 5–6, 61–3, *62*, 168–9
and the body as a hydraulic system 180
Harvey's discovery of the circulation of the blood xii, xxi, 167, 168–73
and Newtonian medicine 183
see also menstruation
bloodletting 3, 61–8
and ancient Greek medicine 10
and barber-surgeons 15, 16, 45, 46, 65
and black slaves 337
calendars 17
and Cardano's description of the death of a patient 54

in eighteenth-century hospitals 159
and gunshot wounds 265
and Harvey's discovery of the circulation of the blood 182
and Helmontianism 125, 132
humanist controversy over 66–8, 79
and learned physicians 15, 46, 64–5
and Malpighi 179, 180, 181
and menstruation 201
and mental illness 242, 252, 253
methods of 63–4
and the nervous system 192
and new models of the body 167
and popular medical books 33
revulsion and derivation 66–8, 72
rules of 63, *65*
and surgeons 15, 44, *45*
and Vesalius 58, 70–3, 80–1, 168
and the zodiac man 63, *64*
see also veins of the human body
bodies *see* human body
'Body Worlds' exhibition (London) xi
Boerhaave, Hermann 133, 180, 181, 187, 360
Bologna
Malpighi's medical practice in 179–80
University of 1, 12, 13–14, 15, 40, 68, 176
bonesetting 3, 10, 30
books
on bloodletting 64, 65–6
on empirical healers 372
Index of forbidden books 98, 115
and itinerant healers 41
on midwifery 214, 218, 220–1
physicians and the publication of 51
and popular medicine 33
and women as healers 37
Borelli, Giovanni Alfonso 174
De Motu Animalium 175
Borgia, Cesare 23
Borjia-Llançol, Cardinal Joan 23
Borromeo, Carlo, bishop of Milan 103
Bostocke, Richard, on Paracelsianism in England 110–11
botany 358, 359
Bourgeois, Louise 218–21, *219*
Boyle, Robert 123, 128, 129, 294
Bracciolini, Poggio 20
Bradford, William 325

Bradwell, Stephen 241
on plague 144–5
brain wounds 266
Brandenburg-Prussia 250, 305
Brereton, John 323
Brissot, Pierre *67*, 67–8, 72
Britain
early modern medicine in xvii
economic growth in the
eighteenth century 344
education of surgeons 364, 370–1
and the Glorious Revolution
(1688) xii
licensed medical practice in
eighteenth-century 345, 346–8,
379
military hospitals 280, 281
voluntary hospitals 155, 156–7
Whig politicians 347, 348
see also England; London;
Scotland
British Medical Journal (BMJ),
survey on the classification of disease
xiv–xv
Brockliss, Laurence xix, xxiii, 37–8,
41, 121, 142
on military hospitals 280–1
on water cures 294
Brueghel, Pieter, *L'Alchemiste 113*
Brunswich, Hieronymus, *The Book of
Wound Dressing* 263
Bugenhagen, Johannes 99, 101–2, *102*
Buisson of Avignon 372–3, 374
burials
cemeteries closed for 307–10
records of 297, 299–300
burns treatment 260, 266–7
Burton, Robert 241, 287–8
The Anatomy of Melancholy
238, *239*
Butterfield, Herbert xii

Caius, John 79–80
calendar reform 14
calendars, medical information on 17
Calvet, Esprit 372, 376
cameralists, and licensed medical
practice 351
Camillans 103–5
see also Lellis, Camillo de
capillaries 169
Capuchins 103, 104
Cardano, Girolamo 47–55, *48*
on the death of a patient 52–5

medical education 48–9
On the Method of Curing 51–2
Caribbean, smallpox and American
Indians 316–17
Carpi, Jacopo Berengario da 78, 198
Castile, licensed medical practice 350
Castle, George 174
Catherine de' Medici 116
Catherine the Great, empress of Russia
303, 305
Catholic church 84
and charitable acts 100
Congregation of Sacred Rites and
Ceremonies 92
and health care reforms 102–5
and holy waters 92–3, 289, 291
and hospitals 149, 154, 360
Jesuits 289
in the Middle Ages 85–6
and Paracelsus 97, 98
and the plague 138–9
post-Tridentine 92, 98
and the study of anatomy 86–8
and the treatment of the insane
245
in German hospitals 246–9,
248
see also Counter-Reformation
cautery 3, 10, 16
cell theory 193
Celsus, Aulus Cornelius 96, 267, 271
cemeteries, closure of 307–10
Chamberlen, Peter 127, 222
Chambon de Montaux, Nicolas 363,
369
Chandler, John 128
Charles I, king of England 124, 142
Charles II, king of England 129, 130
Charles V, Holy Roman Emperor 2, 68,
78, 79
Chauliac, Guy de 19
on the history of surgery 15, 16
chemical medicine xix, 94, 95,
108–33, 166, 358
chemical analysis of mineral
waters 294–5
Society of Chemical Physicians
128–31
see also Paracelsus and
Paracelsianism
chemistry 358, 359
Cheselden, William 363
Chester, smallpox inoculation in 304
Cheyne, George 183–4, 186

childbirth xv–xvi, xxi–xxii, 215–23,
224
birthing chair *216*
and gossips *215*, 216
and mental illness 232
puerperal feasts *218*
use of forceps in 215, 222
see also midwives
children, and madness in early modern
England 232
Christian II, king of Denmark 95
Christian IV, king of Denmark 92, 269
Christianity *see* religion and medicine
Cicero 59, 60
Cipolla, Carlo 142–3
climate
effects on health and illness 286,
287–8, 301
in European colonies
318–21, 322–5
and epidemic diseases 297
Clowes, William 118, 267, 268, 269,
282
Surgery in the Fields 270
Colombo, Realdo 168
colonial medicine xvii, xxiii, 315–41
and climate, place and health
318–21
and hybrid models of government
327
and regimens 319
and slavery 334–41
see also American colonies;
Spanish America
Columbus, Christopher 22, 316, 322,
325, 330
complexion
in Galenic medicine 6–7, 8, 10
and learned physicians 52, 55
conjuring medicine 339, 340–1
consilia
in Galenic medicine 10–11
and medieval medical education
14
contraception 205
Cook, Captain James 318
Cook, Harold 129
Cook, John 127
Cooper, Astley 370
Copenhagen, University of 89, 92
Copernicus, Nicholas xii
Cortés, Hernando 317
Counter-Reformation xix, 84
and health care 100, 103–5, 106
and sacred healing 92–3, 106

criminality, and madness in early modern England 234, 235
Crosby, A.W. 318
Cruso, J. 270
Cullen, Professor William 158, 159, 187–9, 191–2, 244
Culpeper, Nicholas 119, 127
Cunningham, A. 138
> The Anatomical Renaissance 87–8
> 'Fabricius and the "Aristotle Project"' 81–2
> 'William Harvey and the discovery of the circulation of the blood' 170–1
Curtius, Matthaeus 68, 76, 77

D'Alembert, Jean le Rond 310
Daughters of Charity (religious nursing order) 154
Davis, Natalie Zemon 100–1
deaths
> bills of mortality 297–300, *298*, 302
> of black slaves 334, 335, 336
> in childbirth xvi
> and childhood diseases 137
> eighteenth-century decline in mortality rates 284
> of European colonists
>> in North America 322, 325
>> in the tropics 319, 321
> indigenous peoples and virgin soil epidemics 316–17
> and the plague 137, 143
> smallpox 302, 316–17, 318
Defoe, Daniel 172
Democritus 7
Denmark
> healing waters 91–2, 289
> medical reform 89–91, 106
> poor relief and health care 101
Descartes, René 167, 172–6, 177, 180, 187, 191
diagnosis
> and humoral medicine 9, *10*
> and learned physicians 53–4
> and pulmonary auscultation 360
Diderot, Denis 371, 375, 376
diet
> and Galenic medicine 11, 125, 133
> and learned physicians 52, 55
> and Newtonian physicians 184
> and scurvy 261, 276–7, 277–8

and the 'sensible' body 191, 192
digestion
> Descartes on 173–4
> Harvey's discussion of 171, 174, 208
Digges, Leonard, *A Prognostication Everlasting 287*
Dimsdale, Thomas 303–4
Dioscorides 17, 61
diseases
> acute 150, 151
> of the army 261, 279
> *BMJ* survey on the classification of xiv–xv
> chronic 149, 151
> Enlightenment attitudes to 375
> epidemics 136, 137
>> analysis of (London 1661–76) 296–7
>> and religion 99–100
> and European colonialism
>> climate and the environment 319–21, 325, 326
>> indigenous peoples and virgin soil epidemics 316–18
> and Galenic medicine 144, 145
> and Helmontianism 124
> history of 137–8
> Luther on the cause and cure of 88
> and medical police 307
> miasma theory of 141, 285
> and the nervous system 189
> and Paracelsianism 95
> and retrospective diagnosis xv, 138, 229
> scurvy 261, 276–8
> suffocation of the mother 243, 244
> Sydenham and new approaches to understanding 295–7
> *see also* plague; smallpox; syphilis
dissections
> of animals 77, 78
> and the education of surgeons 365, 367–8
> and Galen 79–80
> and medical humanists 60
> and pathological anatomy 160
> public xi, 14, *76*, 358
>> and Christianity 19, 106
>> and Vesalius 58, 73–4, 74–6, 77
> and religion 87
doctrine of signatures 122

Dolben, Sir William, and 'Dolben's Act' (1788) *335*
Doryphorus, statue of 77
drugs
> in the American colonies 323–4, 329–30
> and apothecaries 47
> Aztec medicine 331–4
> and the education of physicians 358
> and eighteenth-century medical practitioners 376, 377
> and empirical healers 39, 40, 55
> and Helmontianism 125
> Luther on 88
> Malpighi's use of 179, 180
> and Paracelsianism 94, 111, 117–18, 119
> pharmacopoeia 118, 119, 339
> in Renaissance hospitals 151
> for syphilis 147, 148
> and women as healers 34
Dubois, Jacques 264
Duchesne, Joseph 111, 117, 118
Duden, Barbara, *The Woman beneath the Skin* 203–4, 205
Dudley, Thomas, deputy governor of New England 325
Dürer, Albrecht *147*

Earlom, Richard, *Sensibility 190*
Edinburgh Royal Infirmary 158–9, 192, 360, *362*
Edinburgh University 158, 187, 329, 345, 359, 363, 369
> medical school 360, 364, 371
education
> and the Reformation 89, 90, 91
> *see also* universities
electric therapy 192
> and madness 254
elixir vitriol 277
empirical healers 55, 372–8
> and Galenic medicine 5, 8
> itinerant 38–43, *42*
> 'Le Grand Thomas' 372, *373*
> and madness 253
> patients of 374–6
> in Spanish America 328
Encyclopédie 310
England
> army surgeons 270
> civil wars 124, 127, 128
> Helmontian revolution in 124–9, 133

holy springs and wells 289
hospitals
    Gloucester Infirmary *156*
    Royal Haslar, Portsmouth
    276, 281, 320
    Winchester County Hospital
    156–7
licensed medical practice in
eighteenth-century 356–7
medical care in 31, 32
medical knowledge and patronage
in eighteenth-century 185–6
mental illness in 231–6, 237–8
    asylums for the insane 245,
    246, 249–54
midwives 127, 215–18, 220,
221–2
Paracelsianism in 110–11,
118–19
plague in 141–2, 143
smallpox inoculation 304–5
Society of Chemical Physicians
128–31
spas 291, 292, 293
theories of conception in early
modern 213–15
see also Britain; London
enlightened despotism 160
Enlightenment xxiii, 378–9
    and changing attitudes to disease
    375
    and man-midwives 222
    and mental illness 230, 244
    and military hygiene 279, 280
    and public health policies 137,
    160–1, 162
    Scottish 191
    and the state 344–5
    and the training of medical
    practitioners 345, 346, 358, 378
environmental medicine xxii–xxiii,
284–310
    and air quality 285–8
    and bills of mortality 297–300,
    298, 302
    and climate 286, 287–8, 301
        in European colonies
        318–21, 322–5
    connections between place and
    disease 284, 286–8
    and hygiene 305–10
    inoculation against smallpox
    301–5
    in the North American colonies
    318–21, 321–7
    and physicians 300–1
    and the plague 285–6, 307, 319

and the understanding of disease
295–7
see also waters and healing
Epicurus 7
epigenesis, and the process of
generation 208–9, 213, 224
epilepsy 19
Erasmus, Desiderius 59, 60, 67, 87,
289
    on health and habitation 284,
    285, 286
Eustachio, Bartolomeo 79, 80
Evenden Nagy, Doreen
    'Lay and learned medicine in early
    modern England' 37
    on midwives in London 221–22
Ewich, Johan 99–100
excretion
    Harvey's explanation of 171–2
    and humoral medicine 181
    measuring 181–2
eyesight, air and the preservation of
288
Eyre, Henry, 'An account of the
mineral waters of Spa' *293*, 294

Fabricius of Aquapendente,
Hieronymous 81–2, *82*, 168, 169, 171,
221
    on the process of generation 208,
    209, 209
facial wounds, sewing of 272, *274*
Fallopia, Gabriele 79, 208, 294
families, and madness in early modern
England 233
feminist history xiii, 196
Ferrara, University of 61, 68, 95
Fett, S.M. 340
fevers
    in the American colonies 326
    and blood flow 62
    diagnosis of 53, 150
    jail or hospital fever 279, 282
    use of milk to treat 179, 180
Ficino, Marsilio, *Theologica Platonica*
22
Fioravanti, Leonardo 38–34, *39*, 51
    Capricci Medicinali 32–3
    Il Tesoro della Vita Humana 38
    La Cirugia 39
    life and medical ideas 38–40
    on syphilis 146
firearms
    gunshot wounds 260, 263–5

technological innovations in
259–60
First World War 275
Fisher, John, bishop of Rochester 284,
285, 286
Florence
    hospitals in Renaissance Florence
    20, 150–1, *152*
    medical practitioners' guilds 3
folk medicine xv, 328
foot rot 275
Fordyce, Sir William 304
Foucault, Michel xiii–xiv, xxi, 150,
229, 245, 250, 254
    on medical police 300
fractures 260, 272, *273*
France
    apothecaries 348, 353–5, 356
    cemetery closures 307–10
    empirical healers 372–5
    and the Holy Roman Empire 2–3
    hospitals 153, 154, 360, 371
        and medical education 360,
        371
        military 280–1
        Paris 20, *21*, 280–1, 364,
        366, 367, *368*, 368, 369
    licensed medical practice 345,
    348–9, 352–7, *353*
    medical training *353*, 356
    military hygiene 278
    Paracelsian ideas in 116–18, 121
    physicians 348–9, 352–7
    plague and health policies 142
    and political arithmetic 299
    smallpox inoculation 303, 305
    surgeons 348, 349, 352–5, 356
        Académie Royale de
        Chirurgie 349
        education of 364–6, 367–70
    water cures and spas 291, 292
    see also Paris
Francis Xavier, St 289
Frank, Johann Peter 161, 162, 306–7
Frederik II, king of Denmark 91, 289
the 'French disease' *see* syphilis
French Revolution (1789) 346, 359,
369, 379
Frontinus, *On the Waters of the City
of Rome* 20
Fuchs, Leonhart 68

Gale, Thomas 263
Galen and Galenic medicine xiv, xvi,
xvii, xviii, 2, 4, 5–8, 24, *120*

and anatomy 58
Arab translations of Galen 12
and Aristotelian philosophy 13
and army surgeons 267
Art of Medicine 8, 13
and Aztec medicine 333–4
The Best Doctor is Also a Philosopher 5
and blood flow 5–6, 61–3, *62*, 168–9
and bloodletting 67, 68, 72, 201
and bodily fluids 176
and Cardano's description of the death of a patient 52–5
challenges to 180, 181
and Christianity 6, 18, 22
definition of medicine 7–8
and Descartes's image of the body 174
diagnosis 9, *10*
and disease 144, 145
and dissections 79–80
and eighteenth-century physiology 184
and European colonialism 319
and fever 53
and Fioravanti 40
and Helmontianism 109, 123–4, 125–6, 128, 131, 133
and the human body 5–8
and the London College of Physicians 130
and the maintenance of health 33
and mental illness 240, 252
and new models of the body 166
On Anatomical Procedures 60, 70
On Critical Days 9
On the Dissection of Veins and Arteries 72
On the Opinions of Hippocrates and Plato 22
On the Use of the Parts 22
and Paracelsianism 93–4, 95, 97, 108, 109, 110, 111, 115, 119–21, 133
in France 117, 118
and Renaissance humanism 60–1, 61
and sense experience 187
and the status of medicine 5
and suppuration 263
treatment (regimen) in 9–11
and university medical education 13, 14, 17, 48, 93
and Vesalius 58, 68, 70, 74–7, 78, 79–80, 87

and water cures 291
and women 6–7
    as healers 35, 37
    male–female differences 197, 198, 199–200, 223
    menstruation 201, 202
    and the process of generation 107, 207–8, 213, 224
    see also ancient Greek medicine; humoral medicine; non-naturals
gangrene 271, 275
gender
    and mental illness 231–2, 233, 244–5
    and users of empirical healers 374
    see also men and medicine; women and medicine
generation, process of 197, 207–15, 224
Gentilcore, David 41, 92
The Gentleman's Magazine 308, 309
George I, king of England 302
George III, king of England 254
Georgiana, duchess of Devonshire 377
Germany
    burials and hygiene in 310
    hospitals for the insane 238, 245–9, *248*
    licensed medical practice 250–1, 345
    medical police 305, 306
    poor relief and health care in sixteenth-century 101–2
    pox hospitals 148, 149
    and public health in the eighteenth century 160–1
    shrine at Altötting, Bavaria 245, *247*
Gersdorff, Hans von 268
Gesner, Conrad 290
Gessner, Johann 367–8
Gilibert, Jean-Emmanuel 372, 379
girdle books 64, *66*
glands, and Malpighi's model of the human body 167, 176–81
Glauber, Johann Rudolph 128
Gondoin, Jacques 365
Goubert, Jean-Pierre 352
Goyen, Jan van, *Village Scene with a Charlatan 42*
Graaf, Régnier de 210, 211
Graham, James, and the Celestial Bed 377–8

Graunt, John, *Natural and Political Observations* 299, 300
'great man' approach to medicine xii, xv, xvi
the great pox *see* syphilis
Greece *see* ancient Greek medicine
guaiac wood (*Guaiacum officinalis*) 330
guilds 3, 29, 31
    apothecaries 30, 46
    hospitals established by 85–6
    and the licensing of medical practitioners 29–30, 346, 347, 348–9
    surgeons 30, 364
Guillemeau, Jacques 268
    La Chirurgie françoise 45
Guinther von Andernach, Johann 60, 61, 68
Gulf War syndrome xiv
gunshot wounds 260, 263–5, 282
    locating bullets in 264–5, *270*
Gustavus Adolphus, king of Sweden 260

Habsburg territories 2
    and public health in the eighteenth century 160–1
    see also Germany; Holy Roman Empire
haemorrhoids, as a form of male menstruation 202
Haen, Anton de 360–1
Hagens, Gunther von xi
Haina, Hesse, Protestant hospital at 246, 247, *248*
Haldane, Isabell 290
Hales, Stephen 183, 307, 308
Haller, Albrecht von 167, 187, *188*, 213, 358, 367
Haly Abbas 12, 13, 15
Hariot, Thomas 322
Harrison, Walter *251*
Harrison, William, *Description of England* 323
Hartlib, Samuel 128–9
Harvey, William 82, 222
    and the circulation of the blood xii, xxi, 167, 168–73, *170*, 200
    On the Motion of the Heart and Blood in Animals 82
Haygarth, Francis 304, 305
head wounds 265–6
health care provision xx, xxi, 136–7

and religion 100–5
see also hospitals; public health
policies
heart
in Galenic medicine 5, 6
and Harvey's discovery of the
circulation of the blood 168–71
Hebrew, and humanists 59
Helmont, Joan Baptista van 108–9,
121–4, *122, 123,* 178
Ortus Medicinae 122
and Paracelsus 121
Helmontianism 108–9, 121–33
and Descartes's image of the body
174
in England 124–9, 133
and Galenic medicine 109, 123–4,
125–6, 128, 131
and the imagination 124
and the medical reform movement
109
and Paracelsianism 109, 121,
123, 125, 126, 127, 128
and the Society of Chemical
Physicians 129–31
treatment 124
Henri IV, king of France 116
Henry VIII, king of England 249
herbal medicine xiv
American 323–4, 329–30
Aztec 331–4
black 240, 339, 341
and female healers 35
hermaphroditism 199, 224
Hermes Trismegistus (mythical sage)
22, 95
hermetic texts 22
Hernández, Francisco 328, 333–4
Heseler, Baldasar 74
Hindu medicine (Ayurveda) 334
Hippocrates and Hippocratic medicine
xvii, 4, 9, 24, *120,* 257, 263, 288
Airs, Waters, Places and
Epidemics 286
and bloodletting 67, 72
and health in the colonies 319
and medical police 307
and menstruation 202
and Paracelsianism 98, 117, 119
and Renaissance humanism 60,
61
and university medical education
13, 15, 17, 48
and Vesalius' *De Humani
Corporis Fabrica* 75
and women as healers 37

Hippocratic oath 18
Hogarth, William, *Scene of Bedlam, A
Rake's Progress* 245, *246*
Holy Roman Empire 2–3, 91
and Paracelsianism 113–14,
115–16
Hooke, Robert 250
hospitals xx, 136–7, 150–60, 162
and Bugenhagen's church orders
102
Catholic nursing orders 103–5,
154
and Christianity 19–20
Counter-Reformation 103
Edinburgh Royal Infirmary 158–9,
192, 360, *362*
and medical education 49, 360–2,
368–9
medieval 85–6
military xxii, 257, 278, 280–1,
282
Moscow 303, 305
physicians and medical knowledge
in 154–5, 159–60
plague hospitals (pesthouses)
140, 141, 142, 144, 151
poor people as patients 157–60
St Caecilia Hospital, Leiden *361*
specialized 151–3
for syphilis sufferers 24, 102,
103, 148–9, 151
ventilation in 307, 310
voluntary 155–7
see also American colonies;
asylums for the insane; England;
France; Italy; London
Houghton, John 292
Howard, John 281
Huguenots, and Paracelsianism 116–17
human body
and ancient Greek medicine 5–9
barber-surgeons and the male
body 44
distinction between inner and
outer body 44
holistic perception of the 167–8
and natural philosophy 86
new models of the 166–93
the skeleton *69,* 70, 78
Vesalius' view of the canonical
body 77–8
see also veins of the human body
human sacrifice, and Aztec culture 333
humanism xviii, 22, 58
and bloodletting 66–8, 79
and the Reformation 87

the Renaissance and medical
humanism 59–61
and Vesalius 68, 70, 74, 76–7, 78
Hume, David 191
humoral medicine xiv, xvi, xix, 6–7
in the American colonies 318–21,
323
and black slaves 337, 338
and herbal medicine 330
and barber-surgeons 44
and bloodletting 61–3
and complexion 6–7, 8
and diagnosis 9
and disease 138, 141
and the environment 286
and excretion 181
the four humours in 7, 319
and Harvey's discovery of the
circulation of the blood 182
and the humoral balance 8, 52,
181, 192
in medieval Europe 17–18
and mental illness 238, 241–2
and Paracelsus 95, 111
and prognosis 9
and scurvy 277
and sex differences 197
treatment 9–11
see also Galen and Galenic
medicine
Hunter, John, *Treatise of the Blood,
Inflammation, and Gun Shot
Wounds* 265
Hunter, William 222, 370
Hutten, Ulrich von 23
hydraulic model of the body 180, 181,
187
hygiene 305–10
and the closure of cemeteries
307–10
and medical police 306–7
military 278–80, 307
and the plague 285–6
ventilators in prisons and
hospitals 307, *308, 309*
hysteria xv, 191, 192, 243, 244–5

iatrochemical revolution 109–33
see also Helmontianism;
Paracelsus and Paracelsianism
imagination
in Helmontianism 124
and madness in early modern
Europe 240–1
India 321, 334
infanticide 217, 233, 235

Innocent III, Pope 19
inoculation
    African techniques of 339
    smallpox xxii–xxiii, 301–5
Inquisition 47, 92, 121
Ireland, licensed medical practice in 347
Italy
    apothecaries 47
    city-states 2
    hospitals
        Renaissance Florence 20, 150–1, *152*
        Rome 4, 19–20, 24, *148*, 151
        for syphilis sufferers 148–9
    itinerant healers 38–43
    licensed medical practice 350
    medical care in xx–xxi, 31–2
    midwives 222
    monastery of Monte Cassino 85
    physicians 48–9, 50–1
    plague in 103, 138–9, 140–1, 142–3
    universities and the medical curriculum 48–9
    see also individual cities and universities
itinerant healers 38–43, *42*

Jamaica, Obeah medicine 340
James I, king of England 118
James II, king of England xii, 348
Jamestown, Virginia 321, 325
Jenner, Edward 301
Jerome, St 60
Jewson, Nicholas, on medical knowledge and patronage in eighteenth-century England 185–6
Johannitius 8–9
Johnson, Samuel 254
Johnson, William 130–1
Jones, Colin 37–8, 41, 121, 142
    on the medical marketplace 373
    on military hospitals 280–1
    on water cures 292, 294
Jones, John 291
Jordanova, Ludmilla 310
Joseph II, emperor of Austria 306
Jourdain, S. 322
Julius II, Pope (Guiliano della Rovere) 23–4
Jurin, James 302–3

Keill, James 181, 183
Kerckring, Theodore *212*
Ketham, Johannes de, *Fasciculus Medicinae 76*
Kupperman, Karen 323

La Mettrie, Julien Offray de 371
Laënnec, Guillaume-François 369–70
Laqueur, Thomas 198, 199, 200
Latin
    and humanists 59, 60
    and Paracelsianism 114
Laurens, André de, 'Air and good health in Renaissance medicine' 288
Lawrence, Christopher 191
lay medical knowledge 33, 55
Le Baillif, Roch 116
Le Dran, Henri-François 363, 367–8
Le Prestre de Vauban, Sébastien 299
Lebrun, François 352
Leeuwenhoek, Antoni van *211*, 211, 212, 213
Leiden, medical education in 360, *361*, 361, 362
Lellis, Camillo de 92–3, 103–5, *104*
    Camillans 103–5
Leonardo da Vinci 59
Leoniceno, Nicolò 61, 68
licensed medical practice (eighteenth century) 344–78
    and attitudes to patients 375
    Britain 345, 346–8
    France 345, 348–9, 352–7
    Germany 350–1
    Italy 350
    Spain 350
licensing of medical practitioners 29–30, 346
    and Paracelsianism 115
    and unqualified healers 344
Lind, James 261, *262*, 276–8, 282
    Essay on Diseases Incidental to Europeans in Hot Climates 319, *320*, 321
Lindemann, M. xvi, 28–9
Linnaeus, Karl 295
literature, novels of sentiment 189–91
lithotomists 30
liver, and Harvey's discovery of the circulation of the blood 172
Locke, John 368
London
    barber-surgeons 43–6
    bills of mortality 297, *298*, 302

'Body Worlds' exhibition xi
College of Physicians 30, 35, 46, 118, *348*
    and Helmontianism 124, 127
    Pharmacopoea Londinensis 119
    and the plague 142
    and the Rose Case (1704) 347–8
    and smallpox inoculation 302
    and the Society of Chemical Physicians 129, 130–1
education of surgeons in 370–1
epidemic diseases in 296–7
female healers in 35–8
hospitals 371
    Bethlem (Bedlam) 245, *246*, 246, 249–53, *250*, 254
    Foundling Hospital 304
    St Bartholomew's Hospital 153–4, 157
    St Luke's Hospital for Lunatics *251*, 251–2, 253
licensed medical practice in eighteenth-century 357
midwives in 221–2
Newgate prison 307, *308*, *309*
plague in 141–2
Royal Society 129, 133, 176, 302, 304
Windmill Street Academy 370
see also Britain; England
Louis XIII, king of France 219
Louis XIV, king of France 112, 299
Louis XV, king of France 365, *366*, 371
Louis XVI, king of France *365*
Louvain, 'trilingual college' at 59
Lucian 60
Lusitanus, Johannes Amatus 80–1
Luther, Martin 68, 101
    and medical reform in Denmark 91
    and medicine 88–90, 106
    and Paracelsus 94, 96, 97, 111
    Vesalius and Lutheran Protestantism 87–8
    'Whether you are allowed to flee the plague' 99
Luton, smallpox inoculation in 304–5

MacDonald, Michael, on madness in early modern England 230, 231–4, 235, 237, 240–1, 243–4
Mackenzie, Henry 189

McLaren, A. 'Popular and learned theories of conception in early modern England' 213–14

Maggi, Bartholomeo 263

magic, and colonial medicine 328, 340

Magni, Francesco 140

Maitland, Charles 302

malaria, and quinine (chinchona bark) 330, 376

Malpighi, Marcello 167, 192
 and anatomical investigation 176–9
 and medical treatment 179–80, 181
 Opera Omnia 177

Manardus, Giovanni 68

Manca, Maria 93

Marburg, University of 115

Mareschal, Georges 364

Maria de' Medici, queen of France 219

Maria Theresa, empress of Austria 160

marital status, and madness in early modern England 232–3

marketplace in medicine xix, xxiii, 254, 345, 372–8

marriage, state intervention in 160–1, 299, 301

Massey, Edmund 302

materia medica 9–10, 47, 330, 359

mathematical models
 of the human body 167
 of the universe 166

Mather, Cotton 301–2

Maurice, landgrave of Hesse-Kassel 114, 115–16

Mayerne, Theodore Turquet de 118, 142

mechanical body 167, *173*, 173–6, *175*, 180, 187

medical pluralism 28–9, 31, 47, 55

medical police 160–1, 300, 305–7

medical semiotics 206

medical training *see* universities

melancholy xv, xxii, 234, 237–8, *239*, 241, 254

Melanchthon, Philip 88

men and medicine
 lactating men 199–200, 204
 and madness in early modern England 233
 male bleeding 201–2, 204
 male practitioners and childbirth 215, 217–18, 219–21
  man-midwives 222–3, 224

patients in hospitals in Renaissance Florence 150, 151

menstruation 200–5, 223–4
 'alternative route' of 202–3
 Aristotelian theories on 197, 207–8
 and the 'flux' 203–4
 Galenic theories on 201
 lack of 205–6
 and male bleeding 201–2, 204

mental illness xiii, xx, 228–54, *247*
 bewitchment and demonic possession 229, 233–4, 240, 242–3
 case study of Richard Napier and his patients 230–45
 contemporary definitions of 228–9, 234–6
 depression 254
 diagnosis and treatment of 240–5
 essentialist view of madness 230
 and the 'golden age' for the insane 229
 and historical and cultural conditions xv, 229–30, 243
 melancholy xv, xxii, 234, 237–9, *239*, 241, 254
 popular and learned responses to xxii, 228
 and war 275, 280
 see also asylums for the insane

Mercurio, Girolamo, *Della Commare o Riccoglitrice 217*

mercury treatment for syphilis 24, 147, 330

Merian, Matthäus 248

Methodists, and mental illness 235

Mexico (New Spain)
 Aztec medicine in 316, 331–4
 European medicine in 328–9
 hospitals in xxiii, 328, 329
 Spanish conquest of 317

miasma theory of disease 141, 285

Michelangelo 59

microscope, discovery of the xxi

Middle Ages
 and ancient manuscripts 59
 Black Death 99, 139, 144
 and bloodletting 63, 64, 65
 consilium 11
 hospitals 150, 155
 medical education and universities 12–18, 85, 86, 93
 medical practitioners and guilds 3
 religion and medicine 85–6
 and water cures 291

Midelfort, H.C.E. 238, 247–9

midwives 197, 206, 215–22
 and Bugenhagen's church orders 101–2
 and the church 19, 85
 clientele 221–2
 licensing of 30, 216–17
 in London 221–2
 male practitioners and childbirth 216, 217–18, 219–21, 224–5
  man-midwives xxii, 222–3
 and medical reform 90, 127
 in Paris (Louise Bourgeois) 218–21, *219*
 popular manuals on midwifery 214
 and the process of generation 213
 public duties of 216–17
 training for 217–18, 222, 359
 see also childbirth

Milan, Maggiore Hospital 105

Mildmay, Lady Grace 34–5, 55

Ministers of the Sick (Catholic nursing order) 104–5

Mithridatum *11*

Molière (Jean Baptiste Poquelin), *Le Malade imaginaire* 372–3

Monardes, Nicolas 330

monasteries 19, 85

Mondeville, Henry of 15

Mondino de' Liuzzi 14

Monro, Alexander I 364

Monro, Alexander II 187, *188*, 364

Monro, John 252, 254

Montaigne, Michel de 291–2

Monte, Giambattista da 49

Montpellier University 1, 12, 14, 116–17, 359, 376

mopishness 234, 237, 238

moral judgements, historians and slavery 338

Morand, Sauveur-François 363, 367

More, Thomas 87

Morgagni, Batista 358, 360

Morris, Lewis 292

Morsing, Christian Torkelsen 89–90

Mouffet, Thomas, *Theatrum Insectorum* 118

muskets 259–60, 263

Muslim medicine (Unani-tibb) 334

nakedness, and madness in early modern England 235, 236

Napier, Richard xxii, 230–45, *231*

and definitions of the insane
234–6
and the diagnosis and treatment
of the insane 240–5
and melancholy 237–9
natural philosophy
and medical education 12–13, 86
and Paracelsus 94, 96–7, 98
naval surgeons xxii, 257–8, 260, 261
and scurvy 276–8
neighbours, and social relations in
early modern England 233
Neoplatonism 22, 24
Neri, Phillipo 104
nervous system
and madness 244–5, 253
and the 'sensible' body 167,
186–92, *188*
von Haller's theories of the
'sensible' body 167
Nestorian Christianity 8
New England 321, 322, 325, 326, 329
New Spain *see* Mexico
Newgate prison, ventilators 307, *308*,
309
Newton, Isaac xii, 166, 181, 187
Newtonian physicians 35, 167,
181–4
Nezel, Siegfried 351
non-naturals 8–9, 11, 52, 133
and environmental themes 288
and healing waters 291
and learned physicians 52
and mental illness 242
and the plague 145
and regimen 288

Obeah medicine 340
obstetrics *see* childbirth
occult sciences 112–13
O'Dowde, Thomas 129–30
Oporinus, Johannes 74
Oribasius 12
ovaries, and the process of generation
210, 210
ovism, and theories of procreation
212, 213

Padua University 1, 12, 14, 48, *49*, 49,
68, 81, 168, 258
Pagano, Giulia 92
papacy 2, 4, 20
syphilis at the papal court 23–4

Paracelsus and Paracelsianism xix, 22,
93–8, *94*, 106, 108, 109–21, 131–3,
166
accusations of heresy against
114–15
and army surgeons 282
concept of the *archeus* 94, 95,
123
and Descartes's image of the body
174
and drugs 94, 111, 117–18, 119
in England 110–11, 118–19
in France 116–18, 121
and Galenic medicine 93–4, 95,
97, 108, 109, 110, 111, 115,
119–21
and Helmontianism 109, 121,
123, 125, 126, 127, 128
in the Holy Roman Empire
113–14, 115–16
the legacy of Paracelsus 109–15
and the medical benefits of travel
96
and mental illness 242
Paracelsiana 109
primary substances 94, 111, 123,
125
published works 98
and spiritual forces 94–5
and water cures 291
Paré, Ambroise 78, *261*, 263–5, 266,
282
and amputations 267, 268, 269,
271–2
and artificial limbs *272*, 272, *273*
and deaths of injured patients 275
and popular medicine 267
sewing of facial wounds 272, *274*
treatment of burns 266–7
treatment of gunshot wounds
263–5
Paris
Cemetery of the Holy Innocents
78, 307–10
hospitals
Hôpital de la Charité 367,
368
Hôtel des Invalides 280–1,
366
Hôtel-Dieu 20, *21*, 364
Salpetrière 369
midwives (Louise Bourgeois)
218–21, *219*
physicians 356
Société Royale de Médecine 309,
310, 349, 372
surgeons 3, 16, 367–70, 371

college of surgery 364–5,
365
University of 3, 12, 60–1, 67, 68,
87
and chemical medicine 108
examination system 363
and Paracelsianism 116,
117, 118
parish registers 297, 299–300
Park, K. 150–1
pathological anatomy 160
patients
Cardano's description of the
death of a patient 52–4
and empirical healers 374–6
and holistic views of health and
sickness 193
and medical pluralism 28–9
and physicians in eighteenth-
century England 185–6
poor people as hospital patients
157–60
power of xiii, xix, 184–6, 223
and traditional therapies 180
and training in clinical medicine
359–61
patristic authors 60
patronage 29, 78, 114, 118
Paul of Aegina 12, 221
Paul of Middleburg 14
Pavia, University of 51
Pelling, Margaret 28, 31, 44
Percy, George 326
Peter of Spain, *Treasury of the Poor*
17
Petit, Antoine 368, 369
Petit, Jean-Louis 268, 363
Petraeus, Heinrich 115–16
Petty, William 299, 301
Peyronie, François Gigot de 364
Philipp, landgrave of Hesse 248
philosophes 303, 310, 378
and empirical healers 375
and the organization of licensed
medical practice 346
physiocrats 371
phlebotomy *see* bloodletting
physicians 27–8
in the American colonies 327–9,
329, 335–6, 337
and apothecaries 47
and astrology 52, 86
and bloodletting 15, 46, 64–5
in Britain 347, 357

and childbirth 214–15, 216, 217–18, 219–21
and Christianity 19
colleges of 15, 30, 40–1, 46, 51
condotta appointments 51
conduct and etiquette 17
critics of xiii, 49–50
in the eighteenth century xxiii, 376
and empirical healers 372
and environmental medicine 300–1
in France 348–9, 352–7
and Galenic medicine 9–11
in Germany 350–1
and Helmontianism in England 124, 128
and hospitals 85, 151, 154–5, 159
and the inner body 44
learned 33, 37, 296, 345, 346
    diagnosis, prognosis and treatment 52–5
    and drugs 376, 377
    and empirical healers 38, 39–40, 40–1, 42–3, 376–7
    and Paracelsus 96
licensing of 30, 50–1
Luther on 88–9
and medical pluralism 28–9, 47, 55
and medical police 161, 306–7
and medical reform in Denmark 90
and midwives 219–21
Newtonian 35, 161, 167, 181–4
and the plague *132*, *139*, 140–1
    Christianity and the duties of 99–100
and pregnancy and childbirth 206
and the process of generation 213
in Rome 3–4
satires on 41
and smallpox inoculation 301–5
Society of Chemical Physicians 128–31
status of xviii, 50, 162, 185–6
and surgeons xxiii, 46, 358, 371–2, 378–9
university education 27–8
    clinical teaching 359–62
    eighteenth-century 185, 357–63
    examinations 362–3
    medieval 12–15, 86
and water cures 290–2, 294
and women as healers 37

see also London, College of Physicians
physiocrats 371
physiology 5, 358
Pico della Mirandola, Gianfrancesco 49, 50
Pietro d'Abano 13
pilgrimages 2, 85, 91, 289
Pinel, Philippe 361–2, 369
Pintor, Pere 23–4
Pistoia, plague in 140–1, 142–3
Pizarro, Francisco de 317
plague xx, *132*, 136, 138–46, *139*, 261
    Black Death 99, 139, 144
    and chemical physicians 131, 132
    and Christianity 99–100
    disappearance from Europe 145–6
    in England 141–2, 143
    and environmental medicine 285–6, 307, 319
    in France 142
    and the history of diseases 137, 138
    hospitals (pesthouses) 140, 141, 142, 144, 151
    in Italy 4, 103, 138–9, 140–1, 142–3
    and public health policies 4, 140–4, 145, 146, 160, 162, 285–6, 307
    and religion 138–9
Plato 6, 22
political arithmetic 299–300, 301
Polycleitus 77
Pomata, G. 200, 201, 202, 203
poor people
    and Bugenhagen's church orders 102
    and the economy of healing 344
    as hospital patients 155, 157–60
    and midwives 217
    and physicians 51
    and the plague 138, 141, 142–4, 143, 145
    and the 'sensible' body 191–2
    and smallpox inoculation 304
    and syphilis 147, 148–50
    and women as healers 34
poor relief xx, 136, 149–50
    and hospitals 153–4, 155, 157, 158
    and the plague 143–4

and the Reformation 89, 100–2, 106
popular medicine 33, 37, 38, 267
population growth 99, 101, 258, 304, 346–7, 356
population records 297, 299–300
Porter, R. xiii, 14, 157, 186, 189, 229, 245, 254, 345, 358
    on James Graham's Celestial Bed 377
    The Greatest Benefit to Mankind 257
power
    Foucault on knowledge and xiii–xiv, xxi
    slavery and medicine 335–6, 337, 338, 341
preformationism, and the process of generation 212–13, 224
pregnancy 205–7
    see also childbirth
Préval, Guilbert de 377
Primrose, James, *Popular Errours* 36–7, 37
Pringle, Sir John 261, *262*, 279–80, 281, 282, 307
printed media xviii 22
    and empirical healers 41, 373–4
    and smallpox inoculation xxii–xxiii, 304, 305
    see also books
prisons, use of ventilators in 307, 308, *309*
Protestantism 84
    and the demand for sacred healing 91–2, 93, 105–6
    and health care 100–2
    and holy wells and springs 289–90, 291
    and hospitals for the insane 245–6
    Lutheran 87–8
    and medical reform in Denmark 89–91
    and Paracelsus 97–8, 110
    and the plague 99–100
    and policing 306
    see also Reformation
public health policies
    in Germany and the Habsburg territories 160–2
    and medical police 160–1, 306–7
    and the plague 4, 140–4, 145, 146, 160, 162, 285–6, 307
    in Russia 305
    and social control 310

pulse-taking 8, 9, *10*, 53
purgatives
  and black slaves 337–8, 339
  and empirical healers 374–5
  and Fioravanti 40
  and the maintenance of health 33
  and Malpighi 179, 181
  and mental illness 242
  metallic medicines as 111, *112*
Pythagoras 18

quacks *see* empirical healers
Quakers 127, 128, 235–6, 245, 254
Quesnay, François 371
quinine (chinchona bark) 330, 376
Quintilian 59

Rakewell, Tom 245, *246*
Ralegh, Sir Walter 321
Rand, William 129
Rau, Wolfgang Thomas 306
Rauschart, Felix 202
Razoux, Jean 301
Reformation xix, 84, 86–91
  and health care 100–2, 106
  and holy waters 289
  and hospitals 148, 149, 154
  and medical reform in Denmark 89–91, 106
  and Paracelsus 97–8, 106, 110
  and the study of anatomy 86–8, 106
  see also Counter-Reformation; Protestantism
Reims University 363
religion and medicine xvii, xix–xx, xx, 84–106
  in the American colonies 317–18, 325–6, 328, 332–3
  in Britain 129, 347
  Christianity and healing xx, 18–20, 21
  and eirenicist aspirations 113
  and epidemics 99–100
  and Galenic medicine 6, 18
  and health care reforms 100–5
  and Helmontianism 125–6, 127–8
  and hospitals 148, 149, 150, 154
  in the later Middle Ages 85–6
  and mental illness 235–6, 240
  Paracelsus and Paracelsianism xix, 22, 93–8, 106, 110–12, 114–15
  and the plague 99–100, 138–9

and popular and sacred healing 85, 91–3, 106, 289–91
Rome as the centre of Christianity xvii, 2
and smallpox inoculation 302
and spiritual medicine 19, 22
and women as healers 34
see also Catholic church; Protestantism; Reformation
Renaissance medicine xi, 1, 20–2, 58
  and bloodletting 65–6
  and male–female bodies 198, *199*
  and Paracelsianism 112–13
  see also humanism; Vesalius
retrospective diagnosis xv, 138, 229
Reuchlin, Johannes 59
Rhazes 12, 13, 24
Richardson, Samuel 189
Richelieu, Cardinal 280
Risse, G.B. 158, 159
  on European medicine in New Spain 328–9
Robinson, Bryan 181–2
Roman Empire 1–2
Rome xvii–xviii, 1–4, 20
  and the classical past xvii, 1–2
  hospitals 19–20, 24, *148*, 151
  midwives 216–17
  University of 4
Rose Case, and the Royal College of the Physicians of London 347–8
Rosicrucian movement 128
Rouelle, Guillaume-François 368
Rudolf II, Holy Roman Emperor 113–14, 115
Rueff, Jacob, *De Conceptu et Generatione Hominis* 207, *215*, 216
Russia, smallpox inoculation 303, 305
Rutherford, John 360

Sahagún, Bernardino de *317*, 331
saints
  healing power of 19, 85, 92–3, 289, 291
  sacred relics and the plague 138, 139
Salamanca, University of 68
Salerno 12
Sanctorius, Sanctorius *182*
  De Statica Medicina 181
Sandrart, Johann Jacob, *Van Helmont's vision of the Sepulchre of Truth 123*

sarsaparilla (*Smilax aristolochiaefolia*) 330
Sbaraglia, Girolamo 178, 179, 180
schizophrenia 236
Schwabe, Johann 350–1
scientific medicine xiii, xiv, 27
scientific revolution xxi, 84, 166, 170
Scotland
  Edinburgh Royal Infirmary 158–9, 192, 360, *362*
  kirk sessions and the visiting of wells and springs 290
Scottish philosophers and physicians, and the 'sensible' body 167, 187–8, 191–2
scurvy 261, 276–8
semen
  and the female body 197
  Galen on the production of 176, 197
  and menstruation 201
  and the process of generation 210, 212
  spermatozoa of animals *211*
Seneca 60
sensibility, the nervous system and the sensible body 167, 186–92, *188*
Seven Years War (1756–63) 265
Severinus, Peter, *Idea Medicinae Philosophicae* 98
sexuality
  female pleasure and the process of conception 208, 213–14, 377
  sex therapy and the Celestial Bed 377–8
Selye, Hans, *The Stress of Life* xv
Sheldon, Gilbert, archbishop of Canterbury 129–30
shell shock 275, 280
Short, Thomas 300
Shorter, Edward 223
shrines, and sacred healing 91–2, 245, 289–90
'sick-building syndrome' 284
Singer, Charles *207*
Siraisi, Nancy 65–6
Sixtus IV, Pope 3, 19
skeleton of the human body, and Vesalius *69*, 70, 78
Slack, Paul 143
slavery and medicine xxiii, 334–41
  and biomedical history 338
  black medicine 338–41
  plantation hospitals 337

and power relations 335–6, 337, 338, 341
transportation of black slaves to the Americas 334, *335*
white medical treatment of slaves 336–8
smallpox xx, 146, 160, 261, 279
and black slaves 335
European colonization and indigenous peoples 316–18, *317*
inoculation xxii–xxiii, 301–5
Smellie, William 215
Smith, Adam 191
Smith, Henrik 89, 90
Smollett, Tobias, *Humphry Clinker* 376
social class/status xiv, 374–5
and mental illness xv, 232–3, 238
and midwives 219–21, 223
and physicians xviii, 50, 162, 185–6
patients of 51, 191–2
and surgeons 46, 346, 363
patients of 43
social constructivist approach to medicine xv, xix
the soul
and Christianity 18–19
in Galenic medicine 6
and mental illness 230, 240, 241
and the 'sensible body' 191
Spa (town of) 292, *293*
Spain 2, 280, 350
Spangenberg, Georg 351
Spanish America xxiii, 2, 327–9
Aztec medicine 316, *331*, 331–4, *332*
conquest of 317
European medicine and indigenous peoples 316
hospitals xxiii, 328
smallpox in *317*
spiritual medicine 19, 22
springs and wells *see* waters and healing
the state and medicine xx, xxi, xxii, 259
and empirical healers 378
and the Enlightenment 344–5
and the environment 285
and licensed medical practice 347, 348–9, 350–1
and medical police 300, 305–6
and political arithmetic 299–300, 301
and scientific medicine 27

see also poor relief; public health policies
Steno, Nicolaus 210
Sterne, Lawrence 189, 190–1
Stoll, Maximilien 360
Stone, Sarah 218
Storch, Johann 203–4
Storey, George 275
Strachey, William 325
stress and stress-related illnesses xv
suicide, and mental illness 236, 254
surgeons xviii, 27, *45*, 46
advances in surgical knowledge 363
and bloodletting 15, 44, *45*
and childbirth 216
education and training 15–17, 43, 346, 357, 363–71
private courses 367–71
in Florentine hospitals 151
in France 348, 349, 352–5, 356
education of 364–6, 367–70
and Galenic medicine 10
in Germany 351
guilds 30, 364
and itinerant healers 39, 43
licensing of 29–30, 346
in London 43–4
and Paracelsianism 118, 120
and physicians xxiii, 46, 358, 371–2, 378–9
social status of 46, 346, 363
in Spain 250
in Spanish America 328
university courses in surgery 358, 359
see also army surgeons; barber-surgeons; naval surgeons
surgical instruments *16*, 265
chests for storing *269*
crochet 216, *217*
'Crowes beake' 271
screw tourniquet *268*, 268
Süssmilch, Johann Peter 300
Sutton, Daniel 303, 304
Sutton, Robert 303
Swammerdam, Jan, and the human ovary *210*
Sweden 280, 299–300
Sydenham, Thomas 295–7, 303
Sylvius, Franciscus (Franz de la Boë) 123, 133
Sylvius, Jacobus 60–1, 68
syphilis 22–4, 136, 146–50

hospitals 24, 102, 103, 148–9, 151
and poor people 147, 148–50
and surgeons 46
symptoms 146
theories on the causes of 146
treatments for 24, 147, *148*, 330
Szasz, Thomas xiii, 229

Tahitians, and the process of deculturation 318
Tenon, Jacques 364
Terence 60
terra sigillata 179
theriac (Greek compound medicine) 10
Thirty Years War (1618–48) 258, 259, 260
Thompson, E.P. xiii
Thomson, George 130–1, 132
Loimotomia: or the Pest Anatomized 132
The Times, report on smallpox inoculation 304, 305
Tissot, Samuel 377, 378
tobacco, medical uses of *324*
Todd, M. 290
Torrella, Gaspar 4, 23–4
Toulouse University 359
Trajan, Roman Emperor 2
Treasury of the Poor 17
Trent, Council of 92
trepanation *45*
Trevor-Roper, Hugh 114, 116
Trithemius, Johannes, abbot of Sponheim 95
Trotter, Dr Thomas 261, 276
Tübingen, University of 68
Tunbridge Wells 291, 292
Turkey, smallpox inoculation in 302

Ulsenius, Theodoricus *147*
Unani-tibb (Muslim medical system) 334
universities
curriculum 12–15, 18, 48–9, 93, 347–62
early modern Italian 48–9
Harvard College 329
Lutheran 88
and medical training 27–8, 126, 185, 357–72
clinical teaching 359–61
examinations 362–3

medicine and Christianity in 105
medieval 12–15, 18, 85, 86, 93
and printed texts 22
in Spanish America 328, 329
see also individual cities
Urbino, Francesco Maria della Rovere,
duke of 14
urine
Galenic medicine and the
examination of 8, 9, *10*, 53
Malpighi's theory of the
production of 176–7
uroscopy 206

vaccination, and inoculation 301
Vallériole, François 286
Vaughan, William, *Directions for
Health* 323
veins of the human body
azygos 72, *73*, 74, 80–1
basilic vein 65
bloodletting points 65
Fabricius and the 'little doors'
81–2, *82*, 168, 169
and Harvey's discovery of the
circulation of the blood 168–71,
172
thoracic 67, 68, 73
vena cava 61, 72, 81
in Vesalius' *Tabulae Anatomicae
Sex* 70–3, *71*
venesection *see* bloodletting
Venice, plague in 138–9
ventilators, in prisons and hospitals
307, *308*, *309*, 310
Vesalius, Andreas xviii, 58, 59, 68–82,
112, 176, 208, 358
and bloodletting 58, 70–3, 80–1,
168
De Humani Corporis Fabrica
58, 74–9, *75*, 87, 88
and the female reproductive
organs 198, *199*
and Fabricius 81, 82
and Galenic medicine 58, 68, 70,
74–7, 78, 79–80, 87
legacy of 79–82
and Lutheran Protestantism 87–8
and public dissections 58, 73–4,
74–6, 77
Tabulae Anatomicae Sex 68–72,
69, *71*
view of the canonical body 77–8

Vicq d'Azyr, Félix 349, 372
Vienna, medical education in 360, 362
Vigo, Giovanni da 263
virgin soil epidemics xxiii, 316–18
Virginia 321, 322–3, 325, 326, 340
Vitruvius, *On Architecture* 20
Voltaire, and smallpox inoculation 303
voluntary hospitals 155–7

war and medicine xxii, 257–82
amputations 267–72, 282
artillery 260, 275
burns treatment 260, 266–7
and the cauterization of wounds
263, 264, 268, 272
and changes in the nature of
warfare 258–60
diseases 261, 279
foot rot 275
fractures 260, 272, *273*
gunshot wounds 260, 263–5, 282
locating bullets in 264–5,
270
head wounds 265–6
medical examination of recruits
278
military hospitals 257, 278,
280–1, 282
field hospitals 281
and military hygiene 278–80, 307
shell shock 275, 280
and surgery in France *366*
and syphilis 146
waters and healing 289–95
chemical analysis of mineral
waters 294–5, *295*
commercialization of spa waters
292–4
holy springs and wells xx, 91–2,
289–90
physicians and water cures
290–2, 294
Webster, Charles 28, 97, 119
Webster, John 126–7
weighing the body 181, *182*
Welde, Thomas 322
welfare state 136
wells *see* waters and healing
Wesley, John 378

West Indies 326, 330, 336, 337, 339,
340
'whiggish' approach to history xii
Whitbourne, Richard 324
Wilberforce, William 335
Williams, Gerhild Scholz 97
Williamson, Janet 158–9, 192
Willis, Thomas 123, 133, 187, 244
Wilson, Adrian 216, 222–3
Winthrop, John 317–18, 325
Wiseman, Richard 266
witchcraft, and mental illness 229,
233–4, 240, 242–3
women and medicine xxi–xxii,
196–225
and childbirth xv–xvi, xxi–xxii,
215–23
churching of new mothers 216
and Galenic medicine 6–7, 35, 37
male–female differences 197,
198, 199–200, 223
and menstruation 201, 202
and the process of
generation 107, 207–8, 213,
224
and hysteria xv, 191, 192, 243,
244–5
and menstruation 197, 200–5,
205–6, 224–5
and mental illness 231–2, 233,
244–5
and the plague 143
and pregnancy 205–7
and the process of generation xxi,
197, 198, 207–15, 224
and sex differences 197–205
and smallpox 301
women as healers 34–8, 54–5
women as patients xv, 150, 151,
196, 223
see also midwives
women's history xiii, 196
Woodall, John 118, *120*
Wortley Montagu, Lady Mary 302
Wotton, Sir Henry 287
Würzburg, Juliusspital 238, 246–7, *248*

Yonge, James 266

zodiac man 63, *64*, *287*
Aztec version of *331*